Surgery in the Multimodal Management of Gastric Cancer

Giovanni de Manzoni • Franco Roviello • Walter Siquini
Editors

Surgery in the Multimodal Management of Gastric Cancer

Foreword by
Keiichi Maruyama

Springer

GIRCG

Editors:
Giovanni de Manzoni
Dept. of Surgery
Upper G.I. Surgery Division
University of Verona
Verona, Italy

Franco Roviello
Dept. of Human Pathology and Oncology
Section of General Surgery and Surgical Oncology
Translational Research Laboratory, University of Siena
Siena, Italy

Walter Siquini
Surgical Clinic, Dept. of Medical and Surgical Sciences
"Ospedali Riuniti" University Hospital
Polytechnic University of Marche
Ancona, Italy

ISBN 978-88-470-2317-8 ISBN 978-88-470-2318-5 (eBook)

DOI 10.1007/978-88-470-2318-5

Springer Milan Dordrecht Heidelberg London New York

Library of Congress Control Number: 2011937633

9 8 7 6 5 4 3 2 1 2012 2013 2014

Cover design: Simona Colombo, Milan, Italy
Typesetting: Graphostudio, Milan, Italy
Printing and binding: Grafiche Porpora S.r.L., Segrate (MI)

Printed in Italy

Springer-Verlag Italia S.r.l. – Via Decembrio 28 – I-20137 Milan
Springer is a part of Springer Science+Business Media (www.springer.com)

Foreword

I am very pleased by the publication of this textbook, "Surgery in the Multimodal Management of Gastric Cancer." The editors, Professor Giovanni de Manzoni, Professor Franco Roviello, and Doctor Walter Siquini, are internationally well known leaders in this field. Moreover, Giovanni de Manzoni and Franco Roviello, respectively President and Secretary General of the International Gastric Cancer Association, are currently organizing the 10th International Congress, to be held in 2013 in Verona. The book's appearance is therefore particularly timely, as it has strongly benefited from the cooperation and support of world-class specialist authors.

Several factors contribute to making this book a valuable reference. Firstly, the editors and authors are actively working specialists, with continuing hands-on experience. Moreover, they are highly engaged not only in communicating their knowledge and preferred surgical techniques but also in seeking out the same from internationally recognized experts, particularly those from Italy, Germany, UK, USA, Brazil, Japan, and Korea. Secondly, this book is not an ordinary textbook, covering all subjects related to this disease, but a unique reference that focuses on the important and practical aspects of gastric cancer. State-of-the-art disease management is presented in detail while emphasizing the need for individualized treatment planning based on the accurate assessment of cancer extension, endoscopic mucosal resection, laparoscopic gastric resection, effective and safe lymph node dissection, neoadjuvant and adjuvant chemotherapy, etc.

I would recommend that you keep this textbook ready on your desk, as you will no doubt find yourself reaching for it time and time again.

September 2011

Keiichi Maruyama, M.D.
Professor of Surgical Oncology
University of Health and Welfare Sanno Hospital
Tokyo

Preface

The Italian Research Group for Gastric Cancer (GIRCG) was established in the mid 1990s as a collaboration among three Italian centers, in Forlì, Siena, and Verona. It now comprises over 20 specialized centers located throughout Italy. In recognition of the current emphasis on a multidisciplinary approach to oncologic diseases the GIRCG's members include not only surgeons and pathologists but also gastroenterologists, medical oncologists, radiologists, and statisticians. The main aims of the GIRCG are the standardization of surgical treatment, pathological assessment, additional therapies and follow-up, surgical, endoscopic and pathological training, as well as the design and completion of clinical studies and cross-discipline research in gastric cancer (GC). Accordingly, since its establishment the group has met regularly and several research protocols covering the many aspects of GC diagnosis and treatment have been evaluated, with the results published in international journals. Among the ongoing research protocols are those addressing a new TNM classification, the validation of prognostic scores, tailored follow-up, HER-2 expression, genetic polymorphisms and GC risk, the *Helicobacter pylori* genome and GC, participation in the National Register of EMR/ESD, randomized controlled trials of neoadjuvant chemotherapy, prophylactic cholecystectomy, and nasogastric tube use after subtotal gastrectomy. A centralized database has been established and adopted, with data prospectively stored and updated every six months. The group has an active web site that serves to coordinate its research activities.

The aim of this book is to summarize the extensive and multidisciplinary work of the GIRCG in order to provide surgical oncologists with state-of-the-art tools and information required for a thoroughly informed approach to GC treatment. In addition to the published and anecdotal experience of the GIRCG, each chapter also extensively refers to the current literature.

Last but not least, this book also serves as a presentation of the GIRCG's research and clinical efforts in advance of its hosting the next International Gastric Cancer Congress, to be held in Verona, Italy, from 19 to 22 June 2013.

September 2011

Giovanni de Manzoni
Franco Roviello
Walter Siquini

Contents

Contributors

William H. Allum, Royal Marsden NHS Foundation Trust, London, UK

Antonella Ardito, Surgical Oncology Unit, IRCCS Istituto Clinico Humanitas, Rozzano (MI), Italy

Gian Luca Baiocchi, Surgical Clinic, Dept. of Medical and Surgical Sciences, University of Brescia, Brescia, Italy

Francesco Bellucci, Dept. of Clinical Pathophysiology, Surgical Unit, University of Florence, Florence, Italy

Lapo Bencini, Oncological Surgery, Careggi University Hospital, Florence, Italy

Emanuele Bendia, Dept. of Gastroenterology, "Ospedali Riuniti" University Hospital, Polytechnic University of Marche, Ancona, Italy

Antonio Benedetti, Dept. of Gastroenterology, "Ospedali Riuniti" University Hospital, Polytechnic University of Marche, Ancona, Italy

Rossana Berardi, Dept. of Medical Oncology, "Ospedali Riuniti" University Hospital, Polytechnic University of Marche, Ancona, Italy

Marco Bernini, Oncological Surgery, Careggi University Hospital, Florence, Italy

Maristella Bianconi, Dept. of Medical Oncology, "Ospedali Riuniti" University Hospital, Polytechnic University of Marche, Ancona, Italy

Alberto Biondi, Dept. of Surgery, General Surgery Unit, Catholic University of Rome, "A. Gemelli" Hospital, Rome, Italy

Alessandro Bittoni, Dept. of Medical Oncology, "Ospedali Riuniti" University Hospital, Polytechnic University of Marche, Ancona, Italy

Maurizio Bossola, Digestive Surgery Unit, Dept. of Surgical Sciences, Catholic University of Rome, "A. Gemelli" Hospital, Rome, Italy

Walter Bugiantella, Dept. of General and Emergency Surgery, University of Perugia, Perugia, Italy

Ferdinando Cananzi, Dept. of Surgery, General Surgery Unit, Catholic University of Rome, "A. Gemelli" Hospital, Rome, Italy

Alessandro Cardinali, Surgical Clinic, Dept. of Medical and Surgical Sciences, "Ospedali Riuniti" University Hospital, Polytechnic University of Marche, Ancona, Italy

Stefano Caruso, Dept. of Human Pathology and Oncology, Surgical Oncology Unit, University of Siena, Siena, Italy

Alessandro Casadei, Gastroenterology and Endoscopy Unit, "GB Morgagni – L. Pierantoni" Hospital, Forli, Italy

Stefano Cascinu, Dept. of Medical Oncology, "Ospedali Riuniti" University Hospital, Polytechnic University of Marche, Ancona, Italy

Filippo Catalano, Surgical Endoscopy Unit, Borgo Trento Hospital, Verona, Italy

Marco Catarci, Dept. of Surgery, "San Filippo Neri" Hospital, Rome, Italy

Emanuel Cavazzoni, Dept. of General and Emergency Surgery, University of Perugia, Perugia, Italy

Arianna Coniglio, Surgical Clinic, Dept. of Medical and Surgical Sciences, University of Brescia, Brescia, Italy

Claudio Cordiano, Dept. of Surgery, University of Verona, Verona, Italy

Giovanni Corso, Dept. of Human Pathology and Oncology, Section of General Surgery and Surgical Oncology, Translational Research Laboratory, University of Siena, Siena, Italy

Andrea Costanzi, General Surgery, Desio Hospital; AIMS Academy, Milan, Italy

Luca Cozzaglio, Surgical Oncology Unit, IRCCS Istituto Clinico Humanitas, Rozzano (MI), Italy

Giorgio Crepaldi, Dept. of Medical Oncology, "Santa Maria della Misericordia" Hospital, Rovigo, Italy

Antonio Crucitti, Dept. of Surgery, General Surgery Unit, Catholic University of Rome, "A. Gemelli" Hospital, Rome, Italy

Giacomo Cusumano, Digestive Surgery Unit, Dept. of Surgical Sciences, Catholic University of Rome, "A. Gemelli" Hospital, Rome, Italy

Domenico D'Ugo, Dept. of Surgery, General Surgery Unit, Catholic University of Rome, "A. Gemelli" Hospital, Rome, Italy

Giovanni de Manzoni, Dept. of Surgery, Upper G.I. Surgery Division, University of Verona, Verona, Italy

Alberto Di Leo, General Surgery Unit, Arco Hospital, APSS of Trento, Trento, Italy

Natale Di Martino, VIII Unit of General Surgery and Gastrointestinal Physiophatology - Second University of Naples, Naples, Italy

Antonio Di Sario, Dept. of Gastroenterology, "Ospedali Riuniti" University Hospital, Polytechnic University of Marche, Ancona, Italy

Giovan Battista Doglietto, Digestive Surgery Unit, Dept. of Surgical Sciences, Catholic University of Rome, "A. Gemelli" Hospital, Rome, Italy

Annibale Donini, Dept. of General and Emergency Surgery, University of Perugia, Perugia, Italy

Luca Faloppi, Dept. of Medical Oncology, "Ospedali Riuniti" University Hospital, Polytechnic University of Marche, Ancona, Italy

Marco Farsi, Oncological Surgery, Careggi University Hospital, Florence, Italy

Orietta Federici, National Cancer Institute "Regina Elena", Rome, Italy

Emilio Feliciotti, Surgical Clinic, Dept. of Medical and Surgical Sciences, "Ospedali Riuniti" University Hospital, Polytechnic University of Marche, Ancona, Italy

Giovanni C. Ferrari, Minimally Invasive and Oncology Surgery, Niguarda Hospital Ca'-Granda; AIMS Academy, Milan, Italy

Aroldo Fianchini, Surgical Clinic, Dept. of Medical and Surgical Sciences, "Ospedali Riuniti" University Hospital, Polytechnic University of Marche, Ancona, Italy

Anna Paola Fraccon, Service of Medical Oncology, "Dott. Pederzoli" Polyspecialist Private Clinic, Peschiera del Garda (VR), Italy

Alfredo Garofalo, National Cancer Institute "Regina Elena", Rome, Italy

Simone Giacopuzzi, Dept. of Surgery, Upper G.I. Surgery Division, University of Verona, Verona, Italy

Riccardo Giampieri, Dept. of Medical Oncology, "Ospedali Riuniti" University Hospital, Polytechnic University of Marche, Ancona, Italy

Francesco Giudici, Dept. of Clinical Pathophysiology, Surgical Unit, University of Florence, Florence, Italy

Stefano M. Giulini, Surgical Clinic, Dept. of Medical and Surgical Sciences, University of Brescia, Brescia, Italy

Luigina Graziosi, Dept. of General and Emergency Surgery, University of Perugia, Perugia, Italy

Ugo Grossi, Dept. of Surgery, General Surgery Unit, Catholic University of Rome, "A. Gemelli" Hospital, Rome, Italy

Monica Gualtierotti, Minimally Invasive and Oncology Surgery, Niguarda Hospital Ca'-Granda; AIMS Academy, Milan, Italy

Giuliano La Barba, Dept. of General Surgery, "G.B. Morgagni – L. Pierantoni" Hospital, Forlì, Italy

Edoardo Landi †, Surgical Clinic, Dept. of Medical and Surgical Sciences, "Ospedali Riuniti" University Hospital, Polytechnic University of Marche, Ancona, Italy

Francesco Lombardo, Surgical Endoscopy Unit, Borgo Trento Hospital, Verona, Italy

Elena Maccaroni, Dept. of Medical Oncology, "Ospedali Riuniti" University Hospital, Polytechnic University of Marche, Ancona, Italy

Dario Maggioni, General Surgery, Desio Hospital; AIMS Academy, Milan, Italy

Gerardo Mangiante, Dept. of Surgery, Upper G.I. Surgery Division, University of Verona, Verona, Italy

Alberto Marchet, Dept. of Oncological and Surgical Sciences, Surgery Section, University of Padova, Padova, Italy

Mario Marini, Gastro-Intestinal Unit "Santa Maria alle Scotte" University Hospital, Siena Italy

Cristina Marmorale, Surgical Clinic, Dept. of Medical and Surgical Sciences, "Ospedali Riuniti" University Hospital, Polytechnic University of Marche, Ancona, Italy

Daniele Marrelli, Dept. of Human Pathology and Oncology, Section of General Surgery and Surgical Oncology, Translational Research Laboratory, University of Siena, Siena, Italy

Marco Marzioni, Dept. of Gastroenterology, "Ospedali Riuniti" University Hospital, Polytechnic University of Marche, Ancona, Italy

Sonia Maurizi, Surgical Clinic, Dept. of Medical and Surgical Sciences, "Ospedali Riuniti" University Hospital, Polytechnic University of Marche, Ancona, Italy

Andrea Mazzari, Dept. of Surgery, General Surgery Unit, Catholic University of Rome, "A. Gemelli" Hospital, Rome, Italy

Simone Mocellin, Dept. of Oncological and Surgical Sciences, Surgery Section, University of Padova, Padova, Italy

Paolo Morgagni, Dept. of General Surgery, "G.B. Morgagni – L. Pierantoni" Hospital, Forlì, Italy

Gianni Mura, Dept. of Surgery, Valdarno Hospital, Arezzo, Italy

Donato Nitti, Dept. of Oncological and Surgical Sciences, Surgery Section, University of Padova, Padova, Italy

Fabio Pacelli, Digestive Surgery Unit, Dept. of Surgical Sciences, Catholic University of Rome, "A. Gemelli" Hospital, Rome, Italy

Felice Pasini, Dept. of Medical Oncology, "Santa Maria della Misericordia" Hospital, Rovigo, Italy

Corrado Pedrazzani, Surgery Division, Rovereto Hospital, Rovereto (TN), Italy

Raffaele Pugliese, Minimally Invasive and Oncology Surgery, Niguarda Hospital Ca'-Granda; AIMS Academy, Milan, Italy

Raffaella Ridolfo, General Surgery Unit, Pergola Hospital, Pesaro, Italy

Luca Rodella, Surgical Endoscopy Unit, Borgo Trento Hospital, Verona, Italy

Fausto Rosa, Digestive Surgery Unit, Dept. of Surgical Sciences, Catholic University of Rome, "A. Gemelli" Hospital, Rome, Italy

Gian Maria Rossi, Dept. of Oncological and Surgical Sciences, Surgery Section, University of Padova, Padova, Italy

Franco Roviello, Dept. of Human Pathology and Oncology, Section of General Surgery and Surgical Oncology, Translational Research Laboratory, University of Siena, Siena, Italy

Luca Saragoni, Dept. of Pathology, "G.B. Morgagni – L. Pierantoni" Hospital, Forlì, Italy

Stefano Scaringi, Dept. of Clinical Pathophysiology, Surgical Unit, University of Florence, Florence, Italy

Mario Scartozzi, Dept. of Medical Oncology, "Ospedali Riuniti" University Hospital, Polytechnic University of Marche, Ancona, Italy

Walter Siquini, Surgical Clinic, Dept. of Medical and Surgical Sciences, "Ospedali Riuniti" University Hospital, Polytechnic University of Marche, Ancona, Italy

Pierpaolo Stortoni, Surgical Clinic, Dept. of Medical and Surgical Sciences, "Ospedali Riuniti" University Hospital, Polytechnic University of Marche, Ancona, Italy

Guido A.M. Tiberio, Surgical Clinic, Dept. of Medical and Surgical Sciences, University of Brescia, Brescia, Italy

Pasquina M.C. Tomaiuolo, Dept. of Surgery, General Surgery Unit, Catholic University of Rome, "A. Gemelli" Hospital, Roma, Italy

Anna Tomezzoli, Pathology Unit, Borgo Trento Hospital, Verona, Italy

Francesco Tonelli, Dept. of Clinical Pathophysiology, Surgical Unit, University of Florence, Florence, Italy

Francesco Torelli, VIII Unit of General Surgery and Gastrointestinal Physiophatology - Second University of Naples, Naples, Italy

Antonio Tortorelli, Digestive Surgery Unit, Dept. of Surgical Sciences, Catholic University of Rome, "A. Gemelli" Hospital, Rome, Italy

Giuseppe Verlato, Unit of Epidemiology and Medical Statistics, University of Verona, Verona, Italy

Carla Vindigni, Division of Pathological Anatomy and Histopathology, University of Siena, Siena, Italy

Andrea Zanoni, Dept. of Surgery, Upper G.I. Surgery Division, University of Verona,Verona, Italy

Epidemiology of Gastric Cancer and Screening Programs

1

Giuseppe Verlato, Alberto Di Leo, Gian Maria Rossi, and Giovanni de Manzoni

Abstract

Despite a major decline in incidence and mortality, gastric cancer is still detected in around one million people every year and accounts for over 700,000 deaths, representing 8% of all cancer cases and 9.7% of all cancer deaths. The incidence is about twice as high in men as in women. In 2008, 60% of new cases occurred in Eastern Asia: 464,439 in China, 102,040 in Japan, and 27098 in South Korea. By comparison, new cases recorded in the European Union as a whole and throughout the United States were 83,120 and 21,499, respectively. High-incidence areas are East Asia, Eastern Europe, Central Asia, and the Pacific coast of South and Central America, while low-incidence areas are Western Europe, North America, Africa, and Australia. Likewise age-adjusted mortality is the highest in South Korea (30.7 and 11.3 per 100,000 person-years, respectively, in men and women in 2004) and the lowest in the USA (3.2 and 1.6 respectively). In Western countries, the decrease in the incidence of noncardia gastric cancers parallels a concomitant increase in the incidence of gastric cardia cancer. Screening programs for gastric cancer are currently ongoing in Japan and South Korea. Two-thirds of Japanese patients survive beyond 5 years, while in Europe 5-year survival does not exceed 25%.

Keywords

Gastric cancer • Incidence • Mortality • Temporal trends • Cardia cancer • Intestinal-type • Diffuse-type • 5-year survival • Primary prevention • Screening

1.1 Incidence of Gastric Cancer and Related Mortality

Despite a major decline in incidence and mortality, gastric cancer remains an important public health burden worldwide. Nearly one million (988,000) new cases of stomach cancer were recorded in 2008, accounting for 7.8% of all cancer cases. At the same time, 736,000 people died from gastric cancer, representing 9.7% of all cancer deaths. Hence gastric cancer is the fourth most commonly occurring cancer after cancer of the lung, breast and colorectum, and the second most common cancer-related cause of death after lung cancer [1]. Gastric cancer is still the most common cancer in several countries of Eastern (South Korea, Japan) and Central (Tadjik-

G. Verlato (✉)
Unit of Epidemiology and Medical Statistics,
University of Verona,
Verona, Italy

G. de Manzoni, F. Roviello, W. Siquini (eds.), *Surgery in the Multimodal Management of Gastric Cancer*,

istan, Afghanistan) Asia and in Ecuador [2-4].

There is a ten-fold variation in the incidence of gastric cancer across the world. In 2008, age-standardized (world) incidence rates ranged from around four new cases per 100,000 person-years in Africa and North America to 30 new cases in Eastern Asia. Incidence rates were rather low also in Australia/New Zealand and South-Central Asia (5 cases), and rather high also in South and Central America (12 and 11 cases, respectively). Large differences were likewise recorded within Europe: incidence rates were the highest in Central and Eastern Europe (15 cases per 100,000 person-years), intermediate in Southern Europe (10 cases), and the lowest in Western and Northern Europe (7 and 6 cases, respectively) [1].

New cases occur twice as often in men (n=640,031 in 2008) as in women (n=348,571), although the geographic pattern is similar. They range from 3.9 per 100,000 person-years in Northern Africa to 42.4 in Eastern Asia for men, and from 2.2 in Southern Africa to 18.3 in Eastern Asia for women [1]. With respect to all cancers, gastric cancer occurs approximately at the same age in men (median age at diagnosis = 66 years) but at older ages in women (median age at diagnosis = 68 years vs. 61 years).

In 2008, around 60% of the gastric cancer cases occurred in Eastern Asia: 464,439 in China, 102,040 in Japan, and 27,098 in South Korea. The corresponding age-standardized (world) incidence rates were, respectively, 41.3 and 18.5 per 100,000 person-years among Chinese men and women, 46.8 and 18.2 among Japanese men and women, and 62.2 and 24.6 among South Korean men and women [1]. For a comparison, the number of new cases recorded in the 27 countries of the European Union and in the US was 83,120 and 21,499, respectively, corresponding to incidence rates of 7.9 and 4.1 per 100,000 person-years [1].

In the period 1998–2002, the age-standardized (world) incidence rate was the highest in South Korea (66.1 per 100,000 person-years in men, 26 in women), followed by Nagasaki and Osaka, Japan (59.5 in men, 22.3 in women and 51.5 in men, 19.8 in women, respectively); Valdivia, Chile (43.1 in men, 15.9 in women); Belarus (35.8 in men, 15.2 in women); and Shanghai, China (34.2 in men, 17.3 in women). The lowest incidence rates (around 7 per 100,000 person-years in men, 3 in women) were reported in Denmark, Sweden, Vaud (Switzerland), and the USA [5]. It should be pointed out, however, that the highest crude rates, which better reflect the socioeconomic burden, occur in Japan: 112 and 50 per 100,000 person-years in Japanese men and women in 2008 vs. 76 and 37 in South Korean men and women. The situation is reversed only after age standardization, which takes into account the marked aging of the Japanese population.

The pattern of mortality from gastric cancer, illustrated in Fig. 1.1, parallels the pattern of incidence [5]. Both in men and in women, the highest rates are observed in Eastern Asia: 30.7 and 11.3 per 100,000 person-years, respectively in South Korea in 2004; 23.4 and 9.2, respectively in Japan. The lowest rates are found in North America: 3.2 and 1.6 per 100,000 person-years, respectively, in US men and women; 4.5 and 2.2 in Canadian men and women. Rather high rates have been recorded for males (M) and females (F) also in the following areas:

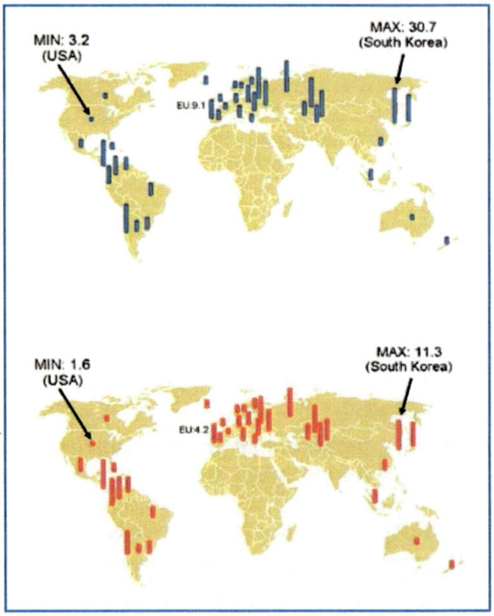

Fig. 1.1 Age-standardized (*world*) mortality rates from gastric cancer in 2004 in men (*upper panel*) and women (*lower panel*). Rates are reported as deaths per 100,000 person-years. *EU*, European Union

- Eastern Europe: Belarus 27.4 (M), 10.5 (F); Russian Federation 27.2 (M), 11.2 (F); Ukraine 21.2 (M), 8.3 (F);
- Central Asia: Kazakhstan 25.7 (M), 10.8 (F); Kyrgyzstan 23.2 (M), 8.3 (F); Tajikistan 14.9 (M) 9.3 (F);
- Pacific coast of South and Central America: Chile 25.4 (M), 9.2 (F); Costa Rica 22.5 (M), 11.2 (F); Ecuador 15.6 (M), 10.8 (F)

1.2 Temporal Trends in Gastric Cancer Incidence and Related Mortality

Until the mid-1990s, gastric cancer was the most common cause of cancer-related death worldwide, although the rates had started to decline much earlier. Between 1980 and 1999, age-adjusted gastric cancer mortality nearly halved in Western and Eastern Europe and decreased by 40% in Russia [6]. In the European Union as a whole, age-standardized mortality from gastric cancer declined by about 30% from 1990–1994 to 2000–2004 in both sexes, from 14.1 to 9.9 per 100,000 person-years in men and from 6.4 to 4.5 in women [7].

In particular, both incidence and mortality have steadily declined in Northern Europe, at least since 1964 [8]. In Eindhoven, The Netherlands, the age-standardized incidence among men decreased from 24 per 100,000 person-years in the beginning of the 1990s to 12 in 2007, and from 10 to 6 in women [9]. In Spain, the age-standardized incidence of gastric cancer declined from 27.2 and 13.4 cases per 100 000 person-years in 1980–1984 to 20.2 and 8.7 in 2000–2004, among men and women, respectively [10]. In Italy, gastric cancer was the site-specific cancer with the largest incidence reduction from 1993–1995 to 2003–2005 (-33.1% in men, -27.4% in women) [11].

In the US, the age-standardized incidence declined from 1977 to 2006 in all races: from 5.9 (95% CI 5.7–6.1) to 4.0 (3.9–4.1) in whites, from 13.7 (12.5–14.9) to 9.5 (9.1–10.0) in blacks, and from 17.8 (16.1–19.4) to 11.7 (11.2–12.1) in other races [12]. In Japan, age-standardized (Japanese population in 1985) mortality from gastric cancer peaked at around 100 per 100,000 person-years in men and at around 50 in women and decreased by more than 60% by 2000 [13]. In the last decade, age-standardized (world) incidence rates declined by 25% in men (from 62.0 per 100,000 person-years in 2002 to 46.8 in 2008) and by 30% in women (from 26.1 to 18.2) [1, 14].

The decline in gastric cancer incidence is partly obscured by population aging. For instance, in Japan the absolute number of new cases has been increasing, as the decreasing age-standardized incidence of gastric cancer is counterbalanced by rapid aging of the Japanese population [13]. In Italy, where 26% of the population is 60 years or older (http://demo.istat.it), the incidence of gastric cancer decreased by one-third from 1986 to 2000–2003, from 59.9 to 39.7 new cases per 100,000 person-years among men and from 40.3 to 27.2 new cases among women; age-standardized incidence, instead, more than halved in the same period, from 56.3 to 27.7 per 100,000 person-years among men and from 27.8 to 13.7 among women [15]. For this reason, GLOBOCAN 2008 predicted that the annual number of new cases will rise from 1 million at present to 1.7 million by 2030 [1].

In developing countries, the decline in gastric cancer has been somewhat delayed and less pronounced than in developed countries. From 1994 to 2004, the annual percentage change in mortality rate was between -3% and -4% for the major European countries, Japan, South Korea, USA, and Australia but only between -1.5 and -2.5% for Latin America [5]. In China, gastric cancer mortality slightly increased from the 1970s to the early 1990s and started to decline thereafter [16]; indeed, an increasing trend continues in rural areas, such as the Gansu province [17]. However, the incidence has not declined in the last decade: age-standardized (world) incidence rates were, respectively, 41.4 and 19.2 per 100,000 person-years among Chinese men and women in 2002, and 41.3 and 18.5 in 2008 [1, 14].

The generalized decline in gastric cancer rates has been attributed to several factors: a more varied and affluent diet, including increased consumption of vegetables and fruit and decreased consumption of cured meat, salt and salt-preserved foods; better food conservation, including refrigeration; control of *Helicobacter pylori* infection [18]; and a decrease in tobacco smoking [5].

1.3 Epidemiology of Gastric Cancer as a Function of Site and Histology

Temporal trends in the incidence of gastric cancer vary as a function of both tumor morphology and organ subsite. The declining incidence of gastric cancer is mainly due to a decreasing incidence of intestinal tumors, while the incidence of diffuse tumor has been generally stable throughout the world [15 Italy; 19 Finland; 20 Japan; 21 United States].

As regards primary tumor site, the decreasing trend mainly concerns tumors arising from the gastric body or antrum, while the incidence of tumors of the cardia and upper third of the stomach has been stable or even increasing. In Norway, age-adjusted rates for distal gastric tumors decreased in both sexes between 1958 and 1992, while the rates of proximal gastric cancer were stable in men and decreased only slightly in females [22]. In the Gansu province of China, the proportion of cardia cancers increased, respectively, from 29.6% in 1993 to 37.1% in 2004, while for body cancers the increase was from 22.6% in 1993 to 31.5% in 2004; within the same period, the proportion of cancers arising from the antrum declined from 41.4% to 21.1% [23].

In particular, cardia cancer reportedly increased in Western countries until the 1990s, remaining stable or declining thereafter. In Spain, the age-adjusted incidence of gastric cardia cancer increased during the 1980s, after which it remained stable in males until 2004 and slightly declined in females [10]. In the US, cardia cancer incidence rates increased from the 1970s to the 1990s [24] and decreased thereafter [21], whereas cancer incidence rates for all other gastric sites steadily declined. A strong increase in cardia cancer was recorded during the 1990s also in Canada: between 1990 and 1999 the incidence of cardia cancer in British Columbia increased by 9.2% per year among women and by 3.8% among men [25]. The most recent studies, performed in the Netherlands from 1990 to 2007 [9] and in South Korea from 1991 through 2000 [26], found no change in the proportion of cardia cancer.

Taking into account the fall in the incidence of esophageal squamous cell carcinoma and the concomitant rise in the incidence of distal adenocarcinoma of the esophagus, we can conclude that upper gastrointestinal tumors are decreasing overall but concentrating around the gastro-esophageal junction. Indeed, when adenocarcinomas of the esophagus and gastric cardia were considered together, their incidence rose in most European countries during the period 1983–1997; the increases were strongest in Northern Europe (1–7% per year), with smaller increases (1–3% per year) seen in the other European regions [27].

1.4 Survival in Gastric Cancer Patients

The prognosis in gastric cancer patients varies enormously across the world, remaining dismal in Europe and the US whereas it has become rather favorable in Japan. In Europe, the average 5-year survival estimate is 25% [28] while in the US median survival is less than 1 year [29]. By contrast, in Japan, 5-year survival is around 66% in patients with primary gastric cancer and 68.2% in resected cases [30].

The good prognosis achieved in Japan is the result of sustained and remarkable improvements in survival in the last decades. For instance, in the Osaka district, 5-year survival improved from 28% in 1975–1977 to 50% in 1990–1992 [31]. In the US [29] and in Europe [32], however, progress in the treatment of gastric cancer has been limited. In 18 European countries, 5-year age-adjusted relative survival for gastric cancer increased from 22% in 1988 to 24% in 2009, an improvement that was clearly lower with respect to all cancers combined (from 34% to 39% in men and from 52 to 59% in women). In the Nordic countries, 5-year survival increased from 10–15% in 1969–1973 to 15–30% in 1999–2003 [8]. Likewise, in Italy, 5-year survival slightly improved from 1986–1989 to 2000–2003, from 22% to 29% in men and from 27% to 32% in women [15, 33].

The lack of remarkable improvements in survival in gastric cancer has been attributed to an increase in the relative proportion of more aggressive cancers [32]. For instance, 5-year survival decreased from 22% in 1990–1993 to 14% in 2002–2006 among Dutch patients with a non-cardia adenocarcinoma, but this decrease was paralleled by a simultaneous increase in the proportion of patients presenting with stage IV tumors, from 31% to 40%. Hence, controlling for stage and other risk factors in multivariable survival analysis, the risk of dying remained stable over time [9].

1.5 Primary and Secondary Prevention of Gastric Cancer

Two strategies are possible to prevent gastric cancer: eradication of *Helicobacter pylori* (primary prevention) or early detection of gastric cancer by mass screening (secondary prevention).

1.5.1 Primary Prevention

Helicobacter pylori is the strongest known risk factor for distal intestinal gastric cancer. Several tests are available to detect *H. pylori* infection, ranging from the most accessible urea breath test to the blood antibody test or stool antigen test, to the most invasive tissue biopsy. The infection is usually eradicated by antibiotics, administered in association with an antisecretory agent. Decision analysis models suggest that preventing *H. pylori* infection via vaccination in childhood could be cost-effective and reduce the incidence of gastric cancer by over 40% [34]. Alternatively, *H. pylori* detection and prophylactic eradication could be offered to high-risk individuals, such as first-degree relatives of patients with gastric cancer, who have double the risk of *H. pylori* infection, gastric atrophy and intestinal metaplasia [35]. The Asia-Pacific Gastric Cancer Consensus Conference recommends a strategy of *H. pylori* screening and eradication only in high-risk populations [36]. As yet, however, no country has adopted public health measures to treat infected individuals or prevent infection in populations at risk.

1.5.2 Secondary Prevention

Screening for gastric cancer is currently ongoing in Eastern Asia, i.e., the area with the highest incidence of the disease. In Japan, a screening system was introduced in the 1960s and extended to all people age 40 years and over in 1983; photofluorography is the procedure recommended [37]. In 2002, as many as 5,843,904 subjects underwent mass screening for gastric cancer, mainly by barium X-ray. Of these, 379,965 underwent further examination, mainly by endoscopy; 5410 subjects were identified as having gastric cancer, yielding a positive predictive value of 1.4% [38]. The total cost for the 2002 screening program in Yen was estimated as 25,393,209,000 (235,748,000 Euros), while the cost in Yen required to find a single case was 4,408,543 (40,928 Euros) [38].

As conventional barium X-ray is able to detect no more than 39% of early gastric cancers, a new screening program has been proposed that combines serum pepsinogen testing and barium digital radiography [39]. This combination is particularly useful as the two methods detect different gastric cancer subgroups: the serum pepsinogen test efficiently detects asymptomatic, small, early cancers with an intestinal-type histology while barium digital radiography is efficient at detecting cancers with a depressed or ulcerated morphology and a diffuse-type histology [39]. With this method, as many as 88% of the detected cancer lesions are still in the early stage, i.e., confined to the mucosa or submucosa.

Also, in South Korea, gastric cancer screening by endoscopy has been implemented since 1999 in people age 40 years and over, and detected gastric adenomas are actively treated. The proportion of early gastric cancer in the screened population was determined to be almost 75%. Diffusion of the screening program was associated with a parallel increase in the percentage of early gastric cancer among surgically treated patients: 28.6% in 1995 and 47.4% in 2004 [3].

In Japan, screening programs for gastric cancer seems to be quite effective. First of all, the proportion of gastric cancers that were localized at diagnosis in 1995–2000 was particularly high (53%) [40], two-fold higher than in the US (27%) [41]. Second, the prognosis of gastric cancer patients has largely improved since the implementation of screening programs: in the Osaka district 5-year survival improved from 28% in 1975–1977 to 50% in 1990–1992 [31].

Clearly, regardless of official screening programs, every case of dyspepsia or unsolved epigastric complaints, especially in patients over 40 years of age and in those who are at high risk, should be investigated promptly by means of endoscopy and biopsy [42].

References

1. Ferlay J, Shin HR, Bray F et al (2010) GLOBOCAN 2008, Cancer Incidence and Mortality Worldwide: IARC CancerBase No. 10 [Internet]. International Agency for Research on Cancer, Lyon, France. Available from: http://globocan.iarc.fr
2. The Research Group for Population-based Cancer Registration in Japan (2004) Cancer incidence and incidence rates in Japan in 1999: Estimates based on data from 11 population-based cancer registries. Jpn J Clin Oncol 34:352–356
3. Kang KJ, Lee JH (2010) Characteristics of Gastric Cancer in Korea - with an emphasis on the increase of the Early Gastric Cancer (EGC). J Korean Med Assoc 53:283-289
4. Moore MA, Eser S, Igisinov N et al (2010) Cancer epidemiology and control in north-western and central Asia - past, present and future. Asian Pacific J Cancer Prev 11:17-31
5. Bertuccio P, Chatenoud L, Levi F et al (2009) Recent patterns in gastric cancer: A global overview. Int J Cancer 125:666-673
6. Levi F, Lucchini F, Gonzalez JR et al (2004) Monitoring falls in gastric cancer mortality in Europe. Ann Oncol 15:338-345
7. La Vecchia C, Bosetti C, Lucchini F et al (2010) Cancer mortality in Europe, 2000-2004, and an overview of trends since 1975. Ann Oncol 21:1323-1360
8. Klint A, Engholm G, Storm HH et al (2010) Trends in survival of patients diagnosed with cancer of the digestive organs in the Nordic countries 1964-2003 followed up to the end of 2006. Acta Oncologica 49:578-607
9. Dassen AE, Lemmens VEPP, van de Poll-Franse LV et al (2010) Trends in incidence, treatment and survival of gastric adenocarcinoma between 1990 and 2007: a population-based study in the Netherlands. Eur J Cancer 46:1101-1110
10. Aragones N, Izarzugaza MI, Ramos M et al (2010) Trends in oesophago-gastric cancer incidence in Spain: analysis by subsite and histology. Ann Oncol 21:69-75
11. Crocetti E, AIRTUM Working Group (2009) Per quali tumori l'incidenza sta cambiando più rapidamente? Epidemiol Prev 33:78
12. Anderson WF, Camargo MC, Fraumeni JF et al (2010) Age-specific trends in incidence of noncardia gastric cancer in US adults. J Am Med Assoc 303:1723-1728
13. Inoue M, Tsugane S (2005) Epidemiology of gastric cancer in Japan. Postgrad Med J 81:419-424
14. Ferlay J, Bray F, Pisani P, Parkin DM (2004) GLOBOCAN 2002: cancer incidence, mortality and prevalence worldwide, Version 2.0. IARC CancerBase No. 5, IARC Press, Lyon
15. Crocetti E, Capocaccia R, Casella C et al (2004) Cancer trends in Italy: figures from the Cancer Registries (1986-1997). Epidemiol Prev 28:S1-S112
16. Yang L (2006) Incidence and mortality of gastric cancer in China. World J Gastroenterol 12:17-20
17. Sun XD, Mu R, Zhou YS et al (2004) Analysis of mortality rate of stomach cancer and its trend in 20 years in China. Chin J Oncol 26:4-9
18. Brown LM (2000) Helicobacter pylori epidemiology and routes of transmission. Epidemiol Rev 22:283-297
19. Laurén PA, Nevalainen TJ (1993) Epidemiology of intestinal and diffuse types of gastric carcinoma. A time-trend study in Finland with comparison between studies from high- and low-risk areas. Cancer 71:2926-2933
20. Kaneko S, Yoshimura T (2001) Time trend analysis of gastric cancer incidence in Japan by histological types, 1975-1989. Brit J Cancer 84:400-405
21. Wu H, Rusiecki JA, Zhu K et al (2009) Stomach carcinoma incidence patterns in the United States by histologic type and anatomic site. Cancer Epidemiol Biomarkers Prev 18:1945-1952
22. Hansen S, Wiig JN, Giercksky KE, Tretli S (1997) Esophageal and gastric carcinoma in Norway 1958-1992: incidence time trend variability according to morphological subtypes and organ subsites. Int J Cancer 71:340-344
23. Zhou Y, Zhang Z, Zhang Z et al (2008) A rising trend of gastric cardia cancer in Gansu Province of China. Cancer Letters 269:18-25
24. Devesa SS, Blot WJ, Fraumeni JF Jr (1998) Changing patterns in the incidence of esophageal and gastric carcinoma in the United States. Cancer 83:2049-2053
25. Bashash M, Shah A, Hislop G et al (2008) Incidence and survival for gastric and esophageal cancer diagnosed in British Columbia, 1990 to 1999. Can J Gastroenterol 22:143-148
26. Lee JY, Kim HY, Kim KH et al (2003) No Changing Trends in Incidence of Gastric Cardia Cancer in Korea. J Korean Med Sci 18:53-57
27. Steevens J, Botterweck AAM, Dirx MJM et al (2010) Trends in incidence of oesophageal and stomach cancer subtypes in Europe. Eur J Gastroenterol Hepatol 22:669-678
28. Sant M, Allemani C, Santaquilani M et al (2009) EUROCARE-4. Survival of cancer patients diagnosed in 1995-1999. Results and commentary. Eur J Cancer 45:931-939
29. Shah MA, Kelsen DP (2010) Gastric Cancer: A Primer on the Epidemiology and Biology of the Disease and an Overview of the Medical Management of Advanced Disease. J Natl Compr Canc Netw 8:437-447
30. Maruyama K, Kaminishi M, Hayashi K-I et al, for The Japanese Gastric Cancer Association Registration Committee (2006) Gastric cancer treated in 1991 in Japan: data analysis of nationwide registry. Gastric cancer 9:51-66
31. Tsukuma H, Oshima A, Murakami R (1999) Effect of stomach cancer screening on reducing the mortality –descriptive data in Osaka. J Gastroenterol Mass Survey 37:53-58
32. Verdecchia A, Guzzinati S, Francisci S et al (2009) Survival trends in European cancer patients diagnosed from 1988 to 1999. Eur J Cancer 45:1042-1066
33. AIRTUM Working Group. New incidence and mortality data: 2003-2005. Epidemiol Prev 2009; 33(1-2): Supplemento 2
34. Ford AC, Axon ATR (2010) Epidemiology of Helicobacter pylori infection and Public Health Implications. Helicobacter 15:1-6
35. Rokkas T, Sechopoulos P, Pistiolas D et al (2010) Helicobacter pylori infection and gastric histology in first-degree relatives of gastric cancer patients: a meta-analysis. Eur J Gas-

troenterol Hepatol 22:1128-1133
36. Fock KM, Talley N, Moayyedi P et al (2008) Asia-Pacific consensus guidelines on gastric cancer prevention. J Gastroenterol Hepatol 23:351-365
37. Hamashima C, Shibuya D, Yamakazi H et al (2008) The Japanese Guidelines for Gastric Cancer Screening. Jpn J Clin Oncol 38:259-267
38. Koga M, Mijakawa K, Ikeda S (2004) Annual Report of Gastroenterological Mass Survey in Japan 2002. Tokyo: Japanese Society of Gastroenterology Mass Survey
39. Ohata H, Oka M, Yanaoka K et al (2005) Gastric cancer screening of a high-risk population in Japan using serum pepsinogen and barium digital radiography. Cancer Sci 96:713-720
40. The Research Group for Population-based Cancer Registration in Japan. Annual reports 1997-2003, 1998-2004. Research Group for Population-based Cancer Registration, Osaka, Japan
41. Ries LAG, Eisner MP, Kosary CL et al (2004) SEER cancer statistics review, 1975-2001. National Cancer Institute, Bethesda, MD. http://seer.cancer.gov/csr/ 1975_2001/
42. Jatzko G, Pertl A, Jagoditsch M (1999) Chirurgische Therapie und Ergebnisse beim Magen-frühkarzinom. Chir Gastroenterol 15:223-226

Etiopathogenesis of Gastric Cancer

2

Giovanni Corso, Daniele Marrelli, and Franco Roviello

Abstract

The introduction of molecular biology into cancer genetics has resulted in the clarification of several crucial aspects in the etiopathogenesis and tumorigenesis of human cancer. However, gastric cancer continues to represent a clinical burden because of its unfavorable prognosis and our poor knowledge of the molecular mechanisms responsible for the early steps in the initiation of gastric tumor development. Progress has been made through the elucidation of different molecular signaling cascades, such as the mitogen-activated protein kinase cascade, in which the mutator phenotype has been ascribed to a deficiency of the mismatch repair system. While this and similar recent discoveries are still being discussed with respect to their scientific implications, it may nonetheless be appropriate to consider potential clinical applications in the management of patients with gastric cancer.

Keywords

Gastric cancer • Tobacco consumption • Helicobacter pylori • E-cadherin • Microsatellite instability • KRAS • PIK3CA • EGFR • MAPK cascade • Prognostic factors • Therapy

2.1 Introduction

Gastric cancer (GC) is the second most common form of cancer in Europe [1]. In 2000, there were 192,000 new cases with 158,000 deaths. In Southern Europe, the highest incidence of GC is found in the Tuscany region of Italy and in Portugal [2]. Despite advances in the prevention and diagnosis of GC; the outcome of these patients has remained poor, with an overall 5-year survival of around 23%.

Several genetic, epigenetic, and environmental factors interact simultaneously in the early steps of gastric carcinogenesis. Among these, human genetic polymorphisms of inflammatory-related genes are thought to be responsible for an increased risk of GC. Other factors, such as tobacco consumption, dietary habits, and *Helicobacter pylori* infection, have been demonstrated to be involved in the multifactorial process of gastric carcinogenesis. Germline inactivating mutations and deletions of the E-cadherin gene (*CDH1*) are well-documented genetic events associated with early-onset GC and with hereditary diffuse gastric cancer (HDGC) syndrome. E-cadherin somatic

G. Corso (✉)
Dept. of Human Pathology and Oncology,
Section of General Surgery and Surgical Oncology,
Translational Research Laboratory,
University of Siena,
Siena, Italy

inactivation correlates with aggressive tumor behavior and a worse prognosis. Conversely, microsatellite instability (MSI) phenotype, which is the hallmark of GC in about 20–25% of cases, is a relatively good prognostic factor. Within MSI patterns, somatic mutations in the oncogenes *KRAS*, *PIK3CA*, and *EGFR* play a crucial role in the genetic instability of GC. In this chapter, we focus on GC etiopathogenesis by exploring its genetic/epigenetic mechanisms.

2.2 Tobacco Consumption and Dietary Habits

Smoking is a major risk factor for adenocarcinomas of the esophagus and gastric cardia, accounting for approximately 40% of cases. Most but not all studies report a higher risk in the cardia than in non-cardia sites in cigarette smokers vs. nonsmokers; conversely, alcohol consumption may be associated with an increased risk of distal and total GC [3, 4]. The risk of gastric cardia adenocarcinomas is increased among current cigarette smokers with a reduction first observed 30 years after smoking cessation; the risk of GC rises with increasing intensity and duration of smoking. Because of the long lag time before the risk of these tumors is reduced among ex-smokers, smoking is thought to affect early-stage carcinogenesis.

In gastric carcinogenesis, diet is also a determinant; salted, smoked, pickled and preserved foods (rich in salt, nitrite, and pre-formed N-nitroso compounds) as well as meat intake are associated with an increased risk of non-cardia GC. However, rather than only a single responsible agent, dietary habits, consumption frequency, amount of exposure to etiologically important agents, traditional food-preparation techniques, and storage methods all play major roles in the etiology of GC. Excessive salt consumption is a confirmed factor whereas in Japan and other Far East countries excessive consumption of fish and other seafood plays the lead role in GC etiology. A reduced consumption of fresh fruits and vegetables is another important etiologic factor. Dietary factors and improvements in food storage, such as refrigeration, which decreases the turnover of nitrosamines to nitrites, have caused a significant decline in the worldwide prevalence of GCs. Interestingly, Palli et al. showed an association between GC and a high consumption of red meat [5]. The etiopathogenesis of gastric cardia carcinoma is related to nitrosamine consumption but also to exposure, as these compounds are present in tobacco and tobacco smoke and their carcinogenic activities have been well established. Similarly, cured fish and meat may contain *N*-nitroso compounds (NOC) such that the mechanism of carcinogenesis due to tobacco consumption and to certain dietary habits may be linked by the common presence of NOC. The role of NOC in GC etiology involves alteration of the pH of gastric juice; specifically, in the presence of NOC the pH of gastric juice is low (1.0–2.5), leading to a phenomenon called "chemical gastric nitrosation," which proceeds as an acid-catalyzed reaction in the normal acidic stomach before premalignant lesions develop. High concentrations of NOC have been identified in vivo also in the inflamed gastric mucosa infected with *H. pylori*, accompanied by a high pH (6.0-8.5). Similarly, high pH induces bacterial gastric nitrosation. This chemical modification results in an increased tolerance to DNA damage, with reduced activity of mismatch repair (MMR) genes leading to an accumulation of errors during DNA replication.

2.3 *Helicobacter pylori* Infection

Several prospective studies have reported a strong association between chronic *H. pylori* infection and GC risk; as such, the World Health Organization's International Agency for Research on Cancer recognized *H. pylori* as a group 1 carcinogen for humans. Chronic gastric inflammation and the interaction between *H. pylori* and gastric epithelial cells have been suggested as mechanisms in gastric carcinogenesis. However, only a few individuals infected by *H. pylori* go on to develop GC. These cases probably also involve environmental factors, host-inflammatory genetic susceptibility, and variation of the bacterial strains. *H. pylori* is a gram-negative bacterium that colonizes the human gastric epithelium. The severity of *H.-pylori*-related disease is correlated with the presence of the *cag* pathogenicity island

(PAI), associated with the production of the *cagA* antigen. The *cagA* gene is a strain-specific *H. pylori* gene located in the right half of the PAI. It encodes the protein CagA, which is secreted via a type IV secretion system and translocated into gastric epithelial cells, affecting host cell physiology. Infection with *cag*-positive *H. pylori* strains has been recognized as a marker for strains that confer increased risk for peptic ulcer disease, gastric mucosal atrophy, and GC. By contrast, the *vacA* gene is present in all *H. pylori* strains. It encodes the vacuolating cytotoxin VacA, which induces epithelial cell injury. *H. pylori* colonizes the atrophic stomach poorly and intestinal metaplasia hardly at all, suggesting that the bacteria creates an environment for intestinal-type gastric carcinogenesis (atrophy and hypochlorhydria) rather than causing the cancer directly. The risk of developing GC for infected persons is estimated to be 2–3 times higher than for non-infected ones. More recently, the role of individual susceptibility has been stressed. In addition, proinflammatory cytokine gene polymorphisms have been demonstrated to interact in the compound process of gastric carcinogenesis [6]. For example, the relationship between interleukin-1 gene polymorphism and GC risk has been investigated. The conclusions support the theory in which host genetic factors affecting the inflammatory and immune response to *H. pylori* infection determine a higher risk of GC development, especially in high-risk areas [7, 8].

In GC, the absence of *H. pylori* infection is related to specific clinico-pathological factors impacting the long-term survival of these patients. Negative *H. pylori* status is associated with cardia tumor location, advanced pT classification, non-curative surgery, and a lower 5-year survival rate after R0 resection. Marrelli et al. demonstrated that *H. pylori* status is a significant prognostic factor, in which negative *H. pylori* status appears to be an indicator of poor prognosis in patients with GC [9].

2.4 E-Cadherin Gene (*CDH1*) and Diffuse Gastric Cancer

The *CDH1* gene maps to chromosome 16q22.1 and consists of 16 exons that encode a 120-kDa protein called E-cad, which is a member of the transmembrane glycoproteins family. E-cad is expressed on epithelial tissues and is responsible for calcium-dependent cell-cell adhesion. Functionally, it is critical for establishing and maintaining polarized and differentiated epithelia through intercellular adhesion complexes. Human E-cad is considered an invasion suppressor, and under-expression of E-cad is correlated with the infiltrative and metastatic ability of the tumor. *CDH1* deregulation has been identified in early tumors of patients with germline mutations and thus may be an initial event in HDGC [10, 11]. In GC, the principal epigenetic and structural mechanisms of *CDH1* inactivation/deregulation are somatic mutations, loss of heterozygosity (LOH), and promoter hypermethylation. About 90% of GC cases appear in a sporadic setting, whereas familial clustering is observed in the remaining 10%; of these cases, only 1–3% are hereditary. Among those with familial aggregation of GC, the most common disease is the HDGC syndrome, which is related to *CDH1* germline mutations. The syndrome was first identified in 1998 by Guilford in Maori kindred from New Zealand. To date, many studies have reported different types of *CDH1* alterations in HDGC families, with 30–40% of these families harboring *CDH1* germline mutations, as reviewed by Pedrazzani and colleagues [12]. In 1999, the International Gastric Cancer Linkage Consortium (IGCLC) defined the following criteria for the identification of HDGC families: (1) two or more documented cases of DGC in first- or second-degree relatives, with at least one of these relatives diagnosed before the age of 50; (2) three or more documented cases of DGC in first- or second-degree relatives, independent of age of onset.

After demonstrating the presence of *CDH1* germline mutations in patients not fulfilling the IGCLC criteria, Brooks-Wilson and colleagues recommended several modifications: (1) two or more documented cases of DGC in first-degree relatives, with at least one diagnosed before age 50; (1A) two or more cases of GC, with at least one case of DGC diagnosed before age 50; (2) three or more documented cases of DGC in first-degree relatives, diagnosed at any age; (2A) three or more cases of GC, diagnosed at any age, with at least one documented case of DGC; (3) isolated individual diagnosed with DGC at less than 45 years of age; (4) isolated individual diagnosed with both DGC and lobular breast cancer (no other criteria met); (5) one family member diagnosed with DGC and another with lobular breast cancer (no other criteria met); (6) one family member diagnosed with DGC and another with signet-ring carcinoma of the colon (no other criteria met) [13]. These novel criteria introduced a new clinical entity called early-onset DGC, in which E-cadherin mutations occur with a frequency of about 6%. The cut-off age for *CDH1* genetic screening is 35 years old at DGC diagnosis [14]. *CDH1* down-regulation plays a specific role in gastric carcinogenesis, and DGC with signet-ring cells (SRCs) is the predominant histological type in carriers of *CDH1* germline mutations. In its early stage, HDGC is characterized by the presence of multiple foci of diffuse-type SRC carcinoma confined to the superficial gastric mucosa [15]. The majority of neoplastic foci observed in the resected specimen after prophylactic gastrectomy are < 1 mm in diameter, and all lie under normal appearing surface epithelium [11]. Multifocal microscopic disease is very common, with a preferential localization along the epithelial wall of the gastric body/fundus. Carneiro and colleagues proposed a histological model for GC development in carriers of E-cad mutation: initially, histopathological analysis shows a pattern of in situ SRC carcinoma with early pagetoid spread and pagetoid proliferation of SRCs followed by invasive SRC carcinoma. *H. pylori* infection is not detected in gastric mucosa obtained from prophylactic gastrectomies [16]. Carriers of E-cad truncating germline mutations have a fairly high lifetime risk of developing GC; the estimated cumulative risk by age 80 years is 67% for men (95% CI, 39–99) and 83% for women (95% CI, 58–99), with a mean age at diagnosis of 40 years (range, 14–85) [17]. Prophylactic total gastrectomy remains the only method to abolish the inherited risk for gastric cancer in carriers of *CDH1* truncating mutation; however, the role of prophylactic gastrectomy in missense mutation carriers remains to be clarified, because to date prophylactic surgery has yet to be performed in these patients [12]. The strategy for clinical management includes a review of the family history, genetic testing, chromoendoscopic surveillance, and prophylactic surgery.

2.5 Microsatellite Instability and Oncogenic Mutations

The mutator or MSI phenotype is caused by a defect in the MMR system, which is responsible for the correction of mismatches that occur during DNA replication. In gastric carcinoma, this phenotype is found in about 15–25% of the cases [18]. To date, no germline mutations involving MMR genes have been described in familial GC; on the other hand, somatic mutations in MMR genes are rare in sporadic GC [19]. Cancers with genomic instability show distinct clinico-pathological features. Most MSI tumors are of intestinal histotype and located in the distal part of the stomach, with limited lymph node involvement; they occur more frequently in older women. Survival analysis of patients with MSI status demonstrated a good prognosis in those with advanced tumors and instability at all markers [18]. In the high-level MSI phenotyope, the mitogen-activated protein kinase (*MAPK*) cascade and phosphatidylinositol 3-kinase (*PI3K*) pathways are frequently activated in the progression of gastrointestinal malignancies. The oncogenes implicated in the MSI subset of GC are *EGFR*, *KRAS*, and *PIK3CA*. While data on *EGFR* alterations as well as mutations (hotspot region) in the gene's downstream targets, namely those belonging to the *MAPK* and *PI3K* pathways, are very limited, alterations of the polyA tract at the 3'-UTR of *EGFR* have been shown to occur with a high frequency (about 50% of cases) [20]. The presence of mutations at the 3'-UTR of *EGFR* is related to a high level of *EGFR* expression [21]. *KRAS* gene mutations occur with a frequency of 3–8% and typically cluster in the MSI subset (~17% of MSI cases). In contrast, several groups, including our own, have found that *BRAF* mutations rarely occur in this type of epithelial cancer. The frequency of *PIK3CA* oncogenic mutations is about 14%; another oncogene albeit one rarely involved (3%) is *MLK3*. Alterations within multiple molecules included in or targeted by the *MAPK* pathway are frequent in MSI GC, with deletions of the A13 repeat of *EGFR* being the most common genetic event followed by *KRAS* and *PIK3CA* mutations. More importantly, this molecular model opens new avenues regarding the stratification of MSI GC patients for anti-*EGFR* therapies and for identifying those patients who are most likely to benefit from a targeted therapeutic approach.

2.6 Conclusions

The etiopathogenesis of GC is complex and multifactorial. This review focused on the principal mechanisms involved in gastric carcinogenesis. Of particular importance are "exogenous" factors, such as tobacco, dietary habits, and *H. pylori* infection, and "endogenous," factors, such as E-cadherin germline mutations and genetic/ epigenetic events. However, endogenous and exogenous factors may not be mutually exclusive; for example, the presence of chronic inflammation resulting from *H. pylori* infection is probably related to the MSI phenotype and thus to alterations in the *MAPK* cascade. For clinical practice, we propose a flow-chart (Fig. 2.1) in which the molecular pathway of GC etiopathogenesis is divided in terms of prognostic and therapeutic biomarkers. Group A includes those patients expressing the prognostic biomarkers MSI and E-cadherin, indicating, respectively, a good vs. a worse prognosis. Moreover, recently we described the CDH1 structural alteration as a novel biomarker of worse prognosis in GC patients [22]. Group B consists of patients who are candidates for a new therapeutic approach, such as *EGFR*-inhibitors, whereas it remains to be determined whether *KRAS/PIK3CA* mutations can also be included in this group.

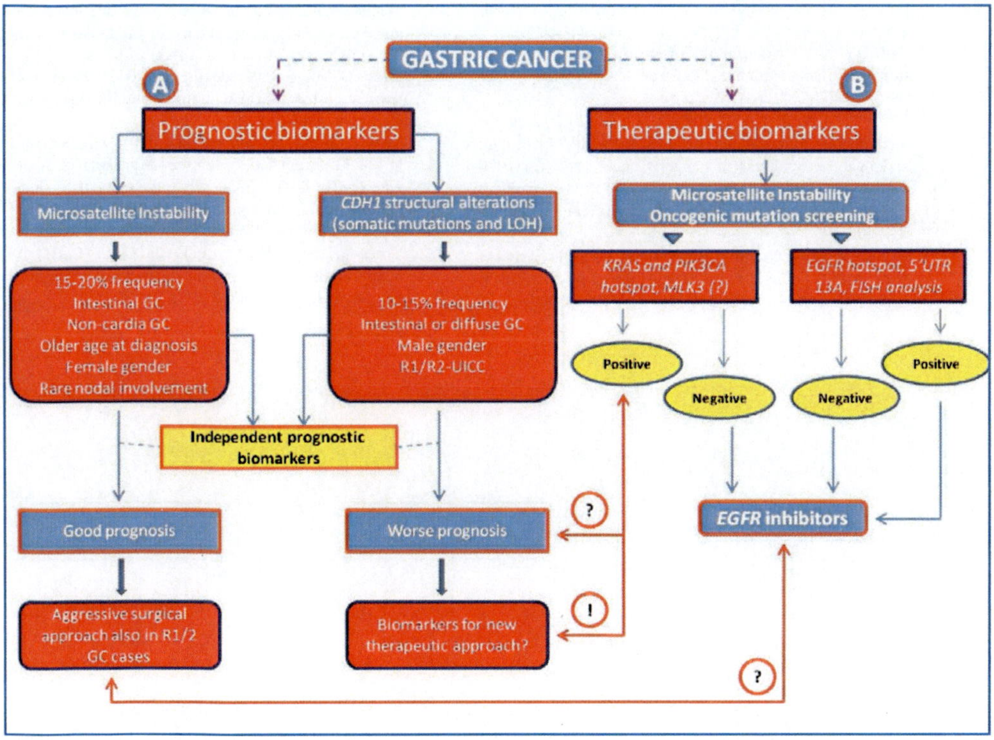

Fig. 2.1 The flow-chart proposes the clinical management of gastric carcinoma with respect to several molecular features of its ethiopatogenesis. Prognostic biomarkers include MSI status and *CDH1* structural alterations. Predictive therapeutic biomarkers consider the *MAPK/PI3K* pathway and oncogenic mutations

References

1. Parkin DM, Bray F, Ferlay J et al (2005) Global cancer statistics, 2002. CA Cancer J Clin 55:74-108
2. Ferlay J, Autier P, Boniol M et al (2007) Estimates of the cancer incidence and mortality in Europe in 2006. Ann Oncol 18:581-592
3. Moy KA, Fan Y, Wang R et al (2010) Alcohol and Tobacco Use in Relation to Gastric Cancer: A Prospective Study of Men in Shanghai, China. Cancer Epidemiol Biomarkers 19:2287-2297
4. Sung NY, Choi KS, Park EC et al (2007) Smoking, alcohol and gastric cancer risk in Korean men: the National Health Insurance Corporation Study. Br J Cancer 97:700-704
5. Palli D, Russo A, Ottini L et al (2001) Red meat, family history, and increased risk of gastric cancer with microsatellite instability. Cancer Res 61:5415-5419
6. El-Omar EM, Rabkin CS, Gammon MD et al (2003) Increased risk of noncardia gastric cancer associated with proinflammatory cytokine gene polymorphisms. Gastroenterology 124:1193-1201
7. Palli D, Saieva C, Luzzi I et al (2005) Interleukin-1 gene polymorphisms and gastric cancer risk in a high-risk Italian population. Am J Gastroenterol 100:1941-1948
8. Palli D (2000) Epidemiology of gastric cancer: an evaluation of available evidence. J Gastroenterol 35 Suppl 12:84-89
9. Marrelli D, Pedrazzani C, Berardi A et al (2009) Negative Helicobacter pylori status is associated with poor prognosis in patients with gastric cancer. Cancer 115:2071-2080
10. Guilford P, Hopkins J, Harraway J et al (1998) E-cadherin germline mutations in familial gastric cancer. Nature 392:402-405
11. Huntsman DG, Carneiro F, Lewis FR et al (2001) Early gastric cancer in young, asymptomatic carriers of germ-line E-cadherin mutations. N Engl J Med 344:1904-1909
12. Pedrazzani C, Corso G, Marrelli D et al (2007) E-cadherin and hereditary diffuse gastric cancer. Surgery 142:645-657
13. Brooks-Wilson AR, Kaurah P, Suriano G et al (2004) Germline E-cadherin mutations in hereditary diffuse gastric cancer: assessment of 42 new families and review of genetic screening criteria. J Med Genet 41:508-517
14. Corso G, Pedrazzani C, Pinheiro H et al (2011) E-cadherin genetic screening and clinico-pathologic characteristics of Early Onset Gastric Cancer. Eur J Cancer 47:631-639
15. Charlton A, Blair V, Shaw D et al (2004) Hereditary diffuse gastric cancer: predominance of multiple foci of signet ring cell carcinoma in distal stomach and transitional zone. Gut 53:814-820
16. Carneiro F, Huntsman DG, Smyrk TC et al (2004) Model of the early development of diffuse gastric cancer in E-cadherin mutation carriers and its implications for patient screening. J Pathol 203:681-687
17. Lynch HT, Grady W, Suriano G et al (2005) Gastric cancer: new genetic developments. J Surg Oncol 90:114-133
18. Corso G, Pedrazzani C, Marrelli D et al (2009) Correlation of microsatellite instability at multiple loci with long-term survival in advanced gastric carcinoma. Arch Surg 144:722-727
19. Pinto M, Wu Y, Mensink RG et al (2008) Somatic mutations in mismatch repair genes in sporadic gastric carcinomas are not a cause but a consequence of the mutator phenotype. Cancer Genet Cytogenet 180:110-114
20. Corso G, Velho S, Paredes J e tal (2011) Oncogenic mutations in gastric cancer with microsatellite instability. Eur J Cancer 47:443-451
21. Yuan Z, Shin J, Wilson A et al (2009) An A13 repeat within the 3'-untranslated region of epidermal growth factor receptor (EGFR) is frequently mutated in microsatellite instability colon cancers and is associated with increased EGFR expression. Cancer Res 69:7811-7818
22. Corso G, Pascale V, Marrelli D et al (2011) CDH1 structural alterations as novel prognostic biomarker in gastric cancer patients. J Clin Oncol 29:(Suppl 4)

Lymphatic Spread, Lymph Node Stations, and Levels of Lymphatic Dissection in Gastric Cancer

3

Giovanni de Manzoni, Franco Roviello, Alberto Di Leo, and Giuseppe Verlato

Abstract

The lymphatic drainage from the stomach is complex and it is difficult to predict the pattern of lymph node metastases from gastric cancer. Nevertheless, there are lymph node stations in which metastases are more frequently observed in relation to the tumor site. Moreover, the frequency of metastasis to various regional node stations depends on the depth of gastric-wall invasion.

The Japanese Gastric Cancer Association (JGCA) guidelines have designated four levels of lymph node dissection. D1 lymphadenectomy is a complete dissection of the N1 lymph node group. D1+α dissection is a D1 lymphadenectomy plus resection of station 7. D1+β dissection is a D1 lymphadenectomy plus resection of stations 7, 8a, and 9. D2 (extended) and D3 (super-extended) dissections remove, respectively, lymph node stations of the N1-N2 and N1-N3 lymph node groups. Recently the JGCA revised the definition of Lymphadenectomy: D1 or D2 are now defined according to the type of gastrectomy performed (total/subtotal).

Keywords

Lymphatic drainage • Regional lymph nodes • Lymph node stations • Lymph node metastasis • Skip metastasis • D1 dissection • D1+α dissection • D1+β dissection • D2 dissection • D3 dissection • Extended lymphadenectomy • Super-extended lymphadenectomy

3.1 Lymphatic Systems of the Stomach

Historically, numerous studies have sought to elucidate the pathways taken by lymph as it flows from the stomach to the regional lymph nodes [1-4], with the study of Rouvière (1938) as one of the major references. More recently, several techniques have been developed and utilized by authors to better investigate the patterns of physiological gastric lymphatic drainage. These include lymphangiography [5], lymph node vital staining with carbon-particle suspensions or dye [6], and lymphoscintigraphy [7]. The results have confirmed that the lymphatic drainage of the stomach is complex and that different pathways exist, depending on the gastric regions.

G. de Manzoni (✉)
Dept. of Surgery,
Upper G.I. Surgery Division,
University of Verona,
Verona, Italy

G. de Manzoni, F. Roviello, W. Siquini (eds.), *Surgery in the Multimodal Management of Gastric Cancer*,

3.1.1 The Anatomy and Regional Lymph Nodes of the Stomach

The lymphatic drainage system of the stomach is strictly dependent on its different anatomical portions. According to the 2nd English edition of the Japanese Classification of Gastric Carcinoma, published in 1998 [8], the stomach is anatomically divided into upper (U), middle (M), and lower (L) parts. If more than one part is involved, they are referred to according to the degree of involvement, with the first letter indicating the part in which the bulk of the tumor is located; for example, LM means a tumor located mainly in the L part and extending to the M part. When a U cancer extends to the esophagus, the case is described as E+. LD means L tumor invading the duodenum. The gastric circumference is divided into the anterior wall (Ant), the posterior wall (Post), the lesser curvature (Less), and the greater curvature (Gre).

The Japanese Gastric Cancer Association (JGCA) classifies the regional lymph nodes draining the stomach into 23 major stations (Table 3.1), consisting of six perigastric and 17 extra-perigastric stations. The latter include lymph nodes along the major vessels in the upper abdomen, those adjacent to the pancreas, and infradiaphragmatic nodes as well as the esophageal hiatus nodes. Stations 4, 8, 11, 12, 14, and 16 are subdivided into smaller stations, for a total of 33 regional lymphatic stations (Fig. 3.1). These are classified into three (N1-N3) groups with respect to the loca-

Table 3.1 Classification of regional lymph nodes (LN) of the stomach. Modified from [8]

Perigastric lymph node stations		Extra-perigastric lymph node stations	
Station	Location	Station	Location
1	Right paracardial	**7**	Along the left gastric artery
2	Left paracardial	**8a**	Along the hepatic artery (anterosuperior group)
3	Along the lesser curvature	**8p**	Along the hepatic artery (posterior group)
4sa	Along the short gastric vessels	**9**	Around the celiac artery
4sb	Along the left gastroepiploic vessels	**10**	Splenic hilum
4d	Along the right gastroepiploic vessels	**11p**	Along the proximal splenic artery
5	Suprapyloric	**11d**	Along the distal splenic artery
6	Infrapyloric	**12a**	Hepatoduodenal ligament (along the hepatic artery)
		12b	Hepatoduodenal ligament (along the bile duct)
		12p	Hepatoduodenal ligament (behind the portal vein)
		13	Posterior surface of the pancreatic head
		14v	Along the superior mesenteric vein
		14a	Along the superior mesenteric artery
		15	Along the middle colic vessels
		16a1	Aortic hiatus
		16a2	Around the abdominal aorta (from the upper margin of the celiac trunk to the lower margin of the left renal vein)
		16b1	Around the abdominal aorta (from the lower margin of the left renal vein to the upper margin of the inferior mesenteric artery)
		16b2	Around the abdominal aorta (from the upper margin of the inferior mesenteric artery to the aortic bifurcation)
		17	On the anterior surface of the pancreatic head
		18	Along the inferior margin of the pancreas
		19	Infradiaphragmatic
		20	In the esophageal hiatus of the diaphragm
		110	Paraesophageal in the lower thorax
		111	Supradiaphragmatic
		112	Posterior mediastinal

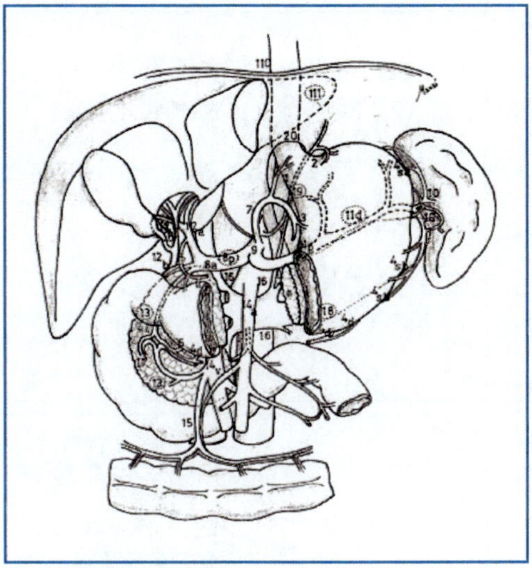

Fig 3.1 Regional lymphatic stations of the stomach according to the JGCA [8]

tion of the primary tumor (Table 3.2). M indicates lymph node stations considered as distant metastases. This grouping system is based on the result of studies of lymphatic flow at various tumor sites, together with the observed survival associated with metastasis at each nodal station [8, 9].

3.1.2 Physiological Lymphatic Drainage from the Stomach

Lymphatic flow from the upper third of the stomach spreads into four major lymphatic channels, running along the left gastric, posterior gastric, splenic, and left inferior phrenic arteries. There are no lymphatic connections with the retropancreatic nodes (station 13) or the mesenteric nodes (station 14).

Lymphatic channels draining the lower third of the stomach run along the common hepatic artery and the root of the superior mesenteric artery, draining into hepatoduodenal ligament nodes (station 12) and the retropancreatic nodes (station 13).

Flow from the gastric lymphatic vessels ultimately drains into the para-aortic nodes (station 16). The perigastric nodes are connected with the nodes of station 16 by four lymphatic pedicles (Fig. 3.2a): (a) the left subdiaphragmatic pedicle

Table 3.2 Lymph node groups (compartments 1–3) by tumor location. The numbers refer to the lymph node stations (see Table 3.1)

Lymph node group	Gastric tumor location		
	Upper third	Middle third	Lower third
Compartment 1 (N1)	1	1	3
	2	2	4d
	3	3	5
	4sa	4sa	6
	4sb	4sb	-
	-	4d	-
	-	5	-
	-	6	-
Compartment 2 (N2)	4d	7	1
	7	8a	7
	8a	9	8a
	9	10	9
	10	11p	11p
	11p	11d	12a
	11d	12a	14v
Compartment 3 (N3)	5	8p	4sb
	6	12b	8p
	8p	12p	12b
	12a	14v	12p
	12b	16a2	13
	12p	16b1	16a2
	16a2	19	16b1
	16b1	20	-
	19	-	-
	20	-	-
M	13	13	2
	14v	14a	4sa
	14a	15	10
	15	16a1	11d
	16a1	16b2	14a
	16b2	17	15
	17	18	16a1
	18	110	16b2
	110	111	17
	111	112	18
	112	-	19
	-	-	20
	-	-	110
	-	-	111
	-	-	112

M, Lymph nodes regarded as distant metastasis.

through the left inferior phrenic artery; (b) the celiac pedicle, which connects with lymph nodes along the left gastric, splenic, and common hepatic arteries; (c) the superior mesenteric pedicle, which receives lymphatics from the infrapyloric nodes (station 6) and passes along the root of the superior mesenteric artery; and (d) the retropancreatic pedicle, which connects with lymphatics from retropyloric nodes (stations 8, 12, and 14).

The left subdiaphragmatic and celiac pedicles receive lymph flow from the upper portion of the stomach. Lymphatic channels from the middle portion are also tributaries to the left subdiaphragmatic pedicle, but they mainly drain through the celiac pedicle. Lymphatic vessels draining the lower region are connected with para-aortic nodes through the celiac, superior mesenteric, and the retropancreatic pedicles.

In the upper half of the stomach (Fig. 3.2b), lymphatic flow from the nodes along the greater curvature (stations 4sa and 4sb) can be directed to nodes at the splenic hilum (station 10) or along the splenic artery (station 11) through the posterior gastric artery, ultimately draining into the para-aortic nodes located above the left renal vein and near the left adrenal gland (station 16a1). Lymphatic vessels from the left paracardial lymph nodes (station 2) drain into the left subdiaphragmatic pedicle connected with para-aortic nodes. In the upper half of the stomach, lymph from nodes along the lesser curvature (station 3) and the right paracardial nodes (station 1) flows to nodes along the left gastric artery (station 7) and around the celiac artery (station 9), which are connected with the para-aortic nodes located around the left renal vein (stations 16a2 and 16b1) through the celiac pedicle.

In the lower half of the stomach (Fig. 3.2c), lymphatics from the nodes along the greater curvature (station 4d) drain mainly into the superior mesenteric pedicle, via the infrapyloric nodes (station 6). Further, they can drain into the retropyloric nodes (stations 8, 12, and 14), which are connected with the para-aortic nodes (stations 16a2 and 16b1) through the retropancreatic pedicle. Lymph can also flow from the nodes along the lesser curvature (stations 3 and 5) to the celiac pedicle and ultimately reach the para-aortic nodes (stations 16a2 and 16b1).

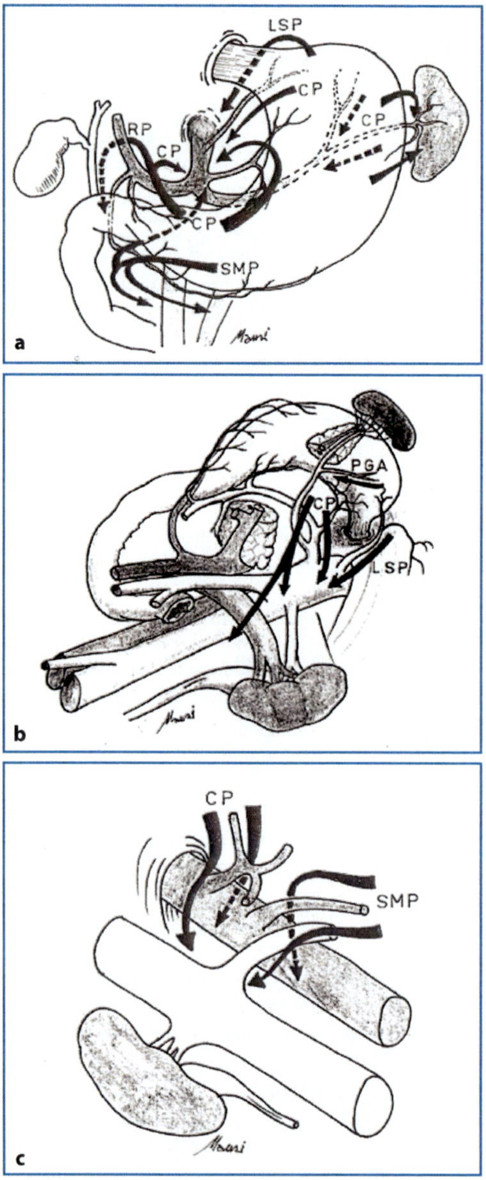

Fig. 3.2 a The connecting lymphatic pedicles between the perigastric and paraaortic nodes: left subdiaphragmatic (*LSP*), celiac (*CP*), superior mesenteric (*SMP*), and retropancreatic (*RP*) pedicles; **b** lymph flow from the upper half of the stomach and posterior gastric artery (*PGA*); **c** lymph flow from the lower half of the stomach

3.2 Patterns of Lymph Node Spread in Gastric Cancer

The presence of a complex and multidirectional lymphatic drainage from the stomach was reported by Maruyama, in a study comprising 1931 patients with gastric cancer [10]. The pattern of lymph node metastasis has been confirmed by recent studies on cancers with single nodal metastasis [11-13] and by analyses of lymph node involvement according to tumor site and T stage [14, 15].

It is difficult to predict the pattern of lymph node metastases from gastric cancer. A study in patients with single perigastric lymph node metastasis has shown that metastatic nodes are usually located on the same side as the tumor, in 87, 83, and 92%, respectively, of upper, middle, and lower tumors, but these ratios decrease and the distribution of metastatic nodes changes to the opposite side of the tumor as the number of metastatic nodes increases [15]. Nevertheless, there are lymph node stations in which metastases are more frequently observed in relation to the part of the stomach in which the bulk of the tumor is located (U, M, or L). Moreover, the frequency of metastasis to various stations depends on the degree of gastric wall invasion [14, 15].

3.2.1 Lymphatic Spread in Adenocarcinoma of the Upper Third of the Stomach

Tumors of the upper third of the stomach are accompanied by nodal metastases in 44–80% of cases [14, 16-20]. In early gastric cancer, the frequency of lymph node metastasis varies from 2% to 5% in intramucosal tumors and from 19% to 50% in submucosal tumors [14, 17, 21]. In advanced gastric cancer, the incidence of nodal metastases is in the range of 65–77% in adenocarcinoma with invasion of the muscularis propria or subserosa and 85–89% if the serosa or adjacent organs are invaded [14, 17].

As shown in Table 3.3, metastatic nodes more frequently occur along the lesser curvature (station 3) and the paracardial stations (1 and 2). Among extra-perigastric nodes, station 7 and 9 are frequently involved, but it is noteworthy that the frequency of infiltration of station 10 and station 16 nodes is higher in upper gastric tumors than in tumors of the middle and lower third of the stomach [8-10, 14].

Table 3.3 Lymph node station involvement by tumor location [8-10, 14]. The values are expressed as range %

Station	Gastric tumor location		
	Upper third	Middle third	Lower third
1	31-51	15-33	5-15
2	13-38	1-11	0-7
3	39-65	39-45	38-42
4	11-25	27-38	29-35
5	2-5	2-9	10-15
6	3-13	15-28	44-49
7	19-39	22-26	22-23
8	7-18	11-15	24-25
9	13-33	8-21	12-13
10	10-26	2-12	0-4
11	12-19	4-11	4-7
12	1-7	2-5	5-9
13	2-12	0-5	8-14
14	0-10	0-9	15-17
15	<1	<1	0-13
16	12-30	7-12	9-13

Table 3.4 reports the frequency of metastatic nodes in each nodal station according to the depth of tumor invasion [14]. The incidence of metastatic nodes at the splenic hilum ranges from 12% to 28% and is related to the depth of invasion; it is null in early cancer, 0–8% in tumors with invasion of muscularis propria or subserosa [14, 18-20], and 22–39% when serosa or adjacent structures are invaded [14, 19, 20, 22]. As described above, lymph from the upper part of the stomach drains into the splenic hilum nodes not only through lymphatic channels along the left gastroepiploic and short gastric arteries, but also through those along the posterior gastric artery. This physiological drainage agrees with the finding that station 10 node metastases are more frequent in tumors located at the greater curvature or posterior wall, and in those with circumferential involvement [10, 18, 20]. Interestingly, from a surgical point of view, this is also the behavior of para-aortic nodes (sta-

Table 3.4 Lymph node stations involvement according to depth of tumor invasion in cancers of the upper third of the stomach [14]. Values are expressed as %

Station	Mucosa	Submucosa	Muscularis propria or subserosa	Serosa	Adjacent structures
1	-	0	52	54	75
2	-	0	38	44	29
3	-	17	59	68	91
4	-	0	13	28	60
5	-	0	0	0	25
6	-	0	6	13	50
7	-	0	31	48	50
8	-	0	10	23	30
9	-	25	18	39	50
11	-	0	4	26	43

tion 16), in which nodal metastases occur in 16–30% of cases [8-10, 14]. Although early gastric cancer does not infiltrate this station, in advanced disease the incidence of metastasis is high: 26% in adenocarcinoma with invasion of the muscularis propria or subserosa, 32% and 38% respectively, when serosa and adjacent organs are invaded [14].

3.2.2 Lymphatic Spread in Adenocarcinoma of the Middle Third of the Stomach

In tumors of the middle third of the stomach, the reported incidence of nodal involvement is 37–65% [14, 16]. Early gastric cancer has metastatic lymph nodes in 0–3% and 19–31%, respectively, of mucosal and submucosal cancers [14, 21]. In patients with advanced gastric cancer, the frequency of metastasis varies from 62% in tumors with invasion of the muscularis propria or subserosa to 90% when the serosa or adjacent structures are infiltrated [14].

Table 3.5 reports the frequency of metastatic nodes in each nodal station according to the depth of tumor invasion [14]. Metastases predominantly occur in perigastric nodes along the lesser curvature (station 3), the greater curvature (stations 4 and 6) and into the right paracardial station (station 1). Indeed extra-perigastric nodes at stations 7 and 9 are frequently involved by tumor [8-10, 14]. The frequency of metastasis into the splenic hilum (station 10) and around the abdominal aorta (station 16) is not as significant as for gastric upper third tumors, but it is noteworthy that these stations are infiltrated, respectively, in 17% and 23% of tumors with invasion of the serosa or adjacent structures [14].

Table 3.5 Lymph node stations involvement according to depth of tumor invasion in cancers of the middle third of the stomach [14]. Values are expressed as %

Station	Mucosa	Submucosa	Muscularis propria or subserosa	Serosa	Adjacent structures
1	0	9	23	52	54
2	0	0	3	17	36
3	0	23	36	93	82
4	0	8	28	61	56
5	0	0	6	15	20
6	0	0	15	51	40
7	0	8	13	43	50
8	0	8	7	28	25
9	0	0	10	33	50
11	0	9	5	16	27

3.2.3 Lymphatic Spread in Adenocarcinoma of the Lower Third of the Stomach

When tumor is located in the lower region of the stomach, lymph node invasion is present in 50–59% of the cases [14, 16]. The incidence of nodal metastases in each level of wall invasion is 2% in intramucosal tumors, 20% in submucosal tumors [21], 57% in cancer with invasion of the muscularis propria or subserosa, and 86% in tumors with invasion of the serosa or adjacent organs [14].

Perigastric metastases from the lower third of the stomach predominantly occur in infrapyloric nodes (station 6) and in nodes along the lesser (station 3) and greater (station 4) curvatures [8-10, 14]. Table 3.6 reports the frequency of metastatic nodes in each nodal station according to the depth of tumor invasion. Among the nodes lying along the greater curvature, the involvement of those associated with short gastric vessels and the left gastroepiploic artery (stations 4sa and 4sb) is rare, even for cancers with infiltration of the serosa or adjacent structures (2%). By contrast, lymph nodes along the right gastroepiploic artery (station 4d) are metastatic in 30% of tumors with invasion of the muscularis propria or subserosa and in 46% if the serosa or adjacent structures are invaded [14].

Among extra-perigastric stations, nodes along the hepatic artery (station 8) and around the celiac artery (station 9) are frequently involved [8-10, 14]; however, infiltration of nodes along the superior mesenteric vein (station 14) is not so rare, especially in tumors with invasion of the subserosa (20%) or serosa (25%) [14].

3.2.1 Skip Metastasis

Gastric adenocarcinoma sometimes spreads to distant lymphatic stations, jumping contiguous nodes. Maruyama reported that in patients with histologically uninvolved perigastric nodes, 2–4% will metastasize to one or more nodes of stations 7–11 and 1% to those of station 12 and to station 16 [10]. In more recent studies, the reported incidence of skip metastasis varied from 5% to 14%, frequently involving extra-perigastric lymph nodes along the left gastric and hepatic arteries (stations 7 and 8) [11-13, 15]. In a GIRCG (Italian Research Group for Gastric Cancer) study, advanced cancers located in the upper and middle parts of the stomach had a higher incidence of skip metastasis. Upper-third gastric tumors were associated with skip metastases to station 9 nodes in 1% of the cases while in 7% there was para-aortic nodal diffusion with a simultaneous involvement only of station 1 or station 3. Advanced tumors in the middle part of the stomach showed skip metastasis within stations 7, 9, or 11 in 2% of the cases; in 1%, there was station 16 metastasis associated with involvement of perigastric stations only. The 1% of advanced cases in the lower portion of the stomach showed metastases at stations 7, 8, and 9, with no involvement of compartment 1 (see below) nodes [14].

The reasons for the occurrence of skip metastasis remain unclear but may include: (a) occult

Table 3.6 Lymph node stations involvement according to depth of tumor invasion in cancers of the lower third of the stomach [14]. Values are expressed as %

Station	Mucosa	Submucosa	Muscularis propria or subserosa	Serosa	Adjacent structures
1	5	8	17	18	40
2	0	0	0	2	0
3	6	15	34	69	87
4	0	0	30	47	50
5	0	0	11	27	20
6	7	22	43	68	50
7	3	3	22	35	28
8	0	7	23	37	50
9	0	0	10	20	67
11	0	0	6	11	0

metastases may remain unseen in a standard histopathological examination; (b) other lymphatic routes in the lesser omentum could be present; (c) there may be only a few perigastric nodes in some patients; (d) the physiological function of these skip metastasis nodes may be the same as the perigastric nodes [11-15].

3.3 Levels of Lymphatic Dissection

The levels of lymphadenectomy in gastric cancer treatment are classified according to the JGCA rules and designated by the letter "D" [8] together with the number 1, 2, and 3 (D1, D2, and D3), depending on the lymph node groups (compartments) dissected for each tumor location (Table 3.2).

In the 2nd English edition of the Japanese gastric cancer treatment guidelines "Guidelines for Diagnosis and Treatment of Carcinoma of the Stomach" issued in April 2004 [23], the JGCA reported two modified D1 dissections (D1+α and D1+β) and classified four levels of lymphadenectomy:

D1 dissection includes only perigastric node stations of the first compartment (N1) according to the tumor location (Table 3.2).

D1+α dissection is a D1 lymphadenectomy plus dissection of extra-perigastric stations along left gastric artery (station 7) irrespective of the location of the lesion and additionally along the common hepatic artery (anterosuperior group, station 8a) in cases in which the lesions are located in the lower area of the stomach.

D1+β dissection is a D1 plus resection of the lymph nodes along the left gastric (station 7), common hepatic (anterosuperior group, station 8a) and celiac (station 9) arteries.

D2 dissection (extended lymphadenectomy) removes all first and second compartments stations (N1 and N2) according to the tumor location (Table 3.2). Consequently, this dissection implies resection of the extra-perigastric nodes along the left gastric (station 7), common hepatic (anterosuperior group, station 8a), celiac (station 9) and proximal splenic (station 11p) arteries. This dissection may also include the lymph nodes in the hepatoduodenal ligament along the hepatic artery (station 12a), except for cancer located in the upper portion of the stomach.

D3 dissection (super-extended lymphadenectomy) includes all stations of the first, second, and third compartments (N1, N2, and N3) according to the tumor location (Table 3.2). This dissection implies excision of additional node stations within the hepatoduodenal ligament (along the bile duct, station 12b and behind the portal vein, station 12p), along the hepatic artery (posterior group, station 8p), and adjacent to the abdominal aorta from the upper margin of the celiac trunk to the upper margin of the inferior mesenteric artery (stations 16a2 and 16b1).

Very recently, the JGCA published the Japanese gastric cancer treatment guidelines 2011 (ver. 3) based on the 3rd English edition of the Japanese Classification of Gastric Carcinoma, which revised the definition of and indications for lymphadenectomy (D). The extent of lymph node dissection is now defined according to the type of gastrectomy indicated. For total gastrectomy, the lymph nodes stations to be dissected in D1 lymphadenectomy are from number 1 to 7, and D2 included D1 plus stations 8a, 9, 10, 11p, 11d and 12a. For distal gastrectomy, the lymph nodes to be dissected in D1 lymphadenectomy are stations number 1, 3, 4sb, 4d, 5, 6, and 7, whereas D2 includes D1 plus stations 8a, 9, 11p, and 12a. Hence, nodes of the second compartment (N2) along the left gastric artery (station 7) has been included in the D1 dissection for any type of gastrectomy [24, 25].

References

1. Rouvière H (1932) Anatomie des lymphatiques de l'homme. Masson, Paris
2. Tanigawa K (1963) A study on the lymphatic system in human stomach, especially on its passage to the thoracic duct. Igaku Kenkyu 1:40-64
3. Hidden G, Hureau J (1978) Les grandes voies lymphatiques des viscères digestifs abdominaux chez l'adulte. Anat Clin 1:167-176
4. Sarrazin R, Pissas A, Dyon JF, Bouchet Y (1979) Le drainage lymphatique dell'estomac. Anat Clin 2:95-110
5. Sasagawa T, Suzuki H, Kitamura Y et al (1995) A study of the area of paraaortic lymph nodes dissection in gastric cancer based on lymphatic flow of the stomach using radioactive isotope. In: Nishi M, Sugano H, Takahashi T (eds) 1st International Gastric Cancer Congress. Monduzzi, Bologna, pp 1301-1307
6. Hagiwara A, Takahashi T, Sawai K et al (1992) Lymph

nodal vital staining with new carbon particle suspension compared with India ink: experimental and clinical observation. Lymphology 25:84-89
7. Yonemura Y (1996) Contemporary approaches toward cure of gastric cancer. Maeda Shoten & CO, Kanazawa
8. Japanese Gastric Cancer Association (1998) Japanese classification of gastric carcinoma, 2nd English edition. Gastric Cancer 1:10-24
9. Aiko T, Sasako M (1998) The new Japanese classification of gastric carcinoma: point to be revised. Gastric Cancer 1:25-30
10. Maruyama K, Gunvén P, Okabayashi K et al (1989) Lymph node metastases of gastric cancer. General pattern in 1931 patients. Ann Surg 5:596-602
11. Kosaka T, Nobuo U, Sugaya J et al (1999) Lymphatic routes of the stomach demonstrated by gastric carcinomas with solitary lymph node metastasis. Surg Today 29:695-700
12. Takunaga M, Ohyama S, Hiki N et al (2009) Investigation of the lymphatic stream of the stomach in gastric cancer with solitary lymph node metastasis. World J Surg 33:1235-1239
13. Liu CG, Lu P, Lu Y et al (2007) Distribution of solitary lymph nodes in primary gastric cancer: a retrospective study and clinical implications. World J Gastroenterol 21:4776-4780
14. Di Leo A, Marrelli D, Roviello F et al (2007) Lymph node involvement in gastric cancer for different tumor site and T stage. Italian Research Group for Gastric Cancer (IRGGC) experience. J Gastrointest Surg 11:1146-1153
15. Kunisaki C, Shimada H, Nomura M et al (2006) Distribution of lymph node metastasis in gastric carcinoma. Hepatogastroenterology 53:468-472
16. Shen KH, Wu CW, Lo SS et al (1999) Factors correlated with number of metastatic lymph nodes in gastric cancer. Am J Gastroenterol 94:104-108
17. Ishikawa S, Shimada S, Miyanari N et al (2009) Pattern of lymph node involvement in proximal gastric cancer. World J Surg 33:1687-1692
18. Mönig SP, Collet PH, Baldus SE e al (2001) Splenectomy in proximal gastric cancer: frequency of lymph node metastasis to the splenic hilus. J Surg Oncol 76:89-92
19. Shin SH, Jung H, Choi SH et al (2009) Clinical significance of splenic hilar lymph node metastasis in proximal gastric cancer. Ann Surg Oncol 16:1304-1309
20. Sasada S, Ninomiya M, Nishizaki M et al (2009) Frequency of lymph node metastasis to the splenic hilus and effect of splenectomy in proximal gastric cancer. Anticancer Res 29:3347-3351
21. Gotoda T, Yanagisawa A, Sasako M et al (2000) Incidence of lymph node metastasis from early gastric cancer: estimation with a large number of cases at two large centers. Gastric Cancer 3:219-225
22. Ikeguchi M, Kaibara N (2004) Lymph node metastasis at the splenic hilum in proximal gastric cancer. Am Surg 70:645-648
23. Japanese Gastric Cancer Association (2004) Guidelines for diagnosis and treatment of carcinoma of the stomach, 2nd English edition. http://jgca.jp/gakkai/foreigner.htlm. Accessed 18 August 2010
24. Japanese Gastric Cancer Association (2011) Japanese classification of gastric carcinoma, 3rd English edition. Gastric Cancer DOI: 10.1007/s10120-011-0041-5
25. Japanese Gastric Cancer Association (2011) Japanese Gastric Cancer Guidelines 2010 (ver. 3). Gastric Cancer DOI: 10.1007/s10120-011-0042-4

Pathologic Classifications and Staging Systems

4

Giovanni de Manzoni, Marco Catarci, Alberto Di Leo, Anna Tomezzoli, and Carla Vindigni

Abstract

Advanced and early gastric carcinomas can be macroscopically and microscopically classified according to different systems. The most widely used are the macroscopic classification proposed by Borrmann and the Lauren histological classification.

The tumor node metastasis (TNM) staging system of the American Joint Committee on Cancer/International Union Against Cancer (AJCC/UICC) is recognized worldwide and its application is simple and reproducible. The seventh TNM staging system for gastric carcinoma is more detailed than the sixth edition. It introduces a clear distinction between tumors invading the muscularis propria (T2) and the subserosa (T3), based on a distinct difference in prognosis. Tumors invading the serosal layer are currently classified as T4a and those invading adjacent organs as T4b. The N groups of the previous edition have been further divided based on the number of involved regional lymph nodes (RLNs). Hence, in the new system, N1 (previously 1–6 RLNs) has been subdivided into N1 (1–2 involved RLNs) and N2 (3–6 involved RLNs), with the former N2 (7–15 involved RLNs) and N3 (> 15 involved RLNs) groups now referred to as N3a and N3b.

Keywords

TNM staging system • Borrmann • Lauren • Japanese classification of gastric carcinoma • Intestinal carcinoma • Diffuse carcinoma • Carneiro classification • Kodama • Lymph node ratio (LNR) • Signet-ring cell carcinoma • Mucinous carcinoma • Adenosquamous carcinoma • Hepatoid carcinoma • Parietal cell carcinoma • Lymphoepithelioma-like carcinoma • Carcinosarcoma • Microsatellite instability (MSI)

4.1 Morphology

4.1.1 Advanced Gastric Cancer

4.1.1.1 Macroscopic Aspects

Advanced gastric carcinomas are the more frequent gastric tumors in Western countries. By definition, these carcinomas infiltrate the gastric wall

G. de Manzoni (✉)
Dept. of Surgery,
Upper G.I. Surgery Division,
University of Verona,
Verona, Italy

G. de Manzoni, F. Roviello, W. Siquini (eds.), *Surgery in the Multimodal Management of Gastric Cancer*,

beyond the submucosa. They are mainly located in the distal stomach, in the antropyloric region, or along the lesser curvature while they are less frequent in the body of the stomach. Carcinomas originating in the cardia are becoming increasingly common and are generally smaller in size than tumors of the distal stomach. Advanced carcinomas are divided into four macroscopic types according to the criteria proposed by Borrmann.

Polypoid tumors consist of soft villous or cauliflower-shaped masses with a low tendency to infiltrate the wall.

Fungating tumors are domed, solid masses, often presenting with central ulceration; they account for about one-third of advanced carcinomas.

Ulcerated tumors are the most common type and are frequently located in the antrum or along the lesser curvature. They resemble a deep ulcer, with a necrotic fundus and irregular, nodous margins, but differ from peptic ulcers, which have a regular shape, thin edges, and a clean fundus.

Infiltrative tumors account for about 10% of advanced carcinomas. This type of cancer does not consist of a real tumoral mass but rather of a considerable plaque-like or tubular thickening of the wall, with flattened mucous plicae. The diffuse variant may affect most of the stomach, giving rise to a *linitis plastica* or *leather bottle* stomach. This variant considerably reduces the volume of the stomach and thoroughly infiltrates the gastric walls, making them thick and rigid.

According to the Japanese classification of gastric carcinoma [1], gastric cancer can be macroscopically categorized into six types (Figs. 4.1, 4.2):

Type 0 are superficial flat tumors with or without minimal elevation or depression. These cancers are also subdivided into type 0 I (protruded; the thickness of the lesion is more than twice that of the normal mucosa), type 0 IIa (superficial elevated; the thickness is up to twice that of the normal mucosa), type 0 IIb (flat), type 0 IIc (superficial depressed), and type 0 III (excavated);

Type 1 comprises polypoid tumors that are sharply demarcated from the surrounding mucosa and usually attached on a wide base;

Type 2 consists of ulcerated carcinomas with sharply demarcated and raised margins;

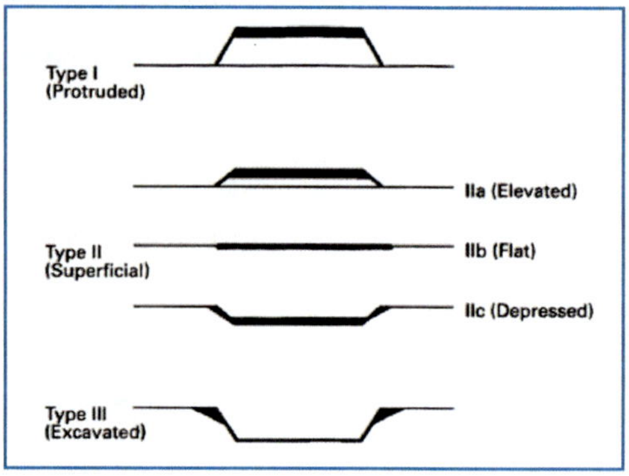

Fig. 4.1 Macroscopic types 1, 2, 3, and 4 according to the JGCA [1]

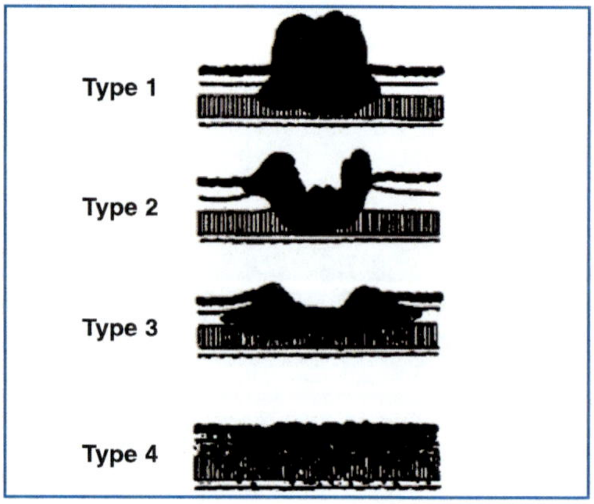

Fig. 4.2 Subtypes of macroscopic type 0 according to the JGCA [1]

Type 3 includes ulcerated carcinomas without definite limits and infiltrating the surrounding wall;

Type 4 are diffusely infiltrating carcinomas in which ulceration is usually not a marked feature;

Type 5 are non-classifiable carcinomas that do not meet any of the above criteria.

4.1.1.2 Histological Types

The most widely used histological classification is that of Lauren, which classifies advanced carcinomas according to three different types [2]: intestinal (Fig. 4.3), diffuse, e.g., signet-ring cell carcinomas (Fig. 4.4a, b), and mixed (due to the presence

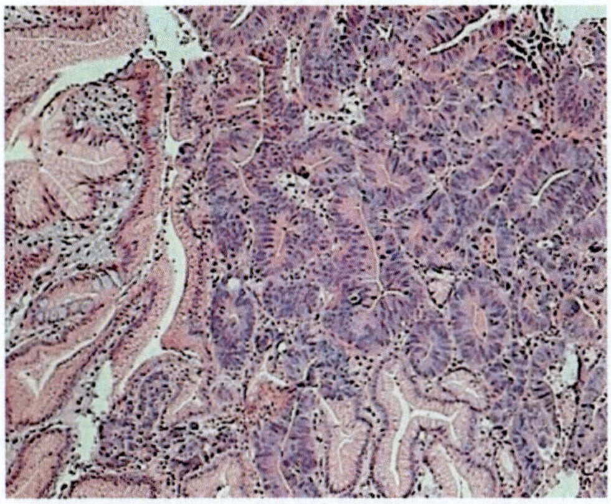

Fig. 4.3 Intestinal adenocarcinoma (H&E staining)

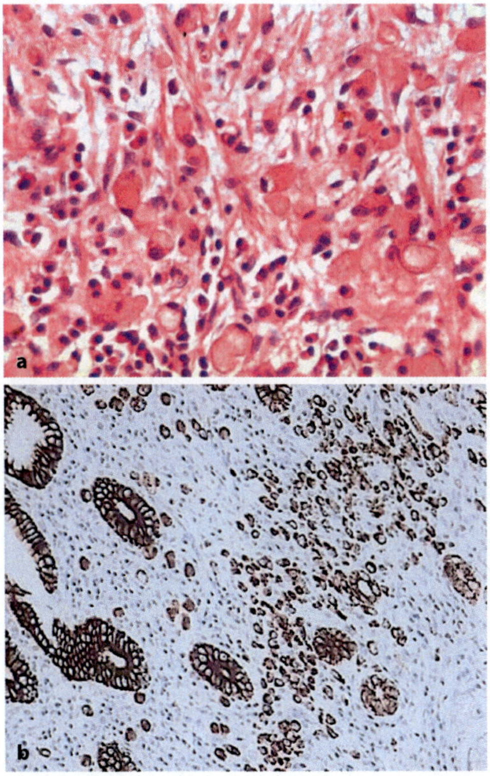

Fig. 4.4 a Diffuse adenocarcinoma (H&E staining); **b** diffuse adenocarcinoma (cytokeratin staining)

of intestinal and diffuse aspects). The frequency of intestinal carcinoma is declining in Western countries, following a reduction in environmentally related risk factors, whereas the frequency of the diffuse type has remained steady.

Intestinal type tumors are the most frequent type in countries with a high incidence of gastric cancer and are usually ascribed to the action of oncogenic factors (*Helicobacter pylori* infection or a high-salt diet). The typical site for this type of carcinoma is the antropyloric region, and its predominant macroscopic appearance is fungating. Intestinal carcinomas have a glandular structure similar to that of carcinomas arising in the small or large intestine. Multifocal chronic gastritis with glandular atrophy and intestinal metaplasia is the gastric pathology that most often gives rise to intestinal carcinoma. The degree of differentiation of these tumors varies considerably from case to case but, generally, in inverse proportion to their size. Sometimes, the carcinoma is so well differentiated that it resembles an intestinal metaplasia of complete type whereas poorly differentiated variants may appear solid.

Diffuse type tumors are usually responsible for the rare cases of gastric carcinoma affecting patients less than 40 years of age and for hereditary carcinomas arising from germinal mutation of E-cadherin. These tumors consist of poorly cohesive cells that infiltrate the gastric wall and do not form glands. The cells are generally small and round, arranged either as single, scattered cells or as clusters in ill-defined, lacy, microglandular, reticular formations. The cells tend to accumulate intracytoplasmic mucin, which shifts the nucleus to either pole of the cell (signet-ring appearance). Diffuse carcinoma is often associated with stromal desmoplasia (stromal production of abundant collagenous fibers) and an inflammatory reaction. However, the most frequent macroscopic appearance of diffuse carcinoma is ulcerated (type 3) or infiltrative (type 4).

4.1.1.3 Carneiro Classification

Carneiro proposed a new classification of advanced gastric carcinoma along the following lines [3]: (a) glandular and (b) isolated cell types that roughly correspond to Lauren's intestinal and diffuse carcinomas, respectively; (c) solid type, formed by clusters, trabeculae, and solid nests of undifferentiated cells without the formation of glands; and (d) mixed type, which is a cross between the glandular and isolated cell types. In a series of Portuguese patients, the glandular type was the most commonly seen, followed by the mixed, solid, and isolated cell types.

4.1.2 Early Gastric Cancer

4.1.2.1 Macroscopic Aspects

Early gastric cancer is a malignant epithelial neoplasm limited to the mucosa and submucosa. It can occur as an intramucosal or submucosal carcinoma, either of which is likely to produce lymph node metastases. In Asian countries, which offer screening for the early diagnosis of gastric cancer, early gastric carcinoma reaches a percentage of 30–50%. In Western countries, by contrast, where screening is not performed, the frequency decreases to 16–24%. The follow-up of dysplastic lesions does not appear to influence the prevalence of early gastric cancer. Like advanced carcinomas, most early carcinomas are located in the distal section of the stomach. These tumors are divided into three main types according to their endoscopic appearance (Fig 4.1):

Type I (protruding) tumors consist of nodular or polypoid masses protruding into the lumen of the stomach;

Type II (superficial) tumors are flat, superficial lesions that may be plaque-like (IIa), flat (IIb), or depressed (IIc);

Type III (excavated) tumors resemble ulcers of various depths.

These types rarely present in pure form but typically in combinations. Consequently, each case is classified according to the prevailing type; for example, IIa+IIc. As reported above, these categories have been adopted into the Japanese classification of gastric carcinoma to describe all macroscopically superficial flat tumors (type 0), irrespective of the depth of wall invasion [1].

4.1.2.2 Histological Types

Histologically, the same histotypes are found in early gastric cancer as in advanced carcinoma. Early carcinomas of type I (protruding) are more often well-differentiated intestinal-type carcinomas with tubular or papillary formations. Type II carcinomas correspond histologically to intestinal carcinomas, ranging from well to poorly differentiated. Early carcinomas of type III can be intestinal or diffuse.

Kodama divided intramucosal carcinomas into Small mucosal carcinomas (< 4 cm) and Super (superficial spreading) carcinomas (> 4 cm) [4]. Both types may be strictly confined to the mucosa (Small mucosal M and Super M) or focally infiltrate the submucosa (Small mucosal SM and Super SM). In the penetrating (Pen) variant (which includes two subcategories, Pen A and Pen B), invasion of the submucosa is more extensive than in the other two variants. Pen A is characterized by infiltration of the submucosa along the entire margin of the neoplasia whereas Pen B, the more frequent of the two, penetrates the muscularis mucosa discontinuously at multiple sites. The prognosis is worse in Pen than in Small mucosal and Super carcinomas, with Pen A associated with the least favorable evolution of all. Kodama's classification agrees with the theory that the frequency of lymph node metastases depends on the depth of tumor infiltration of the mucosa and submucosa. In spite of these probabilities of developing metastases, patients with early carcinomas have a more favorable prognosis than those with advanced carcinomas. In order to understand the favorable clinical evolution of early carcinoma, we must consider two of its biological features: (1) This type of carcinoma tends to grow superficially or radially rather than in depth. (2) Early cancer is not always the precursor of advanced cancer but a completely different disease, with a less aggressive biological potential.

4.1.2.3 Histochemical and Immunohistochemical Aspects

The main secretion of gastric carcinomas, and especially intestinal carcinomas, is an acid mucin that stains positively with Alcian blue. The mucin produced by diffuse carcinomas can be acidic or neutral. On immunohistochemical examination, intestinal carcinoma expresses mainly MUC1 mucin while diffuse and mucinous carcinomas express, respectively, MUC5AC and MUC2. Moreover, gastric carcinomas constitutively express cytokeratin,

CEA, and epithelial membrane antigen. About 70% of gastric carcinomas are positive for cytokeratin 7 (CK7) while only 20% show CK20 positivity. Markers of specific gastric differentiation are pepsinogen 1 (main cells and fundic neck cells), pepsinogen 2 (mucopeptic cells), E cathepsin (an aspartic proteinase), and antigen M1 (a mucin antigen indicative of foveolar differentiation).

4.2 Cytochemical, Genetic, and Molecular Alterations

Examinations of DNA ploidy have revealed that aneuploidy is more frequent in intestinal than in diffuse carcinomas. In about 30% of sporadic diffuse carcinomas, E-cadherin expression is either reduced or abnormal and there are alterations of the E-cadherin gene and its transcripts. Similar changes are seen in the diffuse component of mixed carcinomas but not in intestinal-type carcinomas. Beta-catenin, which together with E-cadherin regulates cellular adhesion, may also be abnormal in diffuse carcinoma.

Microsatellite instability (MSI) is found in 13–44% of sporadic carcinomas. Carcinomas with this genetic alteration tend to be of the intestinal type (often solid-medullary), located in the antrum, of polypoid appearance, and with a lower incidence of lymph node metastases at a lower stage. In general, they are seen more often in elderly patients. Allelic loss of P53 occurs in about 50% of gastric carcinomas. These neoplasias often, but not always, show nuclear accumulation of P53 on immunohistochemical examination. P53 overexpression mainly occurs in intestinal carcinomas, both early and advanced, and is seen in the advanced stage of diffuse and mixed carcinomas. A loss of P16 (the product of the *CDKN2A* gene) occurs in about 25% of gastric carcinomas, especially those located in the body of the stomach and those positive for Epstein-Barr virus (EBV). Somatic mutations of the *APC* gene are present in a high percentage of adenomas and dysplasias but only in a low percentage (4%) of gastric carcinomas. Telomerase is often overexpressed in the advanced stages of gastric carcinomas; the prognosis in these cases is generally unfavorable.

4.3 Other Microscopic Types of Carcinoma

Mucinous carcinoma (mucoid, gelatinous) is characterized by mucin lakes, caused by the abundant production of mucin, which accumulates in the cells, glandular lumens, and interstices. The mucins involved are O-acetylated sialomucins and are immunoreactive for MUC2. The prognosis of mucinous carcinoma is more favorable than that of diffuse carcinoma but the same as intestinal carcinoma.

Adenosquamous and squamous carcinomas are rare (< 1% of gastric carcinomas) and must be distinguished from squamous carcinomas of the esophagus that invade the stomach. They combine a squamous component with a more or less plentiful glandular component. The adenocarcinomatous, glandular component is minimal and is detected only after careful examination of sections of squamous carcinomas.

Hepatoid carcinoma has both a glandular component and a solid or trabecular component consisting of large eosinophilic cells similar to hepatocytes. These cells are always immunoreactive for hepatocyte antigen Hep-Par-1 and often immunoreactive for α-fetoprotein (AFP), which is also a marker of hepatocarcinoma. These neoplasias often exhibit extensive venous invasion and affected patients have an unfavorable prognosis.

Parietal cell carcinomas consist of large cells with an abundant granular, eosinophilic cytoplasm. As seen on electron microscopy, the cells are clustered in glandular or solid formations. These carcinomas also exhibit numerous mitochondria, intracellular canaliculi and tubules.

Lymphoepithelioma-like carcinoma (undifferentiated carcinoma with plentiful lymphoid stroma) is similar to neoplasias that affect the nasopharynx. The tumor cells of many of these gastric carcinomas, like the nasopharyngeal ones, are EBV-positive. By contrast, other gastric carcinomas, rich in lymphoid stroma and with a solid-medullary appearance, are EBV-negative and associated with MSI.

Carcinosarcoma is a biphasic neoplasia, with an epithelial component that is generally glandular and a sarcomatous-like, spindle-cell component. The latter component may contain heterologous elements, such as muscle-derived or osteoid cells.

4.4 The American Joint Committee on Cancer (AJCC)/International Union Against Cancer (UICC) TNM Staging System

According to the 7th edition of the TNM classification [5], all tumors with an epicenter in the stomach > 5 cm from the esophagogastric junction (EGJ) or those within 5 cm of the EGJ without extension into the esophagus are staged using the gastric carcinoma scheme (Table 4.1). Tumors arising at the EGJ or in the stomach within 5 cm from the EGJ and crossing the EGJ are classified and staged using the TNM system for esophageal adenocarcinoma.

4.4.1 Primary Tumor (T)

The staging of primary gastric cancer depends on the depth of wall invasion and is detailed in Table 4.2. A tumor may penetrate the muscularis propria with extension into the gastrocolic or gastrohepatic ligaments, or into the greater or lesser omentum, without perforation of the visceral peritoneum covering these structures. In this case, the tumor is classified as T3. If there is perforation of the visceral peritoneum covering the gastric ligaments or the omentum, the tumor is classified as T4.

The adjacent structures of the stomach include the spleen, transverse colon, liver, diaphragm, pancreas, abdominal wall, adrenal gland, kidney, small intestine, and retroperitoneum. Intramural extension to the duodenum or esophagus is classified by the depth of the greatest invasion at any of these sites, including the stomach.

This classification does not mention the mesocolon as an adjacent structure involved in gastric cancer. A recent study has shown that the clinicopathologic characteristics of tumors with invasion of this anatomical structure more closely resemble those of tumors with infiltration of adjacent structures (T4b) than tumors with serosal infiltration (T4a). Furthermore, the survival rates of patients with tumors characterized by mesocolon invasion are lower than those of patients with T4a tumors but similar to those of patients with T4b tumors [6].

The 7th edition of the TNM staging system [5] incorporated several changes from the 6th edition

Table 4.1 The TNM for gastric carcinoma according to AJCC 7th edn, 2010. (Reproduced from [5], with permission)

Stage 0	Tis	N0	M0
Stage IA	T1	N0	M0
Stage IB	T2	N0	M0
	T1	N1	M0
Stage IIA	T3	N0	M0
	T2	N1	M0
	T1	N2	M0
Stage IIB	T4a	N0	M0
	T3	N1	M0
	T2	N2	M0
	T1	N3	M0
Stage IIIA	T4a	N1	M0
	T3	N2	M0
	T2	N3	M0
Stage IIIB	T4b	N0	M0
	T4b	N1	M0
	T4a	N2	M0
	T3	N3	M0
Stage IIIC	T4b	N2	M0
	T4b	N3	M0
	T4a	N3	M0
Stage IV	Any T	Any N	M1

Table 4.2 Primary tumor categories (T)

TX	Primary tumor cannot be assessed
T0	No evidence of primary tumor
Tis	Carcinoma in situ: intraepithelial tumor without invasion of the lamina propria
T1	Tumor invades the lamina propria, muscularis mucosae, or submucosa
T1a	Tumor invades the lamina propria or muscularis mucosae
T1b	Tumor invades the submucosa
T2	Tumor invades the muscularis propria
T3	Tumor penetrates the subserosal connective tissue without invasion of the visceral peritoneum or adjacent structures
T4	Tumor invades the serosa (visceral peritoneum) or adjacent structures
T4a	Tumor invades the serosa (visceral peritoneum)
T4b	Tumor invades adjacent structures

[7], providing a more detailed classification of prognosis, particularly between T2 and T3 carcinomas [8]. Thus, tumors involving the muscularis propria and those involving the subserosa belong, respectively, to categories T2 and T3, which are now considered part of the stage grouping. In the previous edition, cancer invading the muscularis propria was assigned to subcategory T2a and cancer invading the subserosa to subcategory T2b, but these subcategories have not been maintained in the stage grouping. These changes were justified because patients with gastric cancer that invades the muscularis propria have less nodal involvement, lower recurrence rates, a more favorable prognosis, and longer disease-free survival than patients with cancers invading the subserosa [9-13].

The new staging system [5] better represents the prognosis for patients with muscularis propria or subserosal involvement. In addition, the prognostic impact of the different subclassifications has been investigated for these tumors. The prognosis of patients with T2 tumors invading the outer longitudinal muscle bands of muscularis propria (sMP) is similar to that of patients with subserosal cancer (T3), but significantly poorer than that of patients with T2 cancer invading the inner circular muscle bands of muscularis propria (dMP) [14]. In subserosal tumor (T3), a recent study showed that the infiltrating growth pattern associated with invasion of the subserosal layer and an indistinct border (ssγ), according to the Japanese classification of gastric carcinoma [1], is an independent negative prognostic factor and is closely related to peritoneal recurrence [15]. Moreover, the horizontal width of spread of a T3 tumor in the subserosal layer has a prognostic impact. The prognosis of patients whose tumors show subserosal invasion of < 20 mm width (ss-narrow cancer) is similar to that of patients with T2 cancer, while cancers with subserosal invasion of > 20 mm width (ss-wide cancer) behave very similar to T4a cancers [16].

Compared to the previous edition, the 7th edition includes modifications in the categorization of tumors with serosal or deeper involvement. The subcategory T4a (cancer perforates serosa) was previously category T3, and subcategory T4b (cancer invades adjacent structures) the earlier category T4, but these two subcategories are still maintained in the stage grouping.

4.4.2 Regional Lymph Nodes (N)

Regional lymph nodes are categorized on the basis of the number of metastatic lymph nodes (Table 4.3). Nodal involvement of the hepatoduodenal ligament, retropancreatic, mesenteric, and para-aortic areas is classified as distant metastasis (M1). According to the 6th edition [7], N stage was categorized as N0 (no metastatic lymph nodes), N1 (1–6 metastatic lymph nodes), N2 (7–15 metastatic lymph nodes), N3 (> 15 metastatic lymph nodes). The 7th edition [5] introduces a new grouping of N categories: the former N1 has been subdivided, with N1 (1 or 2 metastatic lymph nodes) and N2 (3–6 metastatic lymph nodes), and the former N2 and N3 categories now referred to as N3a and N3b.

Adequate dissection of regional nodal areas is important to enable appropriate determination of the pN status. Although it is suggested that at least 16 regional nodes should be assessed pathologically, a pN0 determination may be assigned on the basis of the actual number of nodes evaluated microscopically. The extent of lymph node dissection performed by the surgeon strongly influences the number of lymph nodes examined by the pathologist. Anatomical studies [17, 18] identified a median number of 25 lymph nodes per patient after extended lymph node dissection (D2 according to the Japanese Gastric Cancer Association, JGCA [1]) and 43–52 lymph nodes per patient after super-extended lymph node dissection (D3 according to the JGCA). A recent analysis by the Italian Research Group for Gastric Cancer (GIRCG) of quality assessment of lymph node dissection [19] identified a median of 14 examined lymph nodes after D1 lymph node dissection, 29 after D2, and 46.5 after D3. Another study report-

Table 4.3 Regional lymph nodes categories (N)

NX	Regional lymph node(s) cannot be assessed
N0	No regional lymph node metastasis
N1	Metastasis in 1–2 regional lymph nodes
N2	Metastasis in 3–6 regional lymph nodes
N3	Metastasis in seven or more regional lymph nodes
N3a	Metastasis in 7–15 regional lymph nodes
N3b	Metastasis in > 16 lymph nodes

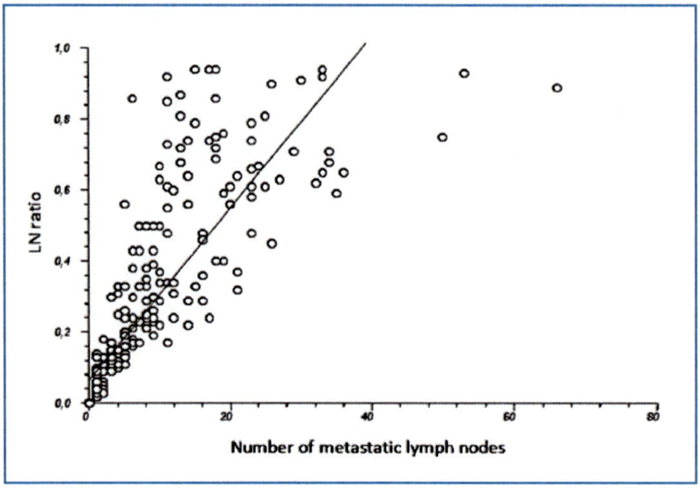

Fig. 4.5 Scatter diagram of linear regression between the number of metastatic lymph nodes and the lymph node ratio (LN ratio; r=0.84; 95% C.I. 0.80–0.87; $p < 0.001$). (Reproduced from [20], with permission)

ed a median of 18 examined lymph nodes per patient after D1α–β lymphadenectomy and 31 after D2 [20]. The incidence of inadequate lymph node examination (< 15 examined lymph nodes per patient) was 54.5% after D1 [19], 34.1% after D1α–β [20], 2.6–6.2% after D2, and 1.4% after D3 lymphadenectomy. These figures are very different from those reported by Western population-based studies [21-23], with a median of 10 examined lymph nodes per patient and the incidence of inadequate lymph node examination exceeding 60% of cases.

Although the TNM staging system, the most widely used, is simple and reproducible, the appropriate classification of nodal status is still debated and different staging systems have been proposed and investigated. The limitations of the TNM system are that it demands the examination of at least 15 lymph nodes, with inadequate staging (under-staging) as a result of limited node dissection [24]. In the Japanese classification of gastric carcinoma (see Chap. 3), the status of regional lymph node metastasis is defined according to the anatomical locations of the involved nodes with respect to the site of the primary tumor (upper, middle, or lower third of the stomach) [1]. In limited lymphadenectomy (D1 dissection), no information is obtained regarding the extra-perigastric nodes and a complete nodal staging is not possible.

To overcome the problem of stage migration induced by extended lymph node dissection [25, 26], a new independent prognostic factor was recently investigated on a large scale and subsequently validated. The lymph node ratio (LNR), defined as the absolute ratio between metastatic and examined lymph nodes, was found to be a strong independent indicator of prognosis [27-30], even in case of inadequate nodal staging (< 15 examined lymph nodes) [31]. The GIRCG defined four prognostic intervals for the LNR: 0, 0.01–0.09, 0.10–0.25, > 0.25. These intervals correspond to a definite different prognosis even within the same pN status, independent of the extent of nodal dissection [29]. It was previously demonstrated that LNR is independently influenced by the number of metastatic lymph nodes (Fig. 4.5) but not by the number of examined lymph nodes [20, 27, 29]. It is therefore suitable as a prognostic factor independent of the stage migration phenomenon. Moreover, LNR reflects the characteristics of both the tumor (number of metastatic nodes) and the surgical treatment (extent of lymph node dissection). Consequently, a tumor-ratio-metastasis (TRM) instead of a tumor-node-metastasis (TNM) staging system was suggested [32].

In the 7th edition of the TNM staging system [5], the UICC elected to retain the pN classification based on the number of metastatic nodes. It seems that this new pN stage grouping is a more accurate prognostic predictor than its precursor [33]. It will be very interesting to investigate the prognostic yield of this new TNM stage grouping in light of the LNR.

Recently, another classification based on the size of lymph node metastasis was proposed. In any TNM stage of patients with lymph node metastasis, this classification yields different prognostic groups. Different cut-offs have been proposed, i.e., 8 mm [34] and 2 cm [35], to define two N subcategories: n1, lymph node metastasis with largest size less than the cut-off, and n2, lymph node metastasis with largest size equal or larger than the cut-off.

4.4.3 Distant Metastasis (M)

The absence and presence of distant metastases are defined, respectively, as M0 and M1. Liver, peritoneal surface, and distant lymph nodes are the most common metastatic sites in gastric cancer. Metastases to the central nervous system and lungs occur but less frequently.

The TNM staging system classifies positive peritoneal cytology as metastatic disease (M1). Although the cytological detection of free cancer cells in peritoneal washings is a marker of poor prognosis and peritoneal recurrence [36], in Japanese [37] and Western [38, 39] series peritoneal lavage cytology did not increase the prognostic information already provided by pathologic T and N staging after curative resection [37]. Moreover, peritoneal lavage cytology is not widely practiced in Western centers [40] and while it has a high specificity in predicting peritoneal recurrence, it retains of low sensitivity [36].

References

1. Japanese Gastric Cancer Association (1998) Japanese classification of gastric carcinoma, 2nd English edition. Gastric Cancer 1:10-24
2. Lauren P (1965) The two histological main types of gastric carcinoma: diffuse and so called intestinal-type carcinoma. An attempt at a histo-clinical classification. Acta Pathol Microbiol Scand 64:31-49
3. Carneiro F, Seixas M, Sobrinho-Simões M (1995) New elements for an updated classification of the carcinomas of the stomach. Pathol Res Pract 191:571-584
4. Kodama Y, Inokuchi K, Soejima K et al (1983) Growth patterns and prognosis in early gastric carcinoma. Superficially spreading and penetrating growth types. Cancer 51:320-326
5. Edge SB, Byrd DR, Compton CC, eds. AJCC Cancer Staging Manual. 7th ed. New York, NY.: Springer, 2010
6. Park JH, Hyung WJ, Choi SH, Noh SH (2010) Should direct mesocolon invasion be included in T4 for the staging of gastric cancer? J Surg Oncol 101:205-208
7. Sobin LH, Wittekind C (2002) TNM classification of malignant tumours. 6th ed. Wiley-Liss, New York
8. Ahn HS, Lee HJ, Hahn S et al (2010) Evaluation of the Seventh American Joint Committee on Cancer/International Union Against Cancer Classification of gastric adenocarcinoma in comparison with the sixth classification. Cancer Epub Aug 24
9. Isozaki H, Fujii K, Nomura E et al (1999) Prognostic factors of advanced gastric carcinoma without serosal invasion (pT2 gastric carcinoma). Hepatogastroenterology 46:2669-2672
10. Kamatsu S, Ichikawa D, Kurioka H et al (2005) Prognostic and clinical evaluation of patients with T2 gastric cancer. Hepatogastroenterology 52:965-968
11. Park DJ, Kong SH, Lee HJ et al (2007) Subclassification of pT2 gastric adenocarcinoma according to depth of invasion (pT2a vs pT2b) and lymph node status. Surgery 141:757-763
12. Lu Y, Liu C, Zhang R et al (2008) Prognostic significance of subclassification of pT2 gastric cancer: a retrospective study of 847 patients. Surg Oncol 17:317-322
13. Nitti D, Marchet A, Mocellin S et al (2009) Prognostic value of subclassification of T2 tumours in patients with gastric cancer. Br J Surg 96:398-404
14. Sun Z, Zhu GL, Lu C et al (2009) A novel subclassification of pT2 gastric cancers according to the depth of muscularis propria invasion. Superficial muscularis propria versus deep muscularis propria/subserosa. Ann Surg 249:768-775
15. Song KY, Hur H, Jung CK et al (2010) Impact of tumor infiltration pattern into the surrounding tissue on prognosis of the subserosal gastric cancer (T2b). Eur J Surg Oncol 36:563-567
16. Soga K, Ichikawa D, Yasukawa S et al (2010) Prognostic impact of the width of subserosal invasion in gastric cancer invading the subserosal layer. Surgery 147:197-203
17. Wagner PK, Ramaswamy A, Ruschoff J et al (1991) Lymph node counts in the upper abdomen: anatomical basis for lymphadenectomy in gastric cancer. Br J Surg 78:825-827
18. Sharma D, Thakur A, Toppo S, Chandrakar SK (2005) Lymph node counts in Indians in relation to lymphadenectomy for carcinoma of the oesophagus and stomach. Asian J Surg 28:116-120
19. Verlato G, Roviello F, Marchet A et al (2009) Indexes of surgical quality in gastric cancer surgery: experience of an Italian network. Ann Surg Oncol 16:594-602
20. Catarci M, Montemurro LA, Di Cintio A et al (2010) Lymph node retrieval and examination during the implementation of extended lymph node dissection for gastric cancer in a non-specialized western institution. Updates Surg 62:89–99

21. Bouvier AM, Haas O, Piard F et al (2002) How many nodes must be examined to accurately stage gastric carcinomas? Results from a population based study. Cancer 94:2862-2866
22. Baxter NN, Tuttle TM (2005) Inadequacy of lymph node staging in gastric cancer patients: a population-based study. Ann Surg Oncol 12:981-987
23. Coburn NG, Swallow CJ, Kiss A, Law C (2006) Significant regional variation in adequacy of lymph node assessment and survival in gastric cancer. Cancer 107:2143-2151
24. de Manzoni G, Verlato G, Roviello F et al (2002) The new TNM classification of lymph node metastasis minimises stage migration problems in gastric cancer patients. Br J Cancer 87:171-174
25. Yoo CH, Noh SH, Kim YI, Min JS (1999) Comparison of prognostic significance of nodal staging between old (4th Edition) and new (5th Edition) UICC TNM classification for gastric carcinoma. International Union Against Cancer. World J Surg 23:492-497
26. De Manzoni G, Verlato G, Guglielmi A et al (1999) Classification of lymph node metastases from carcinoma of the stomach: comparison of the old (1987) and new (1997) TNM systems. World J Surg 23:664-669
27. Cheong JH, Hyung WJ, Shen JG et al (2006) The N ratio predicts recurrence and poor prognosis in patients with node-positive early gastric cancer. Ann Surg Oncol 13:377-385
28. Liu C, Lu P, Lu Y et al (2007) Cinical implications of metastatic lymph node ratio in gastric cancer. BMC Cancer 7:200-207
29. Marchet A, Mocellin S, Ambrosi A et al (2007) The ratio between metastatic and examined lymph nodes (N ratio) is an independent prognostic factor in gastric cancer regardless of the type of lymphadenectomy: results from an Italian multicentric study in 1853 patients. Ann Surg 245:543-552
30. Xu DZ, Geng QR, Long ZJ et al (2009) Positive lymph node ratio is an independent prognostic factor in gastric cancer after D2 resection regardless of the examined number of lymph nodes. Ann Surg Oncol 16:319-326
31. Kulig J, Sierzega M, Kolodziejczyk, Popiela T (2009) Ratio of metastatic to resected lymph nodes for prediction of survival in patients with inadequately staged gastric cancer. Br J Surg 96:910-918
32. Persiani R, Rausei S, Antonacci V et al (2009) Metastatic lymph node ratio: a new staging system for gastric cancer. World J Surg 33:2106-2111
33. Deng J, Liang H, Sun D et al (2010) Suitability of 7th UICC N stage for predicting the overall survival of gastric cancer patients after curative resection in China. Ann Surg Oncol 17:1259-1266. 24
34. Dhar DK, Kubota H, Kinukawa N et al (2003) Prognostic significance of metastatic lymph node size in patients with gastric cancer. Br J Surg 90:1522-1530
35. Cheong O, Oh ST, Kim BS et al (2008) Large metastatic lymph node size, especially more than 2 cm: independent predictor of poor prognosis in node-positive gastric carcinoma. World J Surg 32:262-266
36. Bando E, Yonemura Y, Takeshita Y et al (1999) Intraoperative lavage for cytological examination in 1,297 patients with gastric carcinoma. Am J Surg 178:256-262
37. Abe S, Yoshimura H, Tabara H et al (1995) Curative resection of gastric cancer: limitation of peritoneal lavage cytology in predicting the outcome. J Surg Oncol 59:226-229
38. Bonenkamp JJ, Songun I, Hermans J, van de Velde CJ (1999) Prognostic value of positive peritoneal lavage cytology findings from abdominal washings in patients with gastric cancer. Br J Surg 83:672-674
39. de Manzoni G, Verlato G, Di Leo A et al (2006) Peritoneal cytology does not increase the prognostic information provided by TNM in gastric cancer. World J Surg 30:579-584
40. Bentrem D, Wilton A, Mazumdar M et al (2005) The value of peritoneal cytology as a preoperative predictor in patient with gastric carcinoma undergoing a curative resection. Ann Surg Oncol 12:1-7

Prognostic Factors and Score Systems in Gastric Cancer

5

Daniele Marrelli, Stefano Caruso, and Franco Roviello

Abstract

Several tumor-related, patient-related, and treatment-related prognostic factors have been identified for gastric cancer patients. Tumor stage, surgical radicality, tumor location, and patient age are the most important conventional prognostic variables. Extended lymphadenectomy and higher numbers of removed lymph nodes are also related to a better prognosis. The role of other factors is controversial or not generally validated. The main feature of prognostic scores is the possibility to simultaneously consider a set of potential prognostic variables and thus to assign a risk of recurrence or death to individual patients. A prognostic score was developed by the GIRCG based on a cohort of patients treated by potentially curative surgery and submitted to periodic follow-up examinations. This score can be easily included in database programs and its accuracy verified. The score has been recalculated according to the new TNM classification of gastric cancer and is currently being validated in a prospective multicenter study.

Keywords

Gastric cancer • Prognosis • Survival • Score systems • Prognostic factors • Recurrence • Multivariate analysis • Gastrectomy • Lymphadenectomy • Lauren histotype • TNM classification • R0 resection

5.1 Introduction

Gastric cancer (GC) is a neoplasm with a dismal prognosis. A recent study from EUROCARE, which collects data from 82 cancer registries of 23 European countries, demonstrated a mean age-adjusted 5-year survival of < 25% in patients diagnosed in the period 1995–1999, with only a modest increase in recent years [1]. In Japan and Korea, better survival rates are reported due to earlier diagnosis of the disease by screening programs and a more extended therapy to advanced forms [2, 3]. Fairly good long-term outcomes have been also obtained in patients treated in specialized Western centers by radical surgery with extended lymphadenectomy; however, those results approached but did not reach the survival probability of Asian patients at the same stage [4, 5].

The end-points usually considered in the evaluation of long-term outcomes of patients with GC

D. Marrelli (✉)
Dept. of Human Pathology and Oncology,
Section of General Surgery and Surgical Oncology,
Translational Research Laboratory,
University of Siena,
Siena, Italy

are overall survival (deaths from any cause) and cancer-related survival (deaths from GC progression). Overall and cancer-related survival rates differ greatly according to several prognostic factors. The statistical weight of different variables on survival prediction is also dissimilar. In general, prognostic factors can be included in three broad categories: (1) tumor-related, (2) patient-related, and (3) treatment-related.

5.2 Tumor-related Prognostic Factors

The most important is obviously tumor stage. The recent AJCC/UICC classification of the TNM system (7th edition) modified the definition of pT and pN classifications as well as stage grouping and introduced new parameters for M stage (peritoneal cytology) [3]. Figure 5.1 reports the cancer-related survival rates according to the new TNM stages (7th edition). Survival analysis was conducted on 2320 patients submitted to surgical resection for GC and included in the Italian Research Group for Gastric Cancer (GIRCG) database. Neoplasms involving the esophagogastric junction (EGJ) were excluded. Patients in Asian countries who were diagnosed with early gastric cancer (EGC) had very high survival probabilities [2, 3]; similar results were obtained in large Western series [6]. Survival rates decrease notably in EGC with lymph node metastases, above all when more than six metastatic nodes are involved.

Prognosis worsens progressively with depth of invasion of the gastric wall, with a sharp decrease in survival for patients whose tumor perforates the serosa [3, 6-8]. In patients with tumors involving adjacent organs, the prognosis is poor even after potentially curative surgery; however, a chance of cure can be obtained after R0 combined resections in node-negative cases [9].

Lymph node involvement is a crucial prognostic factor in GC. Patient survival in advanced cases (pT2 and beyond) in the absence of lymph node metastases reaches high rates even in Western patients [10]. The number of involved nodes has a deep impact on prognosis such that cut-off values were modified in the new TNM classification. Nonetheless, an important loss in the new staging system is that the pN3a (7–15 involved nodes) and pN3b (> 15 involved nodes) subgroups were not

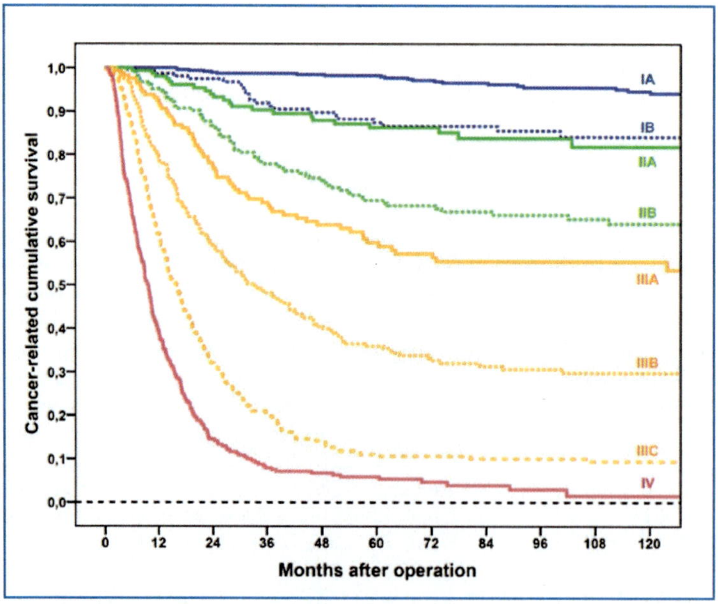

Fig. 5.1 Cancer-related survival curves according to the new TNM stages (7th edition); 2320 patients submitted to surgical resection and included in the Italian Research Group for Gastric Cancer (GIRCG) database were analyzed

differentiated in the stage grouping. This may affect the prognostic power of N status when large numbers of lymph nodes are removed [3].

The presence of distant metastases is generally associated with unfavorable outcome in GC patients, although there are isolated cases of long-term survivors after multimodality treatment of hepatic or peritoneal metastases [11].

The presence of tumor cells in the peritoneal washing is another important prognostic factor. Several series reported very low or no probability of survival in patients with positive peritoneal cytology even after R0 resection [12]. Positive peritoneal cytology is now considered as a distant metastasis (pM1) in the new TNM staging system, and thus included in stage IV.

A proximal location of the tumor in the stomach was found in several reports to negatively influence prognosis [5, 7, 13, 14]; however, as neoplasms involving the EGJ are considered as esophageal tumors in the new TNM classification, this aspect needs to be re-evaluated in future specific studies.

The real association between histological features and the prognosis of patients with GC is controversial. Tumor grading and WHO histological types have been reported to have either no influence, except following univariate analysis, or independent prognostic value [14, 15]. The Lauren histological classification (intestinal, diffuse, or mixed type) seems to be of more useful clinical value. Different epidemiological, clinical, and molecular features have been observed in the intestinal and diffuse histotypes of GC [16]. The main clinical difference is related to the different recurrence patterns, with the diffuse-mixed types more prone to peritoneal dissemination, especially when the serosa is involved, whereas the risk of liver metastases is higher in the intestinal type of GC [8, 16]. However, the high correlation between histotype and the number of involved nodes probably limits the independent prognostic power of the Lauren system.

Tumor size has long been disregarded as an independent prognostic factor in GC, as its prognostic value has been broadly corrected by tumor stage. Large tumors are frequently histologically poorly differentiated or of diffuse histotype, have infiltrative growth, and penetrate the serosa; peritoneal recurrence is also more frequent [16, 17]. Similar considerations can be made for macroscopic type IV of the Borrmann classification.

The prognostic value of venous and lymphatic invasion in GC has also been reported [18] but the main influence of either one on survival probability seems to be restricted to neoplasms involving the muscolaris/subserosal layer or in the absence of lymph node involvement [10, 19]. For unconventional and biological prognostic factors see Chap. 2.

5.3 Patient-related Prognostic Factors

Age is the most important patient-related prognostic factor. Generally, advanced age influences overall survival and, to a lesser extent, cancer-related survival [5, 13, 14]. Some authors have reported younger age (< 45 years) to be associated with worse prognosis [20]. In younger patients, the diffuse histotype is relatively more frequent and neoplasms may present at diagnosis in more advanced stages; however, when matching for tumor stage, young age itself is not an independent prognostic factor.

The prognostic value of gender is unclear. Males usually have a worse prognosis than females, but this may be related to the higher frequency of proximal tumors in the former. In most series, gender shows no independent prognostic value for cancer-related survival [5, 14].

Geographic area and the patient's ethnicity are emerging prognostic factors for GC. Several recent studies from the US have reported a better outcome in Asian Americans than in other ethnicities [21]. The survival advantage of Asian patients with GC seems to be limited to foreign-born individuals, whereas that of US-born Asians and the resident population is similar. This suggests that factors acquired in youth affect gastric cancer development and biology. In a recent paper, we documented the different prognoses of GC patients coming from different risk areas of Italy but treated at the same center [22]. A higher frequency of Lauren diffuse histotype, more advanced stage, and worse outcome were determined in patients from Southern Italy (where the incidence of gastric cancer is very low) than in those from Tuscany (a high-risk area). Differences in survival rates between high-risk and low-risk areas were also observed in epidemiological studies [22].

Other patient-related prognostic factors are related to the immune system. A high preoperative neutrophil/lymphocyte ratio (NLR) in peripheral blood is associated with worse prognosis [23]. An increase in the neutrophil count may be due to the increased number of immature and non-functional neutrophils; alternatively, it may be a result of a relative lymphocytopenia, with a consequent weaker lymphocyte-mediated immune response to the tumor.

5.4 Treatment-related Prognostic Factors

The most important treatment-related prognostic factor is undoubtedly surgical radicality. The UICC criteria define R0 resection as complete tumor removal without microscopic or macroscopic residual disease. This assumes a very accurate preoperative (clinical), intraoperative (peritoneal cytology, biopsies), and postoperative (resection margins) tumor staging. If the definition is accurate, surgical radicality may be one of the most important prognostic factors in GC; however, in many cases there is recurrence of the GC even after R0 resection, reflecting the current limits in the definition of this parameter [5, 7, 13, 14].

The therapeutic role of lymphadenectomy has not been completely established. Despite the negative results of two randomized studies conducted in Europe, a recent re-evaluation of the Dutch trial demonstrated a significant long-term survival benefit of D2 vs. D1 lymphadenectomy [24]. In particular, after a median follow-up of 15 years, there was a lower risk of locoregional recurrence and fewer cancer-related deaths after D2 dissection. These data confirm the results of observational studies from specialized Western centers, where extended lymphadenectomy is currently performed and morbidity and mortality rates are low [25, 26]. Furthermore, it should be noted that extended lymphadenectomy is associated with more accurate pN staging and a more reliable prediction of the patient's prognosis by tumor stage [26].

The number of removed lymph nodes has a prognostic value in GC [4, 27]. The probability of death due to the cancer seems to be reduced as the number of removed lymph nodes increases. This may be due to the therapeutic role of lymphadenectomy or to the well-known Will Rogers phenomenon (stage migration). For this reason, the UICC advises a minimum number of 16 analyzed lymph nodes to obtain adequate pN staging. The ratio of metastatic to examined lymph nodes (N ratio) has been proposed as a novel prognostic factor that may be useful to limit stage migration and identify different prognostic subgroups among N stages [27]. One of the major limits for the clinical application of this factor is the identification of homogeneous and universally validated cut-off limits. In particular, it is unclear whether the prognostic power of the N ratio differs according to the extent of lymphadenectomy [28].

The extent of stomach resection does not affect the patient's prognosis. When performed with negative resection margins and adequate lymphadenectomy, partial gastrectomy offers a chance of cure similar to that achieved with total gastrectomy, even in advanced forms of GC.

A few studies have suggested adverse outcome in GC patients submitted to perioperative blood transfusions. A recent evaluation of a GIRCG large series demonstrated that blood transfusions, although associated with slightly worse prognosis, are not an independent prognostic factor. The need for transfusion was related to several demographic, pathologic, and surgical variables (patient age, tumor location, need for extensive surgery, major postoperative complications), which could explain its correlation with long-term survival [29].

5.5 Prognostic Scores

The utility of prognostic scores is the possibility to simultaneously consider a set of variables in order to assign a risk score to an individual patient. Several mathematical models designed to predict the prognosis of GC patients have been reported to date [5, 13]. Computer software (the Maruyama program) has been developed and applied in the analysis of a large series of patients at the National Cancer Center Hospital in Tokyo, with the aim of individualizing the extent of lymphadenectomy according to the patients' demographic and clinical features. From this model, a Maruyama index of unresected disease (MI) was developed, and subsequently confirmed to be significantly related to patient long-term survival [30]. Kattan et al. recently developed a prognostic nomogram based on a large number of patients treated at Memorial Sloan Kettering Cancer Center [13]. The endpoint of the nomogram was tumor-related death of patients and the estimation of survival probability after R0 resection. This prognostic score was validated in several large series from Asian and Western centers [7, 14].

A prognostic score for the prediction of risk of recurrence after R0 resection was recently calculated based on a large series of patients treated in three centers belonging to the GIRCG [5]. The main methodological characteristics of the GIRCG prognostic score were: (1) a prospective evaluation of patients submitted to radical surgery and periodic follow-up examinations according to a standard protocol, with a long follow-up time for survivors; (2) an analysis of the patient-, tumor-, and treatment-related variables commonly used in clinical practice; (3) the endpoint of the study:clinically assessed tumor recurrence rather than survival time obtained from patient records, family physicians, or demographic services; (4) attribution of the risk of recurrence to individual patients rather than inclusion in a risk category.

The score was developed using a logistic regression model in which the presence of recurrence was the dependent variable, and a set of clinical/pathological variables (age, gender, tumor location, tumor size, Lauren histotype, depth of invasion, nodal status, extent of lymphadenectomy, and extent of resection) as the covariates.

The probability of the event (recurrence) was estimated by the formula:

$$(e^{Z}/1 + e^{Z}) \times 100$$

where e is the base of the natural logarithm and Z is the result deriving from the logistic regression equation:

$$Z = c + B_1X_1 + B_2X_2 + \ldots. B_pX_p$$

c is the constant of the logistic regression model, and X1...p are the independent variables identified by the model, with their regression coefficients (B1...p). With this method, we were able to estimate the probability of recurrence for each patient. The formula was included in a database, and the risk of recurrence calculated automatically. The first GIRCG prognostic score considered pT and pN status according to the 6th edition of the TNM classification [5]. With the introduction of the new TNM classification (7th edition), the scoring system has been recalculated according to the new criteria, excluding EGJ neoplasms and patients with linitis plastica.

The new formula for score calculation is:

Z = – 1.978 – 0.366 (middle third) + 2.123 (upper third) + 0.912 (pT2) + 1.363 (pT3) + 2.307 (pT4) + 1.333 (pN1) + 1.634 (pN2) + 3.616 (pN3a) + 4.728 (pN3b) – 1.290 (D2-D3 dissection)

The most important characteristic of the GIRCG scoring system is the distribution of values in the extreme of the range (Fig. 5.2). Most patients were assigned to low-risk or high-risk categories, and only a few remained in the subgroups with intermediate prognosis. This demonstrates an important clinical feature of the scoring system.

The majority of patients with a high score experienced recurrence during early follow-up whereas only a few patients with low scores had disease recurrence (Fig. 5.3). Figure 5.2 shows the linear correlation between the score and the risk of recurrence.

5.6 How To Easily Calculate The GIRCG Prognostic Score

The formula can be easily included in an Excel file structured as depicted in Fig. 5.4, in the exact position (lines and columns) as indicated. Four parameters are necessary: tumor location, pT and pN stages (TNM 7th edition), and extent of lymphadenectomy. In order to calculate the prognostic score for a patient, the number "0" of different cells should be replaced with "1" depending on the different parameters (i.e. if the TNM stage of the patient is T2N1, the number "1" is included in cell T2 and in cell N1, and so on for other parameters such as tumor location and lymphadenectomy).

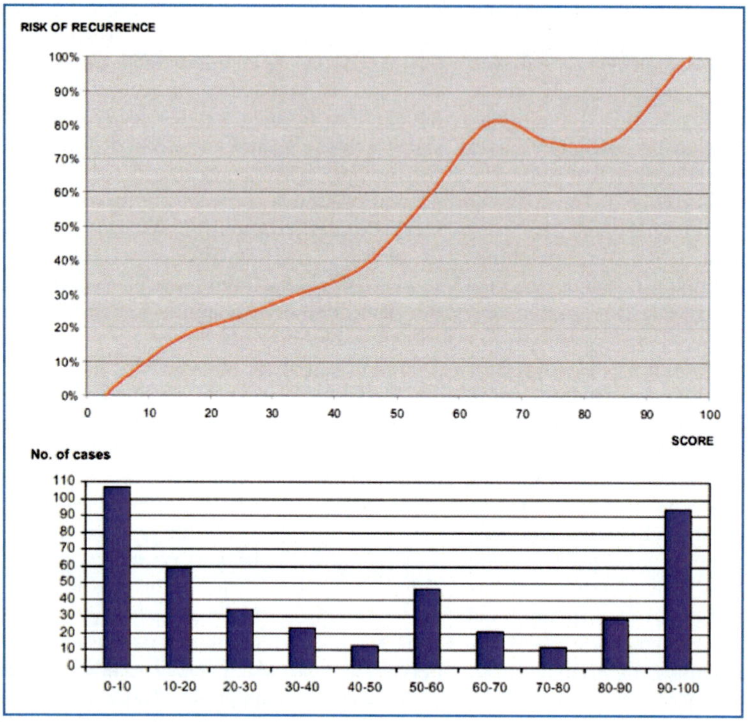

Fig. 5.2 Distribution of patients according to different ranges of the GIRCG prognostic score (*bottom*) and linear correlation with the risk of recurrence (*top*). Most patients were distributed in the extreme of the range (low-risk or high-risk categories). A high correlation between the score and the risk of recurrence was observed

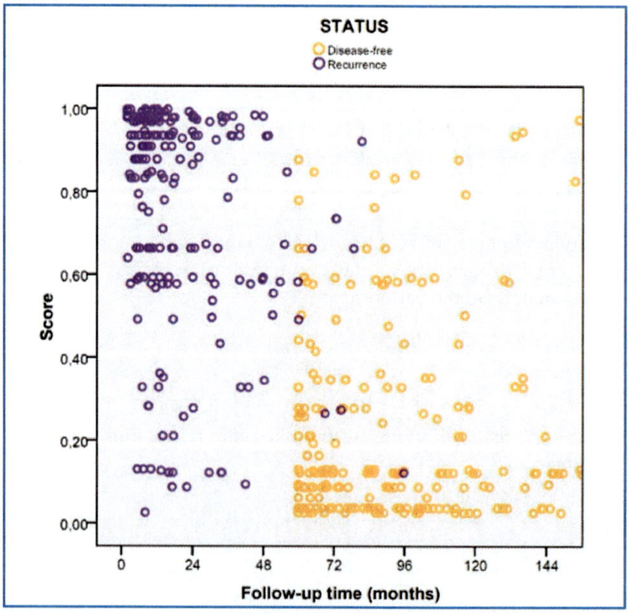

Fig. 5.3 Correlation between GIRCG prognostic score and follow-up time. Most patients with high scores had disease recurrence early in the follow-up period whereas the great majority of patients with low scores were disease-free during long-term follow-up

	A	B	C	D	E	F	G	H	I	J	K	L	M	N	O	P	Q
1	NAME	LOCATION			DEPTH OF INVASION				NODAL STATUS					LYMPHADENECTOMY		EQ	SCORE
2		LOWER	MIDDLE	UPPER	T1	T2	T3	T4	N0	N1	N2	N3a	N3b	LIMITED	EXTENDED		
3	EXAMPLE 1	0	0	0	0	0	0	0	0	0	0	0	0	0	0		
4																	
5																	
6																	

Fig. 5.4 How to easily calculate the GIRCG prognostic score using Excel. See instructions in the text or download the model at the GIRCG website: www.gircg.it

In the cell EQ (P3) insert the formula:

= – 1.978 – 0.366 (C3) + 2.123 (D3) + 0.912 (F3) + 1.363 (G3) + 2.307 (H3) + 1.333 (J3) + 1.634 (K3) + 3.616 (L3) + 4.728 (M3) – 1.290 (O3)

In the cell SCORE (Q3), insert the formula:

=1/(1+1/EXP(P2))*100

The number that appears in the cell SCORE is the estimated risk of recurrence for such patient.

A prospective study has been conducted for several years by the GIRCG in order to validate the prognostic score (manuscript in preparation). External validations by other large series in different geographic areas are necessary for clinical application of the model. The model can be downloaded at the website of the GIRCG: www.gircg.it

References

1. Verdecchia A, Guzzinati S, Francisci S et al (2009) Survival trends in European cancer patients diagnosed from 1988 to 1999. Eur J Cancer 45:1042-1066
2. Japanese Gastric Cancer Association Registration Committee (2006) Gastric cancer treated in 1991 in Japan: data analysis of nationwide registry. Gastric Cancer 9:51-66
3. Ahn HS, Lee HJ, Hahn S et al (2010) Evaluation of the Seventh American Joint Committee on Cancer/International Union Against Cancer Classification of gastric adenocarcinoma in comparison with the sixth classification. Cancer 116:5592-5598
4. Smith DD, Schwarz RR, Schwarz RE (2005) Impact of total lymph node count on staging and survival after gastrectomy for gastric cancer: data from a large US-population database. J Clin Oncol 23:7114-7124
5. Marrelli D, De Stefano A, de Manzoni G et al (2005) Prediction of recurrence after radical surgery for gastric cancer: a scoring system obtained from a prospective multicenter study. Ann Surg 241:247-255
6. Roviello F, Rossi S, Marrelli D et al (2006) Number of lymph node metastases and its prognostic significance in early gastric cancer: a multicenter Italian study. J Surg Oncol 94:275-280
7. Strong VE, Song KY, Park CH et al (2010) Comparison of gastric cancer survival following R0 resection in the United States and Korea using an internationally validated nomogram. Ann Surg 251:640-646
8. Roviello F, Marrelli D, de Manzoni G et al (2003) Prospective study of peritoneal recurrence after curative surgery for gastric cancer. Br J Surg 90:1113-1119
9. Cheng CT, Tsai CY, Hsu JT et al (2011) Aggressive Surgical Approach for Patients with T4 Gastric Carcinoma: Promise or Myth? Ann Surg Oncol 18:1606-1614
10. Baiocchi GL, Tiberio GA, Minicozzi AM et al (2010) A multicentric Western analysis of prognostic factors in advanced, node-negative gastric cancer patients. Ann Surg 252:70-73
11. Glehen O, Gilly FN, Arvieux C et al (2010) Peritoneal carcinomatosis from gastric cancer: a multi-institutional study of 159 patients treated by cytoreductive surgery combined with perioperative intraperitoneal chemotherapy. Ann Surg Oncol 17:2370-2377
12. Mezhir JJ, Shah MA, Jacks LM et al (2010) Positive peritoneal cytology in patients with gastric cancer: natural history and outcome of 291 patients. Ann Surg Oncol 17:3173-3180
13. Kattan MW, Karpeh MS, Mazumdar M et al (2003) Postoperative nomogram for disease-specific survival after an R0 resection for gastric carcinoma. J Clin Oncol 21:3647-3650
14. Novotny AR, Schuhmacher C, Busch R et al (2006) Predicting individual survival after gastric cancer resection: validation of a U.S.-derived nomogram at a single high-volume center in Europe. Ann Surg 243:74-81
15. Adachi Y, Yasuda K, Inomata M et al (2000) Pathology and prognosis of gastric carcinoma: well versus poorly differentiated type. Cancer 89:1418-1424
16. Marrelli D, Roviello F, de Manzoni G et al (2002) Different patterns of recurrence in gastric cancer depending on Lauren's histological type: longitudinal study. World J Surg 26:1160-1165
17. Kunisaki C, Makino H, Takagawa R et al (2008) Tumor diameter as a prognostic factor in patients with gastric cancer. Ann Surg Oncol 15:1959-1967
18. Nozoe T, Iguchi T, Egashira A (2010) Pathological prognostic score as a simple criterion to predict outcome in gastric carcinoma. J Surg Oncol 102:73-76

19. Kooby DA, Suriawinata A, Klimstra DS et al (2003) Biologic predictors of survival in node-negative gastric cancer. Ann Surg 237:828-835
20. Santoro R, Carboni F, Lepiane P et al (2007) Clinicopathological features and prognosis of gastric cancer in young European adults. Br J Surg 2007 94:737-742
21. Al-Refaie WB, Tseng JF, Gay G et al (2008) The impact of ethnicity on the presentation and prognosis of patients with gastric adenocarcinoma. Results from the National Cancer Data Base. Cancer 113:461-469
22. Marrelli D, Pedrazzani C, Corso G et al (2009) Different pathological features and prognosis in gastric cancer patients coming from high-risk and low-risk areas of Italy. Ann Surg 250:43-50
23. Shimada H, Takiguchi N, Kainuma O et al (2010) High preoperative neutrophil-lymphocyte ratio predicts poor survival in patients with gastric cancer. Gastric Cancer 13:170-176
24. Songun I, Putter H, Kranenbarg EM et al (2010) Surgical treatment of gastric cancer: 15-year follow-up results of the randomised nationwide Dutch D1D2 trial. Lancet Oncol 11:439-449
25. Marrelli D, Pedrazzani C, Neri A et al (2007) Complications after extended (D2) and superextended (D3) lymphadenectomy for gastric cancer: analysis of potential risk factors. Ann Surg Oncol 14:25-33
26. Verlato G, Roviello F, Marchet A et al (2009) Indexes of surgical quality in gastric cancer surgery: experience of an Italian network. Ann Surg Oncol 16:594-602
27. Marchet A, Mocellin S, Ambrosi A et al (2007) The ratio between metastatic and examined lymph nodes (N ratio) is an independent prognostic factor in gastric cancer regardless of the type of lymphadenectomy: results from an Italian multicentric study in 1853 patients. Ann Surg 245:543-552
28. Pedrazzani C, Sivins A, Ancans G et al (2010) Ratio between metastatic and examined lymph nodes (N ratio) may have low clinical utility in gastric cancer patients treated by limited lymphadenectomy: results from a single-center experience of 526 patients. World J Surg 34:85-91
29. Pacelli F, Rosa F, Marrelli D et al (2011) Do perioperative blood transfusions influence prognosis of gastric cancer patients? Analysis of 927 patients and interactions with splenectomy. Ann Surg Oncol 18:1615-1623
30. Hundahl SA, Peeters KC, Kranenbarg EK et al (2007) Improved regional control and survival with "low Maruyama Index" surgery in gastric cancer: autopsy findings from the Dutch D1-D2 Trial. Gastric Cancer 10:84-86

Preoperative Work-up: Endoscopy and Endoscopic Ultrasonography

6

Emanuele Bendia, Marco Marzioni, Antonio Di Sario, Walter Siquini, and Antonio Benedetti

Abstract

Since mortality related to gastric cancer correlates with tumor stage at diagnosis, the recognition of early lesions can significantly modify short- and long-term prognoses of patients with these tumors. At present, several methods able to increase diagnostic accuracy are available, such as vital stains and/or high-resolution endoscopic devices. The morphological evaluation of gastric lesions can be improved by performing intragastric ultrasonography, which allows the distinction of non-invasive from invasive lesions and plays an important role in gastric cancer staging. In the absence of signs of deep infiltration and metastases, endoscopic resection of gastric lesions can be performed, especially in patients at high surgical risk.

Keywords

Early gastric cancer • Vital stains • Endoscopic magnification • Endoscopic ultrasonography • Endoscopic mucosal resection • Endoscopic submucosal dissection.

6.1 Introduction

Mortality related to gastric cancer (GC) is very high, even in economically advanced countries, and correlates with tumor stage at diagnosis. The diagnosis of early-stage GC is still less common in Western countries than in Japan [10–15% vs. 50%) [1, 2]. This difference is likely due to differences in the incidence of GC in the two populations and to the existence of screening programs in Japan.

Surgical resection with lymphadenectomy is currently the first-line treatment for patients with GC and achieves a 5-year survival of 90% in those who undergo surgery at an early-stage (IA) of the disease. However, mortality following gastrectomy is in the range of 1–6.5% and morbidity is about 15–20% [3, 4]. Moreover, symptoms such as early satiety, dysphagia, gastroesophageal reflux, diarrhea, vomiting, and increased gastrojejunal transit reduce the quality of life in patients after surgery [5, 6].

In early-stage GC, the tumor is superficial and does not extend beyond the submucosa, regardless of the presence or absence of metastatic lymph nodes [2]. Superficial neoplastic lesions of the stomach have recently been reclassified according to their macroscopic morphology: type 0-I consists of pedunculated or sessile polyps that are easily

E. Bendia (✉)
Dept. of Gastroenterology,
"Ospedali Riuniti" University Hospital,
Polytechnic University of Marche,
Ancona, Italy

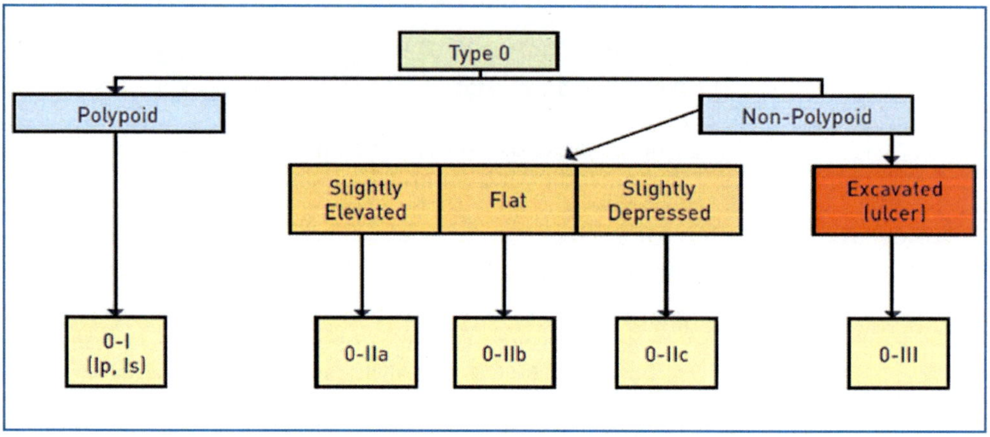

Fig 6.1 Classification of gastric tumors

recognizable endoscopically and resectable by standard techniques; type 0-IIa, 0-IIb, and 0-IIc lesions are non-polypoid and are, respectively, raised, flat, or depressed; type 0-III lesions are cavitary [7] (Fig. 6.1). Superficial non-polypoid tumors are especially difficult to detect and usually require specific resection techniques. Type II lesions are the most frequently diagnosed in Japan (about 96% of all superficial lesions), and about 75% of them are of the depressed type (0-IIc) or mixed with a depressed component. In Western countries, however, about 75% of the early lesions are of the cavitary type (0-III) [7]. The reason for this difference is at present not clear.

6.2 Diagnosis

Several methods that may improve the diagnostic endoscopic examination are available, such as vital stains, often associated with endoscopic magnification, high-resolution and/or high-definition endoscopic devices, narrow-band imaging, virtual staining, or confocal microendoscopy.

Mucosal staining increases the recognition of type II superficial lesions by more clearly defining the margins and extension of the tumor and by allowing targeted biopsies. The combined use of vital stains and endoscopic magnification, as well as the use of virtual confocal microendoscopy, has a high sensitivity in diagnosing gastric tumors and in discriminating differentiated from undifferentiated cancers.

Staining with indigo carmine in combination with endoscopic magnification results in a better definition of the margins of the lesion and improves structural identification of the mucosal and vascular patterns. Alterations in those patterns in differentiated tumors vs.undifferentiated tumors can be distinguished. In the former, glandular folds are regular and the vessels are of variable size whereas in the latter there is a loss of glandular structure but small and irregular vessels are evident [8]. Similar results were obtained using narrow-band imaging, which has a high sensitivity (89–96%) and specificity (83–95%) [9].

A few data are currently available on the roles of high-definition endoscopy and virtual staining. Preliminary studies show that these devices better define the margins of the lesion in approximately 50% of cases, suggesting that they have a better diagnostic yield than conventional endoscopy [10], especially through the identification of irregularities in the vascular pattern, which are present in about 50% of lesions [11].

In the evaluation of early GC, confocal microendoscopy is, unlike the other diagnostic endoscopic methods, currently the only one that can provide a histological evaluation "in vivo" and thus discriminate differentiated from undifferentiated tumors

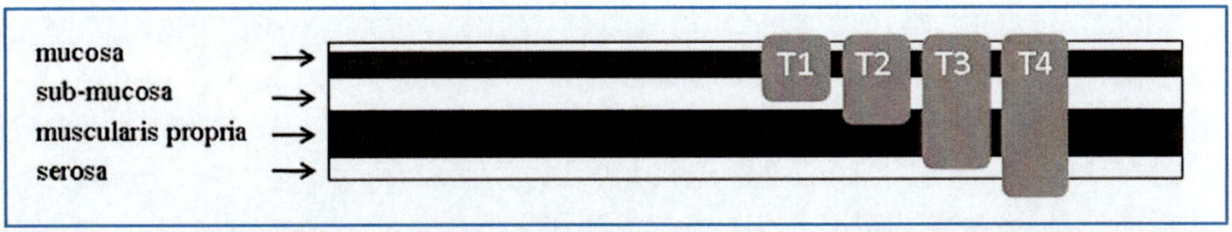

Fig. 6.2 Endoscopic ultrasonography (EUS) easily distinguishes the five layers of the gastric wall on the basis of their alternating hyper- and hypo- echogenicities. Thus, the first two layers, the superficial and deep mucosa are hyper- and hypo-echoic, respectively; the third layer, the submucosa, is hyper-echoic, the fourth layer, the muscularis propria, is hypo-echoic, and the fifth layer, the serosa, is hyper-echoic. Therefore, EUS well identifies the T stage of gastric cancer: T1 (limited to the submucosa), T2 (extending to the muscularis propria), T3 (growing into the subserosa), and T4 (invading the serosa and extending outside the organ)

[12] and neoplastic from non-neoplastic lesions, with high sensitivity, specificity, diagnostic accuracy, and positive and negative predictive values (90, 99, 97, 86, and 97%, respectively) [13].

6.3 Staging

The size of the gastric lesion is directly related to the risk of submucosal invasion, although small type 0-IIc lesions frequently infiltrate the submucosa [7]. The morphological evaluation of gastric lesions can be improved by performing intragastric ultrasonography with 20- to 30-MHz mini-probes, which distinguish non-invasive from invasive lesions [14]. Submucosal invasion is correlated with the risk of metastases to regional lymph nodes, which are not always detectable by ultrasonographic or radiological methods, since both endoscopic ultrasonography (EUS) and computed tomography (CT) have a low diagnostic accuracy (50–87% and 52–71%, respectively) [15, 16]. However, if the submucosa is deeply infiltrated, the risk of lymph node metastases is extremely high.

Excellent spatial resolution is obtained with EUS, which allows the study of the gastric wall in five different layers (Fig. 6.2). Those layers are easily distinguishable from each other on the basis of their alternating hyper- and hypo-echogenicities. The first two layers are hyper- and hypo-echoic, respectively, and define the superficial and deep mucosa; the third layer is hyper-echoic and identifies the submucosa; the fourth layer, the muscularis propria, is hypo-echoic and the fifth, the serosa, hyper-echoic [17].

The major role played by EUS in GC is in disease staging (Fig. 6.3), as accurate staging is one of the main factors affecting prognosis [18]. Although EUS is generally well accepted by clinicians due its importance in GC staging, there is currently a lack of solid and definitive data that support its use in that setting. Many studies suffer from different types of bias; in particular, very few have compared EUS with CT or other techniques. Those which are available are often rapidly left behind by the development of new techniques or methods, such as fine-needle aspiration (FNA) that are being introduced into the staging work-up. Other biases arises from the recent changes in the lymph node staging of the TNM system and the fact that several studies have assessed the specificity and sensitivity of a technique in determining either the T or N or M status, but rarely have all three been examined together [19-20].

Nevertheless, the contribution of EUS has increased in response to the demand for precise locoregional staging of GC. From a theoretical point of view, the main clinical decision in the management of GC is the detection of distant metastases, as only those patients are excluded from direct surgical resection, thus making the local invasiveness an issue of secondary consideration. However, the precise determination of parietal invasion (T) and lymph node extension increases in importance with time, since definition of that stage may be crucial in determining whether the patient is a candidate for endoscopic or laparoscopic treatment, to establish the extent of nodal resection, and eventually for laparoscopy in the staging work-up in specific cases. Hence the growing value of EUS

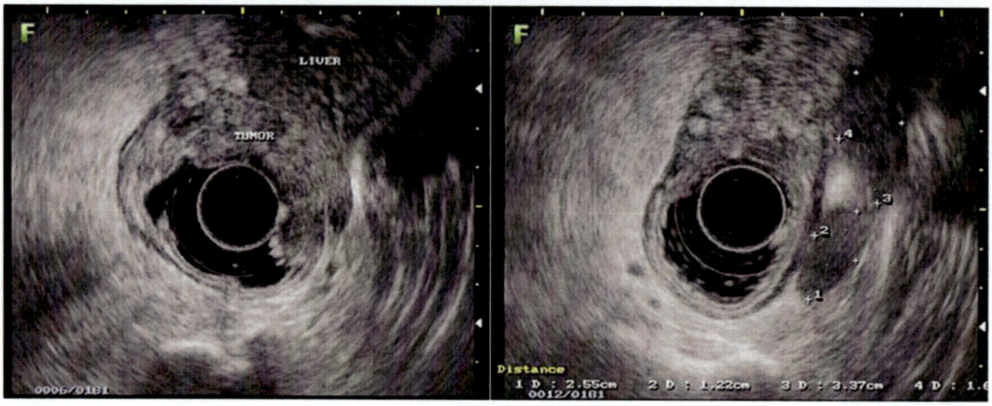

Fig. 6.3 A case of gastric cancer staged by EUS. The tumor originates from the 2nd layer and infiltrates the entire gastric wall, extending outside the organ to reach the inferior liver margin (*left*). Eight positive lymph nodes around the stomach were found (*right*). EUS staged the disease in this patient as a T4N2

in this field is coupled to its essential support of clinical trials establishing the effectiveness of neoadjuvant protocols [21-23].

In addition, EUS has a good diagnostic accuracy in studies of parietal invasiveness (T stage): overall sensitivities for the diagnosis of particular T stages ranged from 0.82 to 0.99 [18, 21]. The lowest value refers to the staging of T3 tumors, in which the problems of differentiating between subserosal and serosal infiltration and thus T3 from T4a are well known. EUS sensitivity for T stage increases in advanced disease, especially compared to early-stage tumors; in contrast, specificity is high at all disease stages. This provides EUS with a very high odds ratio, which means that at a given T stage established by EUS there is a very high probability that the tumor is indeed at that stage, as determined by anatomical inspection after resection [18]. This is of major relevance for clinicians, since it provides the basis for offering endoscopic submucosal resection to patients with very early disease [18, 24].

The opposite side of the coin is the fact that EUS has a low likelihood ratio for advanced disease, lower than in early disease. The likelihood ratio measures the ability of a test to exclude the disease; in other words, EUS performs better in excluding the disease at T4 than at T1. For example, if EUS finds that the patient has stage T3 disease, then it can substantially be ruled out that the disease is at T4. Such a concept is, again, important in offering the patient a specific treatment option. Following the above example, a patient with T3 disease is still a candidate for radical rather than palliative treatment. Similarly, if a patient's disease is staged at T2 by EUS, even if there has been a mis-staging the worst that may happen is that the correct stage is actually T1, which will not change the treatment options.

It is currently difficult to establish how well EUS performs in defining N stage; this is mostly due to changes in the TNM classification (1997), which introduced four rather than the previous three N stages. Overall, however, it is known that EUS does not perform as well in N as in T staging. This may be due to the fact that approximately 55% of metastatic lymph nodes from GC are < 5 mm in diameter [21, 25], and thus, although they are visible, will be considered negative. Experts also believe that the performance deficiencies of EUS in N staging are due to the staging system per se. The current staging system is based on the number of pathologic nodes [17], a count that is difficult to make with precision using an imaging technique [21]. As a result, the overall accuracy of EUS in N staging according to the new system is estimated, in some studies, to be as low as 30% [20, 21]. This limitation might be overcome by the extensive application of FNA of the lymph nodes, as examined in studies that systematically evaluated EUS-

FNA in GC staging [19, 21, 26].

Conceptually, EUS may represent an advantage in the staging of early GC compared with other techniques employed for disease staging. Early GC can be studied by two different approaches: (1) conventional ultrasound endoscope with the radial scan transducer at the tip of the endoscope, and (2) an ultrasound probe with a small radial scan transducer at the tip of the catheter, which can be used through the working channel of the endoscope (mini-probes) [27]. Diagnosis of a mucosal lesion, which is a good indication for endoscopic mucosectomy, is 90% accurate. This is one of the most important diagnostic abilities of EUS, i.e., to evaluate the indications for endoscopic treatment in early GC. Another tool is the recently introduced 3D reconstruction of EUS images, which allows not only a more specific definition of the lesion but also quantification of its volume, which is useful to evaluate therapeutic effect [27]. One study assessed the sensitivity and specificity of mini-probes in the detection of submucosal invasion, obtaining values of 0.71–0.95 and 0.64–0.91, respectively [21, 28].

Results of systematic reviews indirectly comparing EUS, multi-slice detector CT (MDCT), and MRI showed that they achieved a similar accuracy in T and N staging, whereas FDG-PET was insensitive in the detection of lymph node metastases. However, experts stress the concept that, despite the similar results, the most experience has been gained with EUS, which justifies its use as the first-choice imaging modality in the staging of GC [21, 29].

6.4 Endoscopic Treatment of Early Gastric Cancer

6.4.1 Endoscopic Mucosal Resection

Histopathological studies conducted in Japan on large series of patients who underwent surgery for early GC have shown that small differentiated intramucosal cancers have a risk of lymph node metastases that is lower than the risk of mortality from gastric surgery. Usually, larger lesions are associated with a higher risk of submucosal invasion and lymph node metastases, both of which correlate with the degree of differentiation of the tumor and with mucosal and submucosal infiltration. These observations validate use of endoscopic mucosal resection (EMR) to remove superficial, non-ulcerated neoplastic lesions ≤2 cm in diameter (Table 6.1). EMR allows resection of the inner part of the gastric wall, including the mucosa, muscularis mucosa, and part of the submucosa (Fig. 6.4) [30]. The current limit of the technique is the impossibility to remove the entire lesion in about 25% of cases. In addition, excision of the lesion is incomplete in 25–30% of cases, especially using the piecemeal EMR technique.

Local recurrence is seen only in 2% of patients treated with complete EMR, but it is significantly higher (10–37%) in case of incomplete resection [31]. Accordingly, a careful histological examination of the resected mucosa is essential.

Table 6.1 Indications for gastric mucosectomy

•	Adenocarcinoma G1, 2
•	Intramucosal tumor
•	Elevated lesion with a diameter ≤20 mm
•	Depressed lesion with a diameter ≤10 mm
•	Absence of ulceration

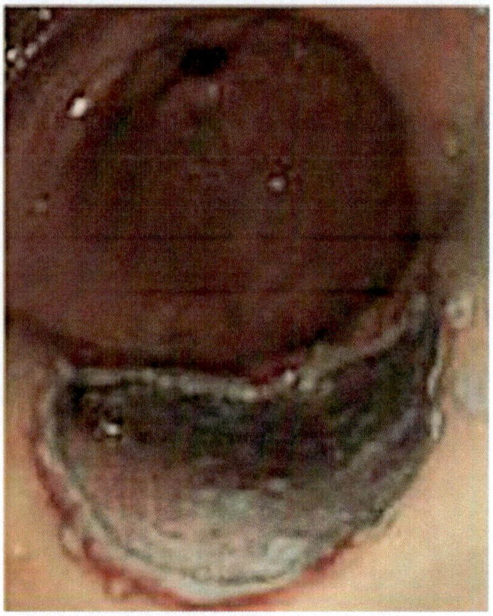

Fig. 6.4 Appearance of gastric mucosa after endoscopic mucosal resection in a patient with early gastric cancer

6.4.2 Endoscopic Submucosal Dissection

Histological data derived from studies of patients who underwent gastrectomy for early GC have shown that some large neoplastic lesions are associated with a low risk of lymph node metastases [32]. The following lesions may benefit from endoscopic treatment: (1) intramucosal lesions without superficial ulceration; (2) lesions with a diameter ≤3 cm and with only superficial ulceration; (3) well differentiated tumors with a diameter 3 cm, submucosal infiltration 0.5 cm (sm1), and without lymphatic and vascular invasion (Table 6.2) [32]. However, the treatment of these lesions by EMR is not suitable due to the size of the lesion itself, to the possibility of leaving residual tumor tissue, and to the high risk of local recurrence.

Table 6.2 Indications for submucosal dissection

• Intramucosal tumor without ulceration
• Ulcerated tumor with a diameter ≤ 3 cm
• Well differentiated tumors with a diameter ≤ 3 cm, without a deep submucosal infiltration (at least 500 μm; sm1) and without lymphatic and vascular invasion

By contrast, submucosal dissection (ESD) allows the complete removal of large lesions, with rates of complete excision of 95–100% and 79–97% for lesions 20 and > 20 mm in diameter, respectively [33]. A recent study comparing EMR and ESD confirmed that ESD is better than EMR for the treatment of lesions > 10 mm in diameter, although the rate of local recurrence seems to be similar [33]. The major limitations of ESD involve lesions > 3 cm in diameter, a location in the proximal stomach, and the presence of ulceration (odd ratio 4.6, 5.3, and 3.2, respectively) [34].

6.4.3 Long-term Results

The 5- and 10-year survival rates following EMR are similar (99%) to those reported for radical surgery [35]. The risk of lymph node metastases is extremely low when the tumor is not ulcerated and does not infiltrate the submucosa; if neither of these conditions are met (sm1 stage), then lymph node metastases can be expected in 3–4% of patients [36].

Another problem is the occurrence of metachronous tumors. Therefore, follow-up should be addressed not only at the prevention of local recurrence but also at the detection of novel tumors, which after 3 years occur with a frequency of about 5.9% [37].

6.5 Conclusions

Although in Western countries early GC is less important from an epidemiological point of view than colorectal cancer, the number of early diagnoses of GC is likely to significantly increase due to the availability of more sensitive endoscopic techniques, which will also allow the adequate treatment of patients at high surgical risk.

References

1. Ferlay J, Bray F, Pisani P, Parkin M (2004) GLOBOCAN 2002: Cancer Incidence, mortality and prevalence Worldwide. IARC Press, Lyon
2. Nakamura K, Ueyama T, Yao T et al (1992) Pathology and prognosis of gastric carcinoma. Findings in 10000 patients who underwent primary gastrectomy. Cancer 70:1030-1037
3. Bonenkamp JJ, Songun I, Hermans J et al (1995) Randomised comparison of morbidity after D1 and D2 dissection for gastric cancer in 996 Dutch patients. Lancet 345:745-748
4. Cuschieri A, Fayers P, Fielding J et al (1996) Postoperative morbidity and mortality after D1 and D2 resection for gastric cancer: preliminary results of the MRC randomised controlled surgical trial. Lancet 347:95-99
5. Davies J, Johnston D, Sue-Ling HM et al (1998) Total or subtotal gastrectomy for gastric carcinoma? A study of quality of life. World J Surg 22:1048-1055
6. Jentschura D, Winkler M, Strohmeier N et al (1997). Quality of life after curative surgery for gastric cancer: a comparison between total gastrectomy and subtotal gastrectomy resection. Hepatogastroenterology 44:1137-1144
7. Anonymous (2003) The Paris endoscopic classification of superficial neoplastic lesions: esophagus, stomach, and colon. Gastrointest. Endosc 58:S3-S43
8. Otsuka Y, Niwa Y, Ohmiya N et al (2004) Usefulness of magnifying endoscopy in the diagnosis of early gastric cancer. Endoscopy 36:165-169
9. Nakayoshi T, Tajiri H, Matsuda K et al (2004) Magnifying endoscopy combined with narrow band imaging system for early gastric cancer: correlation of vascular pattern with histopathology. Endoscopy 36:1080-1084
10. Mouri R, Yoshida S, Tanaka S et al (2009) Evaluation and validation of computed virtual chromoendoscopy in early gastric cancer. Gastrointest Endosc 69:1052-1058
11. Yoshizawa M, Osawa H, Yamamoto H et al (2009) Diagno-

sis of elevated type early gastric cancers by the optimal band imaging system. Gastrointest Endosc 69:19-28
12. Kitabatake S, Niwa Y, Miyahara R et al (2006) Confocal endomicroscopy for the diagnosis of gastric cancer in vivo. Endoscopy 38:1110- 1114
13. Zhang J, Li YQ, Zhao YA et al (2008) Classification of gastric pit patterns by confocal endomicroscopy. Gastrointest Endosc 67:843-853
14. Yanai H, Matsumoto Y, Harada T et al (1997) Endoscopic ultrasonography and endoscopy for staging depth of invasion in early gastric cancer: a pilot study. Gastrointest Endosc 46:212-216
15. Rosch T (1995) Endosonographic staging of gastric cancer: a review of literature results. Gastrointest Endosc Clin N Am 5:549-557
16. Polkowski M, Palucki J, Wronska E et al (2004) EUS versus helical tomography for locoregional staging of gastric cancer. Endoscopy 36:617-623
17. Kah TJ, Wang TC (2002) Tumors of the Stomach. In: Feldman M, Friedman LS, Slesinger MH (eds) Slesinger & Fordtran's Gastrointestinal and Liver Disease. Saunders, Philadelphia, pp 829-858
18. Tsendsuren T, Jun SM, Mian XH (2006) Usefulness of endoscopic ultrasonography in preoperative TNM staging of gastric cancer. World J Gastroenterol 12:43-47
19. Puli SR, Bechtold ML, Reddy JB et al (2009) How good is endoscopic ultrasound in differentiating various T stages of rectal cancer? Meta-analysis and systematic review. Ann Surg Oncol 16:254-265
20. Polkowski M, Palucki J, Wronska E et al (2004) Endosonography versus helical computed tomography for locoregional staging of gastric cancer. Endoscopy 36:617-623
21. Polkowski M (2009) Endosonographic staging of upper intestinal malignancy. Best Pract Res Clin Gastroenterol 23:649-661
22. Allum WH, Griffin SM, Watson A et al (2002) Guidelines for the management of oesophageal and gastric cancer. Gut 50:1-23
23. Moehler M, Galle PR, Gockel I et al (2007) The multidisciplinary management of gastrointestinal cancer. Multimodal treatment of gastric cancer. Best Pract Res Clin Gastroenterol 21:965-981
24. Bhandari S, Shim CS, Kim JH et al (2004). Usefulness of three-dimensional, multidetector row CT (virtual gastroscopy and multiplanar reconstruction) in the evaluation of gastric cancer: a comparison with conventional endoscopy, EUS, and histopathology. Gastrointest Endosc 59:619-626
25. Monig SP, Zirbes TK, Schroder W et al (1999) Staging of gastric cancer: correlation of lymph node size and metastatic infiltration. Am J Roentgenol 173:365-367
26. van Vliet EP, Eijkemans MJ, Kuipers EJ et al (2007) Publication bias does not play a role in the reporting of the results of endoscopic ultrasound staging of upper gastrointestinal cancers. Endoscopy 39:325-332
27. Yasuda K (2006) Early gastric cancer: diagnosis, treatment techniques and outcomes. Eur J Gastroenterol Hepatol 18:839-845
28. Kwee RM, Kwee TC (2008) The accuracy of endoscopic ultrasonography in differentiating mucosal from deeper gastric cancer. Am J Gastroenterol 103:1801-1809
29. Kwee RM, Kwee TC (2007) Imaging in local staging of gastric cancer: a systematic review. J Clin Oncol 25:2107-2116
30. Japanese Gastric Cancer Association (2004) Treatment Guideline for Gastric Cancer in Japan (2nd edn). Kanehara, Tokyo
31. Ono H, Kondo H, Gotoda T et al (2001) Endoscopic mucosal resection for treatment of early gastric cancer. Gut 48:225-229
32. Gotoda T, Yanagisawa A, Sasako M et al (2000) Incidence of lymph node metastasis from early gastric cancer: estimation with large number of cases at two large centers. Gastric Cancer 3:219-225
33. Nakamoto S, Sakai Y, Kasanuki J (2009) Indications for the use of endoscopic mucosal resection for early gastric cancer in Japan: a comparative study with endoscopic submucosal dissection. Endoscopy 41:746-750
34. Takenaka R, Kawahara Y, Okada H et al (2008) Risk factors associated with local recurrence of early gastric cancers after endoscopic submucosal dissection. Gastrointest Endosc 68:887-894
35. Mochiki E, Yanai M, Toyomasu Y et al (2010) Clinical outcomes of double endoscopic intralumenal surgery for early gastric cancer. Surg. Endosc 24:631-636
36. Jee YS, Hwang SH, Rao J et al (2009) Safety of extended endoscopic mucosal resection and endoscopic submucosal dissection following the Japanese Gastric Cancer Association treatment guidelines. Br J Surg 96:1157-1161
37. Nakajima T, Oda I, Gotoda T et al (2006) Metachronous gastric cancer after endoscopic resection: how effective is endoscopic surveillance? Gastric Cancer 9:93-98

Preoperative Work-up and Assessment of Resectability

7

Luigina Graziosi, Walter Bugiantella, Emanuel Cavazzoni, and Annibale Donini

Abstract

Radical surgery consisting of gastrectomy and D2 lymphadenectomy remains the standard procedure in the treatment of gastric cancer. To improve outcome, neoadjuvant treatment strategies with chemo- and/or radiotherapy regimes are employed. The optimal treatment plan and overall prognosis are critically dependent on accurate assessment of local invasion, tumor size, lymph node involvement, and the presence or absence of distant metastases. Total body computed tomography (CT), gastroduodenal endoscopy, and endoscopic ultrasonography have all been used in the diagnosis and initial staging of gastric cancer, showing a moderate sensitivity and specificity for the detection of lymph node metastases. ^{18}-FDG-positron emission tomography (PET)-CT has no role in the primary detection of gastric cancer due to its low sensitivity, but better accuracy than CT in the evaluation of lymph node metastases. A key staging modality in patients with gastric cancer is staging laparoscopy, which has high accuracy in detecting occult metastases and avoids the need for laparotomies.

Keywords

Gastric cancer • Pre-operative staging • Computer tomography • Endoscopic ultrasonography • ^{18}-FDG-PET-CT • Laparoscopy • Intraperitoneal lavage • Primary tumor • Lymph nodes metastases • Distant metastases

7.1 Introduction

The prognosis of gastric cancer patients depends on the metastatic potential of the tumor, even after curative resection. Thus, early detection and accurate staging of this disease can improve survival.

A. Donini (✉)
Dept. of General and Emergency Surgery,
University of Perugia,
Perugia, Italy

The mainstay of treatment of gastric cancer is radical surgery, but even with optimal surgical resection the prognosis remains poor. Currently, most therapeutic efforts are directed toward an individualization of treatment protocols involving surgical resection integrated with the administration of perioperative chemotherapy [1]. The goal is to improve prognosis by achieving a complete resection, reducing the tumor's dimensions and the spreading of neoplastic cells. Accurate preoperative staging is critical to define the most suitable therapeutic strategy and to consider whether a

G. de Manzoni, F. Roviello, W. Siquini (eds.), *Surgery in the Multimodal Management of Gastric Cancer*,

tumor is surgically resectable.

Clinical staging of gastric cancer has steadily improved through technical advances in endoscopic ultrasound (EUS), computed tomography (CT), positron emission tomography (PET), combined PET-CT, magnetic resonance imaging (MRI), and laparoscopy. The different settings for the use of these various modalities are discussed in the following.

7.2 Endoscopic Ultrasound

Echoendoscopes are available in radial and linear configurations. Radial devices are used for diagnostic imaging, whereas linear ones also facilitate image-guided tissue sampling (tumor and/or pathological lymph nodes).

EUS has become indispensable in the local preoperative staging of gastric cancer, as its high resolution yields detailed images of the gastric wall and perigastric lymph nodes. Compared to CT, EUS is the most reliable method to evaluate tumor depth and lymph node metastases [2-11].

The accuracy of EUS for gastric cancer according to different reports ranges from 64.8 to 92% with respect to T stage and from 50 to 90% with respect to N stage (with a sensitivity ≤ 66% and a specificity of 90%), with a few cases of over- rather than under-staging. Accuracy in the T staging of early gastric cancer is about 83% (67–90%) for T1 but decreases to 77% (64–97%) for T1m, and 46% (18–65%) for T1sm since a distinction between these two stages is difficult, especially in determining invasion of the second and third layers of the submucosa [4, 9-11]. T over-staging is mainly due to thickening of the gastric wall as part of a perifocal inflammatory reaction, which is easily mistaken for cancer. A sharpening or absence of the serosal layer in the lesser curvature, posterior wall of the fundus, and anterior wall of the antrum may also lead to over-staging, typically of pT3. This stage is defined as infiltration of the subserosal fat tissue; however, sonographically, the muscularis propria appears hypoechoic and the subserosal fat tissue and serosa itself hyperechoic, leading to staging by EUS as uT4a.

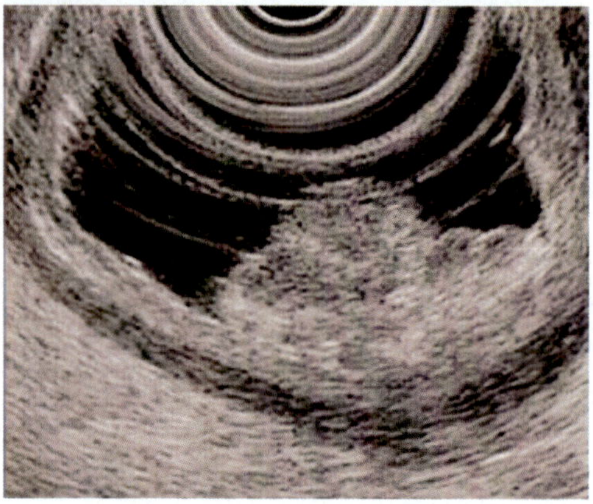

Fig. 7.1 Endoscopic Ultrasound (EUS) image of early gastric cancer: polypoid thickening of the gastric mucosa not involving the submucosa. (Courtesy of the General and Emergency Surgery department, University of Perugia, Italy)

Moreover, staging accuracy is influenced by endoscopic tumor type, histological type, and tumor size. The accuracy in determining depth of invasion is significantly higher for elevated (91%) than for depressed (56%) types of early gastric cancer [4-11]. Staging based on histological type is significantly more accurate for differentiated (86%) than for undifferentiated (18%) gastric cancer and decreases as tumor size increases. The relatively low accuracy and sensitivity in N staging are related to the absence of standard differential echoendoscopic criteria for benign and malignant lymph nodes. The echoendoscopic features of metastatic lymph nodes used by various groups include size > 10 mm or largest diameter/smallest diameter ratio < 2, rounded structure, sharp borders, and hypoechoic pattern [4-6]. The high frequency (> 12 Mhz) but limited depth (< 6 cm) of the transducer prevents satisfactory visualization of distant lymph nodes (second-level stations) (Figs. 7.1-7.2) [9-11].

7.3 Computed Tomography

Chest-abdomen-pelvis CT, using contrast-enhanced three-phase scanning, is fundamental in the preoperative staging of gastric cancer for evaluating the

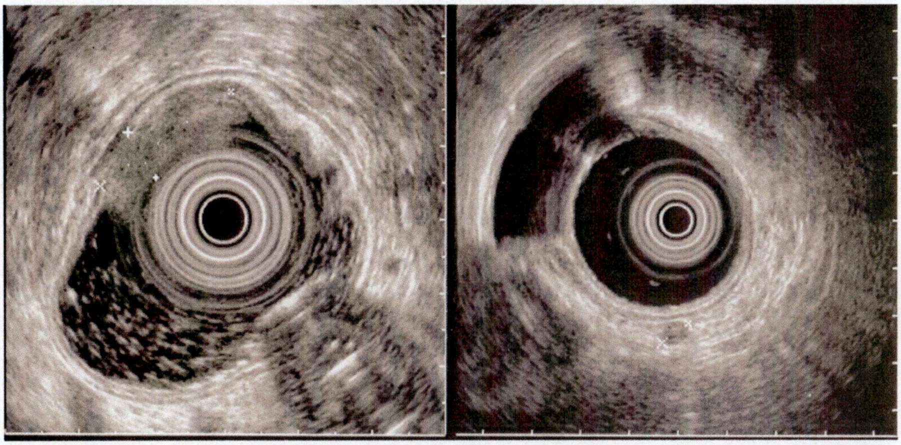

Fig. 7.2 EUS image of an advanced gastric cancer revealing thickening of the mucosa, submucosa and muscular layers, not involving the fifth layer (serosa). A peri-gastric lymph node is also evident. (Courtesy of the General and Emergency Surgery Department, University of Perugia, Italy)

local extent, nodal involvement, and metastatic spread of the disease. Multi-detector row CT allows thinner collimation and faster scanning. The addition of three-dimensional image reconstruction improves imaging resolution and provides accurate information regarding the space-occupying and hemodynamic features of the tumor, thus improving the accuracy of preoperative staging.

The accuracy of CT in the T staging of a gastric tumor is 69–89% but is very low, only 20–53%, in early gastric cancer (Figs. 7.3-7.4) [6, 7-16]. To improve imaging definition, the patient should be prepared by overnight fasting or fasting for at least 5 h to empty the stomach. Since the collapsed gastric wall can obscure disease or simulate pathology, optimal gastric distention and visualization are achieved using oral contrast agents: neutral (water), or negative (air) contrast, or both. The low staging accuracy of CT is caused mainly by over-staging of T1 and T2 and under-staging of pathological T4a and T4b, mostly due to the difficulty in observing the multilayered pattern of the gastric wall where it is thinner (pre-pylorus) or in areas scanned obliquely (gastric angle) because of partial volume-averaging effects [15, 16].

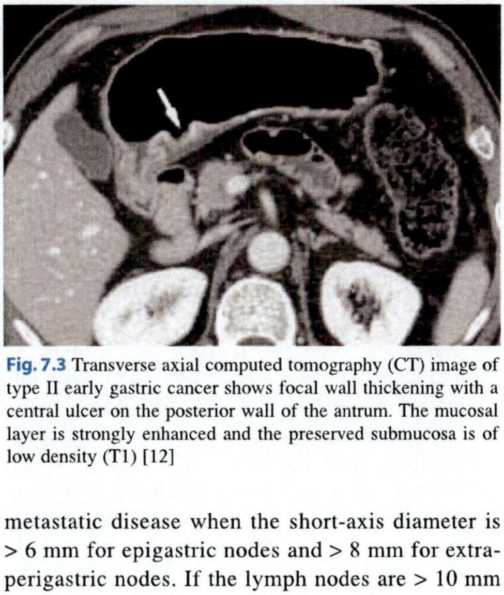

Fig. 7.3 Transverse axial computed tomography (CT) image of type II early gastric cancer shows focal wall thickening with a central ulcer on the posterior wall of the antrum. The mucosal layer is strongly enhanced and the preserved submucosa is of low density (T1) [12]

N staging using CT has an accuracy of 71–82%. According to more recent experiences, regional lymph nodes are considered to be involved by metastatic disease when the short-axis diameter is > 6 mm for epigastric nodes and > 8 mm for extra-perigastric nodes. If the lymph nodes are > 10 mm in diameter, they are considered positive if CT attenuation values are > 100 HU [13-16]. However, there is no worldwide consensus regarding pathological lymph nodes in terms of measuring method, size, shape, or enhancement patterns. CT limitations in the nodal staging of gastric cancer are a product of the high frequency of microscopic nodal

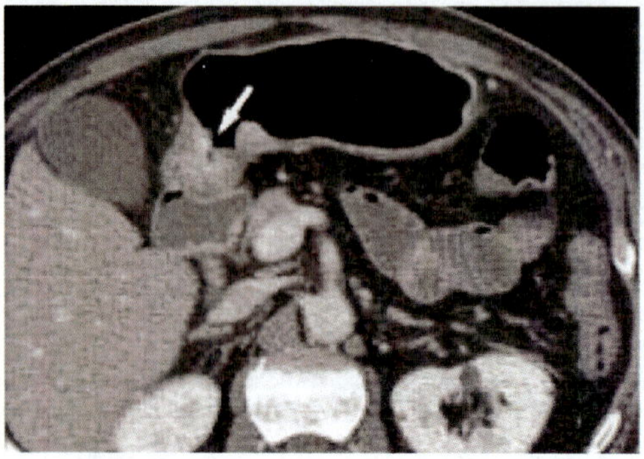

Fig. 7.4 Transverse axial CT image of an advanced gastric cancer, with an irregularly enhanced thickening of the antrum wall but without perigastric fatty infiltration (T2) [12]

invasion, with normal-size nodes, and poor differentiation between reactive or inflammatory and metastatic nodal enlargement.

The accuracy of CT in M staging is 91–100%. Although CT has a high sensitivity (100%) and specificity (99%) in detecting liver, splenic, and lung metastases, its accuracy in diagnosing peritoneal carcinomatosis is very low because of its low resolution (≥ 5 mm) [6, 7, 12, 13].

7.4 Fluorodeoxyglucose Positron Emission Tomography

Imaging with ^{18}F-fluoro-2-deoxyglucose PET (^{18}FDG-PET) is based on the increased glucose uptake of neoplastic cells, which over-express the main cell-membrane glucose transporter GLUT-1, resulting in higher uptake of ^{18}FDG as well. More than visual analysis, an often-used semi-quantitative method to assess tumor ^{18}FDG uptake is the standard uptake value (SUV), which is the measurement of ^{18}FDG uptake in a tumor volume normalized on the basis of a distribution volume. ^{18}FDG-PET is a well-established method in detecting and staging a variety of solid malignancies, including lung, esophageal, and colorectal cancers and lymphomas. However, despite the clinical importance of gastric cancer, ^{18}FDG-PET is currently not a standard procedure in the staging of this tumor.

In addition, most studies show that ^{18}FDG-PET is not an accurate imaging technique for the primary diagnosis of a gastric tumor, based on its high specificity but low sensitivity [17-24]. Indeed, in about 20% of patients with gastric cancer, the tumors are non-assessable by ^{18}FDG-PET. The sensitivity for detecting the primary tumor ranges from 58 to 94% (median 81.5%), and the specificity from 79 to 100% (median 90%).

Technical difficulties in performing ^{18}FDG-PET for gastric cancer are: (a) background signaling, due to the high physiological uptake of ^{18}FDG in the normal gastric wall because of its dense blood flow; (b) difficulty in wall distension, which is achieved by water ingestion after the patient has fasted for at least 5 h; and (c) the low spatial resolution (> 5 mm) of this technique. Furthermore, ^{18}FDG-PET is influenced by several other factors. The first is tumor location, i.e., whether the cancer is located in the upper, middle, or lower third of the stomach. The second is tumor size, as sensitivity is only 26–63% in early gastric cancer but increases to 93–98% in locally advanced gastric cancer. The third is the histological type, as the intestinal pattern has a higher SUV than the diffuse pattern (and also mucinous adenocarcinoma or signet-ring cell types) because of their high content of metabolically inert mucus and low cellular densities.

^{18}FDG-PET has a lower sensitivity than CT for metastases to N1 lymph nodes (17.6–46.4%; mean 27.5% vs. a mean sensitivity of 68%) because of its relatively low spatial resolution (> 5 mm). Consequently, perigastric lymph nodes often cannot be distinguished from the primary tumor or the normal stomach wall. For the detection of N2/N3 lymph nodes, ^{18}FDG-PET has low sensitivity (33–46.2%) but high specificity (91–100%) [18-24]. The positive predictive value of ^{18}FDG-PET for lymph node metastasis is higher than that of CT, allowing a tailored palliative therapy when N3 lymph nodes are metastatic and patients are not eligible for curative surgery. A combination of anatomy-based CT imaging and metabolically based ^{18}FDG-PET imaging might increase the detection of nodal involvement (Fig. 7.5).

^{18}FDG-PET has little value in diagnosing peritoneal carcinomatosis, again hampered by its low sensitivity (9–50%; mean 32.5%) but relatively high specificity (63–99%; mean 88.5%). Some

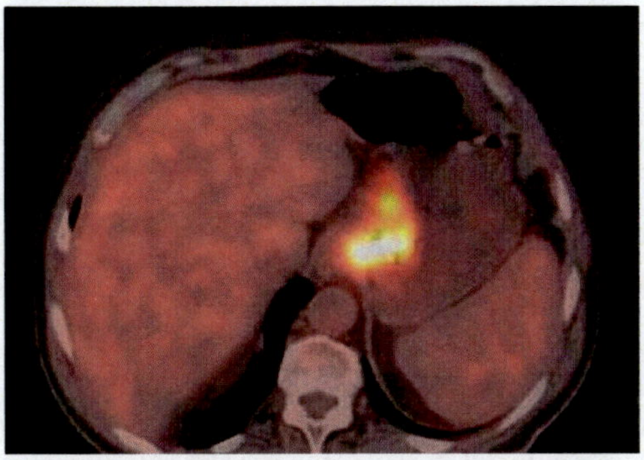

Fig. 7.5 ^{18}FDG- positron emission tomography image of esophagogastric junction cancer, showin perigastric nodal uptake. (Courtesy of the General and Emergency Surgery Department, University of Perugia, Italy)

authors have reported that peritoneal lesions show an extensive fibrosis around relatively few malignant cells, which could explain the low sensitivity of this imaging modality [17, 19-21]. The small size of peritoneal nodules (< 5 mm) may be another reason for the low detection rate.

The role of PET-CT in detecting distant metastases is not clear. In the few series reported thus far, sensitivity was 85% and specificity 74% for the detection of liver metastases, 67% and 88% for lung metastases, 24% and 76% for ascites, 4% and 100% for pleural carcinomatosis, and 30% and 82% for bone metastases, respectively [18, 19]. The low number of tumor cells in ascites, pleural, and bone metastases accounts for the low sensitivity.

However, ^{18}FDG-PET has a significant role in monitoring the response to neoadjuvant chemotherapy, showing chemo-responders at early stage.

It is anticipated that the use of new tracers, such as C-11-choline, will improve the sensitivity of PET-CT for gastric cancer.

7.5 Magnetic Resonance Imaging

In the diagnosis of gastrointestinal cancer, MRI has become an important technique following improvements in imaging quality, such that high resolution of soft-tissue contrast is currently possible. However, the results are poor in T staging, as the detection of early or small gastric cancers is difficult because of the inconspicuous thickness of the cancerous gastric wall [25-27]. Additionally, benign lesions, such as gastric ulcers, that are accompanied by marked inflammatory changes or perilesional edema may appear as wall thickening and thus misdiagnosed.

MRI is helpful in evaluating the extraserosal invasion of gastric cancer based on the irregular changes in low-signal-intensity bands at the fat–water interface, unlike CT, in which extraserosal invasion may be difficult to visualize due to interference by partial volume-averaging effects or associated perigastric inflammation.

However, MRI tends to underestimate the involvement of lymph nodes, and the accuracy of N staging is only 52–65%, inferior to that achieved with CT or EUS [25-27]. The low detection rate is due not only to frequent microscopic nodal invasion but also to reactive-inflammatory nodal enlargement. The use of lymph-node selective contrast agents reportedly improves the N staging accuracy of MRI [26].

Contrast-enhanced MRI is very helpful in detecting liver metastases and in defining suspected malignant hepatic lesions diagnosed by other imaging procedures.

7.6 Laparoscopy

A key aspect of tumor staging in patients with gastric cancer is staging laparoscopy. Important studies have demonstrated the efficacy of laparoscopy as a highly accurate technique in the detection of occult metastases, thereby avoiding unnecessary laparotomies in a significant number of patients [28-33].

Compared to CT, laparoscopy can show serosal malignant involvement, lymph node enlargement, small surface liver metastases, and small peritoneal lesions, even those < 5 mm. The sensitivity and specificity of videoscopy for gastric cancer are, respectively, 90% and 86% for stage II and 94.5% and 100% for stage III [28, 30, 31, 33]. Indeed, diagnostic laparoscopy obviates the need for surgical procedures in up to 67% of advanced gastric cancer patients, in whom radical surgery cannot be performed.

Videoscopy is also very important in re-staging an initially unresectable gastric cancer after neoadjuvant therapy, in order to evaluate tumor response and thus the feasibility of surgery.

During laparoscopy, peritoneal liquid can be withdrawn for cytological examination, either ex tempore or later. Positive malignant cytology is a contraindication of curative resection and could indicate the need for neoadjuvant chemotherapy or merely supportive care. The Japanese classification considers gastric cancer with positive peritoneal cytology as stage IV disease, i.e., not surgically resectable.

In addition, ultrasonography can be performed at the same time as the laparoscopy. This is of interest because diagnostic laparoscopy is limited in the assessment of retroperitoneal structures and lymph node involvement whereas laparoscopic ultrasound provides clear information regarding liver metastases, lymph node involvement, and local extension of the primary gastric cancer.

References

1. Biondi A, Persiani R, Cananzi F et al (2010) R0 resection in the treatment of gastric cancer: room for improvement. World J Gastroenterol 16:3358-3370
2. Kwee RM, Kwee TC (2007) Imaging in local staging of gastric cancer: a systematic review. J Clin Oncol 25:2107-2116
3. Chen CH, Yang CC, Yeh YH (2002) Preoperative staging of gastric cancer by endoscopic ultrasound: the prognostic usefulness of ascites detected by endoscopic ultrasound. J Clin Gastroenterol 35:321-327
4. Godfrey EM, Rushbrook SM, Carroll NR (2010) Endoscopic ultrasound: a review of current diagnostic and therapeutic applications. Postgrad Med J 86:346-353
5. Tsendsuren T, Jun SM, Mian XH (2006) Usefulness of endoscopic ultrasonography in preoperative TNM staging of gastric cancer. World J Gastroenterol 12:43-47
6. Tsujimoto H, Sugasawa H, Ono S et al (2010) Has the accuracy of preoperative diagnosis improved in cases of early-stage gastric cancer? World J Surg 34:1840-1846
7. Kim JH, Eun HW, Goo DE et al (2006) Imaging of various gastric lesions with 2D MPR and CT gastrography performed with multidetector CT. Radiographics 26:1101-1116; discussion 1117-1118
8. Yanai H, Noguchi T, Mizumachi S et al (1999) A blind comparison of the effectiveness of endoscopic ultrasonography and endoscopy in staging early gastric cancer. Gut 44:361-365
9. Akahoshi K, Chijiwa Y, Hamada S et al (1998) Pretreatment staging of endoscopically early gastric cancer with a 15 MHz ultrasound catheter probe. Gastrointest Endosc 48:470-476
10. Ohashi S, Segawa K, Okamura S et al (1999) The utility of endoscopic ultrasonography and endoscopy in the endoscopic mucosal resection of early gastric cancer. Gut 45:599-604
11. Yoshida S, Tanaka S, Kunihiro K et al (2005) Diagnostic ability of high-frequency ultrasound probe sonography in staging early gastric cancer, especially for submucosal invasion. Abdom Imaging 30:518-523
12. Kim AY, Kim HJ, Ha HK (2005) Gastric cancer by multidetector row CT: preoperative staging. Abdom Imaging 30:465-472
13. Pan Z, Zhang H, Yan C et al (2009) Determining gastric cancer resectability by dynamic MDCT. Eur Radiol 20:613-620
14. Lakadamyali H, Oto A, Akmangit I et al (2003) The role of spiral CT in the preoperative evaluation of malignant gastric neoplasms. Tani Girisim Radyol 9:345-353
15. Lee IJ, Lee JM, Kim SH et al (2009) Helical CT evaluation of the preoperative staging of gastric cancer in the remnant stomach. AJR Am J Roentgenol 192:902-908
16. Chen CY, Hsu JS, Wu DC et al (2007) Gastric cancer: preoperative local staging with 3D multi-detector row CT–correlation with surgical and histopathologic results. Radiology 242:472-482
17. Bilici A, Ustaalioglu BB, Seker M et al (2011) The role of (18)F-FDG PET/CT in the assessment of suspected recurrent gastric cancer after initial surgical resection: can the results of FDG PET/CT influence patients' treatment decision making? Eur J Nucl Med Mol Imaging 38:64-73
18. Sun L, Wan Y, Lin Q et al (2011) Multiple primary malignant tumors of upper gastrointestinal tract: a novel role of 18F-FDG PET/CT. World J Gastroenterol 16:3964-9
19. Kim EY, Lee WJ, Choi D et al (2010) The value of PET/CT for preoperative staging of advanced gastric cancer: Comparison with contrast-enhanced CT. Eur J Radiol Mar 10 [Epub ahead of print]
20. Nakamoto Y, Togashi K, Kaneta T et al (2009) Clinical value of whole-body FDG-PET for recurrent gastric cancer: a multicenter study. Jpn J Clin Oncol 39:297-302
21. Sim SH, Kim YJ, Oh DY et al (2009) The role of PET/CT in detection of gastric cancer recurrence. BMC Cancer 9:73
22. Dassen AE, Lips DJ, Hoekstra CJ et al (2009) FDG-PET has no definite role in preoperative imaging in gastric cancer. Eur J Surg Oncol 35:449-455
23. Gananadha S, Hazebroek EJ, Leibman S et al (2008) The utility of FDG-PET in the preoperative staging of esophageal cancer. Dis Esophagus 21:389-394
24. Sun L, Su XH, Guan YS et al (2008) Clinical role of 18F-fluorodeoxyglucose positron emission tomography/computed tomography in post-operative follow up of gastric cancer: initial results. World J Gastroenterol 14:4627-4632
25. Kim IY, Kim SW, Shin HC et al (2009) MRI of gastric carcinoma: results of T and N-staging in an in vitro study. World J Gastroenterol 15:3992-3998
26. Tokuhara T, Tanigawa N, Matsuki M et al (2008) Evaluation of lymph node metastases in gastric cancer using magnetic resonance imaging with ultrasmall superparamagnetic iron oxide (USPIO): diagnostic performance in post-contrast images using new diagnostic criteria. Gastric Cancer 11:194-200
27. Wu JG, Fang GE, Luo TH et al (2008) Value of dynamic subtraction technique of magnetic resonance imaging in pre-

operative TNM-staging assessment of gastric carcinoma 11:533-536
28. Hur H, Lee HH, Jung H et al (2010) Predicting factors of unexpected peritoneal seeding in locally advanced gastric cancer: Indications for staging laparoscopy. J Surg Oncol 102:753-757
29. Togonel RD, Muntean V, Fabian O (2010) The role of laparoscopic peritoneal cytology in the diagnosis and treatment of gastric cancer. Chirurgia (Bucur) 105:113-117
30. Shimizu H, Imamura H, Ohta K et al (2010) Usefulness of staging laparoscopy for advanced gastric cancer. Surg Today 40:119-224
31. Muntean V, Mihailov A, Iancu C et al (2009) Staging laparoscopy in gastric cancer. Accuracy and impact on therapy. J Gastrointestin Liver Dis 18:189-195
32. Fagotti A, Ferrandina G, Fanfani F et al (2008) Prospective validation of a laparoscopic predictive model for optimal cytoreduction in advanced ovarian carcinoma. Am J Obstet Gynecol 199:642-646
33. Roviaro GC, Varoli F, Sonnino D et al (2000) Can routine laparoscopy help to reduce the rate of explorative laparotomies for gastric cancer? Diagn Ther Endosc 6:125-131

Resection Margins in Gastric Cancer

8

Paolo Morgagni, Giuliano La Barba, and Luca Saragoni

Abstract

The margins of the surgically resected gastric specimen are distinguished as proximal and distal, while deep and lateral margins are determined only after endoscopic resection. Several clinicopathological features of the tumor have been reported as risk factors for resection margin involvement. The most important of these is poorly differentiated carcinoma, large size of the tumor (minimum diameter > 5 cm), and macroscopic Borrmann's type III or IV. The diffusion of the disease is related to the primary tumor site and differences exist between the esophageal and duodenal margins. In the resected specimen, the distance from the tumor and the resection margins must always be checked by the surgeon, and frozen sections are required when infiltration is suspected. When the resection margins are infiltrated, patients must be re-treated to achieve radical resection whenever possible, except in cases of very advanced cancer. Based on the good prognosis of some early gastric cancers, age and associated diseases also must be taken into consideration before proposing a second treatment in these patients.

Keywords

Resection margins • Frozen sections • Palliative surgery • Prognosis

8.1 Background

Residual disease at the resection margins (RMs) is reported to adversely affect survival in gastric cancer patients. For this reason, particular attention should be paid by surgeons and pathologists, who must provide specific information regarding these margins [1-4]. The margins of the surgically resected gastric specimen are referred to as proximal and distal, while deep and lateral margins are determined only after endoscopic resection.

According to the UICC/AJCC criteria, R0 (curative resection) is defined as en bloc resection of the primary tumor without microscopic or macroscopic residual disease, and R1 resection as microscopic residual disease after surgery. R2 resection is used in the presence of macroscopic infiltration [5].

Several clinicopathological features of the tumor have been reported as risk factors for RM involvement. The most important of these is poor-

P. Morgagni (✉)
Dept. of General Surgery,
"G.B. Morgagni – L. Pierantoni" Hospital,
Forlì, Italy

ly differentiated carcinoma or mucin-producing gastric cancer, such as signet-ring cell cancer and mucinous adenocarcinoma. These kinds of cancers, even at an early stage, have a tendency to be larger and to spread superficially to the mucosal and submucosal layers, with a higher rate of RM invasion [6, 7]. Furthermore, large tumors (minimum diameter > 5 cm) [8] and those judged to be macroscopic Borrmann's type III or IV have a predisposition for positive margins. It has also been observed that cancers with deep invasion at stage III or IV are often associated with Borrmann's type III or IV and more undifferentiated tumor types. Such cancers are significantly correlated with positive margins [9, 10].

As far as the diffusion of the disease in relation to the primary tumor site is concerned, differences exist between the esophageal and the duodenal margin. Some authors have described, albeit infrequently, a lymphatic submucosal diffusion of as much as 8 cm from the cardia cancer margin into the esophagus [11]. Some authors consider a tumor-free margin of at least 2 cm as safe in well-defined tumor types, but if tumor margins are not well defined then as much of the esophagus as possible should be resected, with a tumor-free distance of at least 4 cm considered sufficient [12]. In the event of esophageal lymphatic involvement, proximal disease-free margins are more difficult to achieve without thoracic access.

Duodenal margins pose different problems. Duodenal Brunner's glands and dense connective fibers in the subepithelial mucosal layer seem to act as a protective barrier against cancer invasion. However, duodenal invasion, when present, is often a result of infiltration through the submucosal and subserosal layers. Although Kakeji et al. reported that 76% of patients with duodenal invasion had transpyloric extension limited to < 2 cm, 4-cm invasion has also been described [13]. In such patients, radical resection cannot generally be performed.

All these aspects of tumor distance from the resection margins must be taken into account to reduce the risk of submucosal skip metastases after an area of normal tissue. Such metastases can only be suspected and confirmed after histologic examination of the RMs.

8.2 Treatment Options

Infiltrated RMs detected after an endoscopic dissection require a new round of treatment, for which different options have been described. If the criteria for endoscopic resection are satisfied but the deep margin is involved, surgical resection is generally proposed. If the lateral margins are infiltrated, a new round of endoscopic treatment associated with follow-up may be an option.

The problems associated with surgery, widely accepted as the gold standard for first-line treatment of gastric cancer, are different. The incidence of a positive RM in surgically treated gastric cancer patients varies widely, ranging between 0.8 and 20% of cases.

To reduce problems that arise due to infiltrated RMs, after gastric resection the stomach is opened along the greater curvature and examined from the mucosal side. The tumor size and its distance from the surgical margins are measured, with intrasurgical frozen sections always obtained when infiltration is suspected. This precaution, however, may not be sufficient to exclude cancer infiltration. Some authors have reported an incidence of false-negative intrasurgical histopathologic diagnoses in about 21% of cases.

One of the problems that can lead to an incorrect intrasurgical diagnosis is the presence of a histologically diffuse type of tumor according to Lauren's classification. In these cases, a rapid immunostaining procedure is required to avoid false-negative intrasurgical results [14].

The presence of RM involvement has consistently been reported to adversely affect prognosis [2-4,9-13, 15]. However, when the involvement is associated with limited lymphatic dissection (D0, D1), the primary tumor may be understaged and the prognostic impact of the infiltrated RMs difficult to assess. Conversely, the prognostic impact of positive margins is better defined in patients who undergo surgery with radical intent. Large-series studies have reported that the survival rate of patients with positive RMs was significantly poorer than that of patients with negative margins, especially when lower tumor stages were considered. For patients with very advanced cancer and/or node-positive disease, survival was not significantly affected by RM involvement and most of these patients died from peritoneal recurrence or distant metastases [2, 9, 10, 15].

If the presence of a positive margin after macroscopic radical resection of advanced cancer (T2-T3-T4a) without nodal involvment (N0) generally indicates the need for surgical retreatment, when technically feasible and when radical resection can be achieved, there is no general consensus regarding patients with lymphatic involvement or early lesions.

Literature sources indicate that the decision to re-treat is sometimes based on the extension of lymph node diffusion, especially when infiltration is limited to N1–2 lymphatic stage [9, 15]. A particular condition is that of early gastric cancer: while some studies have reported poorer survival especially in N0 patients with RM involvement [2, 16], others have described 100% 5-year survival in the absence of re-intervention for these patients [17, 18]. For these patients, re-treatment is a difficult decision and age or associated diseases must be taken into consideration.

In conclusion, there are no absolute indications that guide decision-making in re-treatment. The distance between the tumor and the resection margins must always be defined, considering the tumor's pathological characteristics, and frozen sections must be obtained when infiltration is suspected. When RMs are infiltrated, patients must be re-treated to achieve radical resection whenever possible, except in very advanced cancer. Based on the good prognosis reported by some studies for early gastric cancers, age and associated diseases must additionally be taken into consideration in these patients.

References

1. Cunningham SC, Kamangar F, Kim MP et al (2005) Survival after gastric adenocarcinoma resection: eighteen-year experience at a single institution. J Gastrointest Surg 9:718–725
2. Cho BC, Jeung HC, Choi HJ et al (2007) Prognostic impact of resection margin involvement advanced gastric cancer: a 15-year experience at a single institute. J Surg Oncol 95:461–468
3. De Gara CJ, Hanson J, Hamilton S (2003) A population-based study of tumor-node relationship, resection margins, and surgeon volume on gastric cancer survival. Am J Surg 186:23-27
4. Kim SH, Karpeh MS, Klimstra DS et al (1999) Effect of microscopic resection line disease on gastric cancer survival. J Gastrointest Surg 3:24-33
5. Sobin LH, Wittekind CH (2002) TNM classification of malignant tumor, 6th edn. Wiley, New York
6. Park JM, Jang YJ, Kim JH et al (2008) Gastric cancer histology: clinicopathologic characteristics and prognostic value. J Surg Oncol 98:520-525
7. Piessen G, PhD, Messager M, Leteurtre E et al (2009) Signet ring cell histology is an indipendent predictor of poor prognosis in gastric adenocarcinoma regardless of tumoral clinical presentation. Ann Surg 250:878-887
8. Yokota T, Sawai K, Yamaguchi T et al (1993) Resection margin in patients with gastric cancer associated with esophageal invasion: clinicopathological study. J Surg Oncol 53:60-63
9. Zhe S, De-ming L, Zhen-ning W et al (2009) Prognostic significance of microscopic positive margins for gastric cancer patients with potentially curative resection. Ann Surg Oncol 16:3028-3037
10. Shang-Yu W, Chun-Nan Y, Hsiang-Lin L et al (2009) Clinical Impact of positive surgical margin status on gastric cancer patients undergoing gastrectomy. Surg Oncol 16:2738-2743
11. Bozzetti F, Bonfanti G, Bufalino R et al (1982) Adequacy of margins of resection in gastrectomy for cancer. Ann Surg 196:685–690
12. Tsujitani S, Okuyama T, Orita H et al (1995) Margins of resection of the esophagous for gastric cancer with esophageal invasion. Hepatogastroenterology 42:873-877
13. Kakeji Y, Tsujitani S, Baba H et al (1991) Clinicopathologic features and prognostic significance of duodenal invasion in patients with distal gastric carcinoma. Cancer 68:380-384
14. Yokota T, Yamaguchi T, Sawai K et al (1989) Intraoperative immunostaining for detection of invasive cells at the resection margin of Borrmann type 4 gastric carcinoma using monoclonal antibody S202. Br J Surg 76:690-692
15. Morgagni P, Garcea D, Marrelli D et al (2008) Resection line involvement after gastric cancer surgery: clinical outcome in nonsurgically retreated patients. World J Surg 32:2661-2667
16. Cascinu S, Giordani P, Catalano V et al (1999) Resection line involvement in gastric cancer patients undergoing curative resections: Implication for clinical management. Jpn J Clin Oncol 29:291-293
17. Morgagni P, Garcea D, Marrelli D et al (2006) Does resection line involvement affect prognosis in early gastric cancer patients? An Italian multicentric study. World J Surg 30:585-589
18. Nakamura K, Ueyama T, Yao T et al (1992) Pathology and prognosis of gastric cancer: Findings in 10,000 patients who underwent primary gastrectomy. Cancer 70:1030-1037

Gastric Cancer: Standard or Extended Lymphadenectomy?

9

Giovanni de Manzoni, Alberto Di Leo, and Giuseppe Verlato

Abstract

Gastrectomy with extended (D2) lymphadenectomy is the standard surgical approach not only in advanced gastric cancer but also in submucosal early gastric cancer. D2 lymphadenectomy can improve the survival of patients with gastric cancer, but it requires surgical expertise to keep post-operative morbidity and mortality at low levels. The Japanese Clinical Oncology Group (JCOG) trial showed that extension of lymphadenectomy to para-aortic nodes does not improve the survival of patients with advanced gastric cancer. Nevertheless, whether para-aortic node dissection is of benefit in selected groups of patients remains a matter of debate, since the 5-year survival of patients with metastases to para-aortic nodes is not negligible.

Keywords

Limited (D1) lymphadenectomy • Extended (D2) lymphadenectomy • Superextended (D3) lymphadenectomy • Dutch trial • British trial • Taiwanese single-institution trial • Para-aortic nodal dissection (PAND)

9.1 Standard or Extended Lymphadenectomy?

Few diseases have varied as greatly in therapeutic approach as gastric cancer. Indeed, the largest expertise in gastric cancer surgery has been achieved by Japanese surgeons, mainly because the incidence of the disease is particularly high in Japan, with about 100,000 new cases per year [1]. During the 1970s and 1980s, Japanese surgeons developed an aggressive strategy to prevent lymphatic spread of the tumor, based on extended (D2) and superextended (D3) lymphadenectomy [2-4]. At the same time, the most widely used intervention in Europe and the USA was a limited (D1) lymphadenectomy.

Thus, a scientific conflict arose. On the one hand, overall 5-year survival achieved the impressive value of 74% in Japanese gastric cancer patients [5] whereas in Europe during the 1990s survival was three-fold lower (24%) [6]. On the other, Japanese surgery, in spite of these outstanding achievements, was not considered the benchmark either in the USA or in Northern Europe, i.e., in those countries considered as the scientific leaders in medicine. Western surgeons and scientists argued that the Japanese results came from retrospective observational studies and attributed the good prognosis recorded in those series to the benign biological behavior of gastric cancer in Japan [7].

G. de Manzoni (✉)
Dept. of Surgery,
Upper G.I. Surgery Division,
University of Verona,
Verona, Italy

G. de Manzoni, F. Roviello, W. Siquini (eds.), *Surgery in the Multimodal Management of Gastric Cancer*,

During the 1990s, a huge effort was made to base the surgical approach to gastric cancer on sound evidence. Dutch [8] and British [9] surgeons organized large trials in which patients were randomly assigned to either D1 or D2 lymphadenectomy. However, the latter trials, despite the recruitment of a large number of patients, were of rather low surgical quality, as they were carried out by surgeons who lacked previous training in extended lymphadenectomy, performing less than five interventions per year. The limited surgical experience yielded a very high post-operative mortality after extended lymphadenectomy (9.7% in the Dutch trial and 13.5% in the British trial) as well as a high percentage of splenectomies (37% and 65%, respectively) and pancreatectomies (30% and 56%) and a low number of nodes retrieved (median of 17 nodes in the British trial) [10]. By comparison, at the same time, mortality after D2 dissection was < 2% in the nationwide Japanese registry [11] and < 1% in specialized institutions [12] and the median number of retrieved nodes was 54 [12].

After 5 years of follow-up, these studies showed no evidence of overall survival benefit after extended lymphadenectomy [13, 14], but the comparison was likely biased by the poor surgical performance in the D2 group [15]. In the Dutch trial, a moderate survival advantage tended to emerge in patients undergoing extended lymphadenectomy after longer follow-up: indeed, 15-year overall survival was 29% after D2 and 21% after D1 ($p = 0.34$) [16]. D2 lymphadenectomy was associated with a decrease in gastric-cancer-related mortality (37% vs. 48%), Interestingly, the difference in overall survival became significant after excluding patients undergoing pancreatico-splenectomy (35% in D2 vs. 22% in D1, p = 0.006) [16, 17].

In the meantime, another randomized trial, performed in Taiwan [18], showed a mild but significant survival advantage after D2 compared to D1; 5-year survival was 59.5% vs. 53.6%, respectively (p=0.041).

A re-evaluation of these trials was reported in a paper recently published in the New England Journal of Medicine, whose first author was Sasako, the Japanese surgeon who supervised the Dutch trial: "The excessive number of early deaths in these studies (Dutch and British trials) may have obscured any potential difference in long-term survival between patients undergoing D1 and D2 gastrectomy." In the Dutch trial "the limited experience of the surgeons made it difficult for them to learn how to perform the procedure safely and effectively, and the small volume of cases limited the ability of the hospitals to manage major surgical complications. By contrast, in a Taiwanese single-institution trial comparing D1 gastrectomy with D2 or more extensive gastrectomy, all the sur-

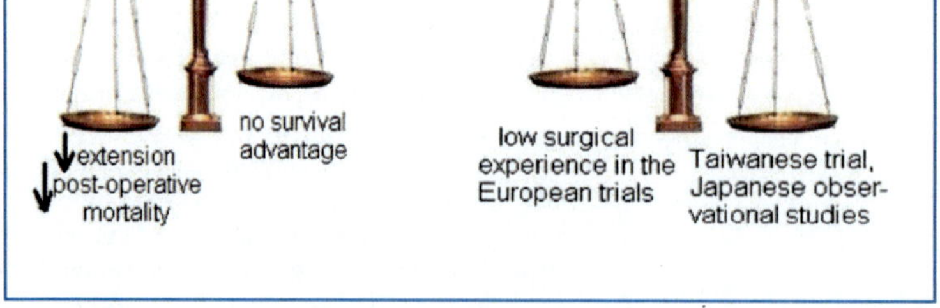

Fig. 9.1 Relative balance between standard (*D1*) and extended (*D2*) lymphadenectomy at the end of the 1990s (*left*) and in 2010 (*right*)

geons had performed at least 80 D2 procedures before participating in the study, and there were no deaths in either group" [19].

In addition, several studies [20-22] showed that D2 lymphadenectomy is necessary to harvest at least 15 lymph nodes, i.e., an adequate number for accurate pathologic tumor staging.

Thus, the balance between D2 and D1 lymphadenectomy has shifted in favor of D2 (Fig. 9.1). Nowadays, gastrectomy with D2 lymphadenectomy is not only the standard of care for advanced curable gastric cancer according to the Japanese Guideline (2004) [23] but it is also recommended by the European Union Network of Excellence for Gastric Cancer (II EUNE Gastric Cancer International Workshop, Madrid, March 2010).

9.2 Surgical Quality of Lymphadenectomy: Post-operative Morbidity and Mortality, and Number of Retrieved Nodes

An implicit message, provided by the debate over the appropriate extension of lymphadenectomy in gastric cancer surgery is that D2 lymphadenectomy can improve prognosis only if an acceptable surgical quality is achieved.

As already mentioned, post-operative mortality after extended lymphadenectomy (D2) varies widely across the world: it is as low as 0.8% [12, 24] or even absent [25] in randomized trials from East Asia, and < 2% in the Japanese nationwide registry [11], but increases to 2–5% in Western observational studies [21, 26-30] or phase II trials (3.1%) [31], and is as high as 5–13% in European clinical trials [8, 9, 32].

Similar differences were observed regarding post-operative morbidity after extended lymphadenectomy, which was again the lowest (17–21%) in East Asian trials [12,25], intermediate (21–35%) in European observational studies [21, 28-30] or phase II trials [31], and highest in European phase III trials (43–46%) [8, 9].

The number of excised lymph node also varies widely. Indeed, while the number of nodes removed by D1 lymphadenectomy remained rather constant, around a median value of 12–13 [9, 21, 28], the median number harvested by D2 lymphadenectomy ranged from 17 in a European trial [9] to 54 in a Japanese trial [12], with 25–26 in Western observational studies [21, 28]. Accordingly, after D2 dissection, the proportion of patients with a sufficient number of excised nodes for adequate staging, i.e., at least 15, varied from to 86% [21] to 95% [28] in Western observational studies, but included virtually all patients in a Japanese trial [12].

Recently, the following indexes of surgical quality have been proposed for gastric cancer surgery: number of retrieved nodes, avoidance of concomitant spleno-pancreatectomy, and post-operative morbidity and mortality [22]. The results achieved in a GIRCG series comprising 1032 patients are shown in Table 9.1 and in Fig. 9.2 [22].

Hence, while acknowledging that the achievements of Japanese surgery are still beyond the possibilities of most European surgeons, the results of the above-mentioned paper could be assumed as a benchmark for European surgeons.

Table 9.1 Indexes of surgical quality in a GIRCG series of 1032 patients, according to the extension of lymphadenectomy (from [22])

	D1	D2	D3
N. of retrieved nodes Median (interquartile range)	14 (9-18.75)	29 (21-38)	46.5 (37-57)
Splenectomy	6.1	10.1	11.4
Spleno-pancreatectomy	1.8	2.4	11.4
Surgical complications	18.4	19.2	21.4
Non-surgical complications	11.0	16.3	11.8
Post-operative mortality	5.7	3.6	2.7

Adjacent organ removal, post-operative morbidity and mortality are reported as percentage, and the number of retrieved nodes as median (interquartile range).

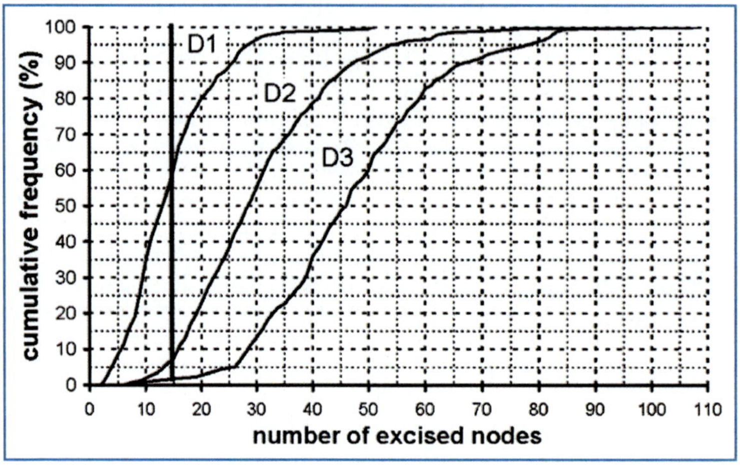

Fig. 9.2 Cumulative distribution of the number of excised nodes according to extension of lymphadenectomy. The gray area represents inadequate staging, i.e., < 15 nodes retrieved by the pathologist. (Modified from [22], with permission)

9.2 And What About Superextended Lymphadenectomy?

The final lymph node station of gastric lymphatic drainage is station 16, the para-aortic lymph nodes. Once metastatic cells manage to surpass this point, they reach the lymphatic duct and the bloodstream.

Metastases to these nodes are already considered distant metastases (M1) by the TNM classification [33]. Nevertheless, para-aortic nodal dissection (PAND) has been practiced since the late 1980s in specialized Japanese and Western centers, with the unproven hope of improving the survival of patients with advanced gastric cancer. Excellent surgical expertise was achieved in this procedure, as endorsed by the rather low rate of operative complications and hospital deaths. In Japan, morbidity after D2 lymphadenectomy + PAND ranges from 28% to 38% and mortality is < 1% [19, 24]. Western specialized centers have managed to achieve similar results, with a morbidity and mortality ranging from 21% to 35% and 1% to 4%, respectively [22, 29, 34, 35].

However, a recent randomized controlled trial, organized by the Japan Clinical Oncology Group (JCOG), showed that extending lymphadenectomy to para-aortic nodes does not improve survival in T2b, T3, and T4 gastric cancer [19]. Consequently, D2 + PAND is no longer indicated as a first-choice treatment in patients with curable gastric cancer according to Japanese guidelines.

Nevertheless, the latter study does not completely exclude the possibility that superextended lymphadenectomy could be of benefit in selected groups of patients with advanced gastric cancer [36, 37]. Indeed, in the JCOG trial, patients with macroscopic metastases to station 16 lymph nodes were excluded, leading to a low incidence of nodal metastases at this site in patients who underwent D2 + PAND (8.5%: 22 out of 259). Moreover, some results were unexpected, such as the paradoxical better survival rates registered among patients with histologically negative nodes assigned to D2 + PAND (96.8%) than in those assigned to D2 alone (78.4%).

In addition, it must be pointed out that survival in patients with metastases to para-aortic nodes is not negligible: 5-year survival in these patients was rather high both in the JCOG trial (18%) [19] and in a series of the Italian Research Group on Gastric Cancer (17.1%) [36]. Median survival in the Italian series was 19.4 (95% CI 15.6–23.2) months.

9.3 Conclusions

Hence, what can we suggest for the sake of our patients? In a recent international meeting, held in March 2010 in Madrid, the EUNE for Gastric

Cancer defined D2 gastrectomy as the standard surgical approach not only in advanced gastric cancer but also in early types with submucosal invasion. Whenever it is not possible to pre-operatively differentiate between mucosal and submucosal early gastric cancer, the preferred surgical approach should be D2 lymph node dissection.

The debate on para-aortic node dissection has yet to reach its conclusion. In some GIRCG centers, as further studies on the usefulness of this procedure are awaited, D2 + PAND is still performed in patients with a high risk of metastases to station 16 nodes, with risk defined according to cancer site, depth of tumor invasion, histology, and perigastric nodal status [38].

References

1. The Research Group for Population-based Cancer Registration in Japan (2004) Cancer incidence and incidence rates in Japan in 1999: Estimates based on data from 11 population-based cancer registries. Jpn J Clin Oncol 34:352-356
2. Maeta M, Yamashiro H, Saito H et al (1999) A prospective pilot study of extended (D3) and superxtended para-aortic lymphadenectomy (D4) in patients with T3 or T4 gastric cancer managed by total gastrectomy. Surgery 125:325-331
3. Kunisaki C, Shimada H, Yamaoka H et al (2000) Indications for paraortic lymph node dissection in gastric cancer patients with paraortic lymph node involvement. Hepatogastroenterology 47:586-589
4. Gunji Y, Suzuki T, Kobayashi S et al (2003) Evaluation of D3/D4 lymph node dissection for patients with grossly N2 positive advanced gastric cancer. Hepatogastroenterology 50:1178-1182
5. Nakajima T (2002) Gastric cancer treatment guidelines. Gastric Cancer 5:1-5
6. Berrino F, De Angelis R, Sant M et al (2007) Survival for eight major cancers and all cancers combined for European adults diagnosed in 1995-99: results of the EUROCARE-4 study. Lancet Oncol 8:773-783
7. Jatzko G, Pertl A, Jagoditsch M (1999) Chirurgische Therapie und Ergebnisse beim Magenfrühkarzinom. Chir Gastroenterol 15:223-226
8. Bonenkamp JJ, Songun I, Hermans J et al (1995) Randomised comparison of morbidity after D1 and D2 dissection for gastric cancer in 996 Dutch patients. Lancet 345:745-748
9. Cuschieri A, Fayers P, Fielding J et al (1996) Postoperative morbidity and mortality after D1 and D2 resections for gastric cancer: preliminary results of the MRC randomised controlled surgical trial. Lancet 347:995-999
10. Guadagni S, Catarci M, de Manzoni G, Kinoshita T (1995) D1 versus D2 dissection for gastric cancer (letter). Lancet 345:1517
11. Fujii M, Sasaki J, Nakajima T (1999) State of the art in the treatment of gastric cancer: From the 71st Japanese Gastric Cancer Congress. Gastric Cancer 2:151-157
12. Sano T, Sasako M, Yamamoto S et al (2004) Gastric Cancer Surgery: Morbidity and mortality results from a prospective randomized controlled trial comparing D2 and extended para-aortic lymphadenectomy – Japan Clinical Oncology Group Study 9501. J Clin Oncol 22:2767-2773
13. Bonenkamp JJ, Hermans J, Sasako M, van de Velde CJH, for the Dutch Gastric Cancer Group (1999) Extended lymph node dissection for gastric cancer. N Engl J Med 340:908-914
14. Cuschieri A, Weeden S, Fielding J et al, for the Surgical Co-operative Group (1999) Patients survival after D1 and D2 resections for gastric cancer: long term results of the MRC surgical trial. Br J Cancer 79:1522-1530
15. de Manzoni G, Verlato G (2005) Gastrectomy with extended lymphadenectomy for primary treatment of gastric cancer (letter). Br J Surg, 92:784
16. Songun I, Putter H, Meershoek-Klein Kranenbarg E et al (2010) Surgical treatment of gastric cancer: 15-year follow-up results of the randomised nationwide Dutch D1D2 trial. Lancet Oncol 11:439-449
17. Hartgrink HH, van de Velde CJH, Putter H et al (2004) Extended lymph node dissection for gastric cancer: who may benefit? Final results of the randomized Dutch Gastric Cancer Group trial. J Clin Oncol 22: 2041-2042
18. Wu C, Hsiung C, Lo S et al (2006) Nodal dissection for patients with gastric cancer: a randomised controlled trial. Lancet Oncol 7:309-315
19. Sasako M, Sano T, Yamamoto S et al, for the Japan Clinical Oncology Group (2008) D2 lymphadenectomy alone or with para-aortic nodal dissection for gastric cancer. N Engl J Med 359:453-462
20. de Manzoni G, Verlato G, Roviello F et al, for the Italian Research Group for Gastric Cancer (2002) The new TNM classification of lymph node metastasis minimizes stage migration problems in gastric cancer patients. Br J Cancer 87:171-174
21. Smith BR, Stabile BE (2006) Aggressive D2 lymphadenectomy is required for accurate pathologic staging of gastric adenocarcinoma. Am Surgeon 72:849-852
22. Verlato G, Roviello F, Marchet A et al (2009) Indexes of surgical quality in gastric cancer surgery: experience of an Italian network. Ann Surg Oncol 16:594-602
23. Japanese Gastric Cancer Association (2004) Gastric cancer treatment guideline, 2nd edn. Kanehara, Tokyo
24. Yonemura Y, Wu CC, Fukushima N et al, for the East Asia Surgical Oncology Group (2006) Operative morbidity and mortality after D2 and D4 extended dissection for advanced gastric cancer: A prospective Randomized trial conducted by Asian surgeons. Hepatogastroenterology 53:389-394
25. Wu CW, Hsiung CA, Lo SS et al (2004) Randomized clinical trial of morbidity after D1 and D3 surgery for gastric cancer. Br J Surg 91:283-287
26. Pacelli F, Doglietto GB, Bellantone R et al (1993) Extensive versus limited lymph node dissection for gastric cancer: a comparative study of 320 patients. Br J Surg 80:1153-1156
27. Siewert JR, Bottcher K, Roder JD et al (1993) Prognostic relevance of systematic lymph node dissection in gastric carcinoma. Br J Surg 80:1015-1018

28. de Manzoni G, Verlato G, Guglielmi A et al (1996) Prognostic significance of lymph node dissection in gastric cancer. Br J Surg 83:1604-1607
29. Marrelli D, Pedrazzani C, Neri A et al (2007) Complications after extended (D2) and superextended (D3) lymphadenectomy for gastric cancer: Analysis of potential risk factors. Ann Surg Oncol 14:25-33
30. Danielson H, Kokkola A, Kiviluoto T et al (2007) Clinical outcome after D1 vs D2-3 gastrectomy for treatment of gastric cancer. Scand J Surg 96:35-40
31. Degiuli M, Sasako M, Ponti A, Calvo F (2004) Survival results of a multicentre phase II study to evaluate D2 gastrectomy for gastric cancer. Br J Cancer 90:1727-1732
32. Kulig J, Popiela T, Kolodziejczyk P et al (2007) Standard D2 versus extended D2 (D+) lymphadenectomy for gastric cancer: an interim safety analysis of a multicenter, randomized, clinical trial. Am J Surg 193:10-15
33. AJCC (American Joint Committee on Cancer) (2010) Cancer staging manual. Springer-Verlag New York, 7th edition, pp. 117-121
34. Günther K, Horbach T, Merkel S et al (2000) D3 lymph node dissection in gastric cancer: evaluation of postoperative mortality and complications. Surg Today 30:700-705
35. Bostanci EB, Kayaalp C, Ozogul Y et al (2004) Comparison of complications after D2 and D3 dissection for gastric cancer. Eur J Surg Oncol 30:20-25
36. Roviello F, Pedrazzani C, Marrelli D et al (2010) Super-extended (D3) lymphadenectomy in advanced gastric cancer. Eur J Surg Oncol 36:439-446
37. Kodera Y (2010) Para-aortic lymph node dissection revisited: Have we been neglecting a promising treatment option for gastric carcinoma? (letter). Eur J Surg Oncol 36:447-448
38. de Manzoni G, Di Leo A, Roviello F et al (2011) Tumor site and perigastric nodal status are the most important predictors of para-aortic nodal involvment in advanced gastric cancer. Ann Surg Oncol 18:2273-2280

Reconstruction After Gastrectomy

10

Francesco Tonelli, Stefano Scaringi, Francesco Giudici, and Francesco Bellucci

Abstract

There are several different techniques for restoring the digestive tract after gastrectomy but the goal in all of them is to obtain effective food intake with a low postoperative morbidity. Three reconstruction techniques are commonly performed after gastric resection: gastro-duodenostomy (Billroth I or Péan reconstruction), gastro-jejunostomy between the remnant stomach and the first jejunal loop (Billroth II), and gastro-jejunostomy with Roux-en-Y reconstruction. A Roux-en-Y reconstruction is the preferred technique after distal gastrectomy because the functional and endoscopic results are better than those achieved with Billroth I or II, while there are no differences in mortality and morbidity. Billroth II is preferred over Billroth I reconstruction because of the latter's low morbidity. It is also suitable for patients with advanced gastric cancer. After total gastrectomy, the following reconstruction techniques are possible: Roux-en-Y with esophago-jejunostomy, jejunal interposition (Longmire's procedure), and reservoir reconstructions. Roux-en-Y reconstruction is the technique of choice rather than jejunal interposition based on its simplicity and the satisfactory nutritional results. Reservoir reconstruction may improve patients' quality of life over the long term and should be discussed with as potentially improving prognosis.

Keywords

Gastrectomy • Gastric cancer • Distal gastrectomy • Total gastrectomy • Roux-en-Y • Billroth • Gastro-jejunostomy • Esophago-jejunostomy • Jejunal interposition • Longmire • Reservoir reconstructions

10.1 Distal Gastric Resection

Different techniques for restoring the digestive tract are possible after gastrectomy [1-3]. In each one, the goal is to obtain an effective food intake with a low postoperative morbidity. After gastric resection three reconstruction techniques are possible: gastro-duodenostomy (Billroth I or Péan

F. Tonelli (✉)
Dept. of Clinical Pathophysiology,
Surgical Unit,
University of Florence
Florence, Italy

reconstruction), gastro-jejunostomy between the remnant stomach and the first jejunal loop (Billroth II), and gastro-jejunostomy with Roux-en-Y reconstruction.

10.1.1 Gastro-duodenostomy (Billroth I or Péan Procedure)

An end-to-end anastomosis, performed manually or mechanically, connects the gastric remnant and the duodenum (Figs. 10.1, 10.2). The advantage of gastro-duodenostomy is that it restores the physiological gastro-duodenal circuit, with the possibility for further endoscopic procedures. Nevertheless, there is a higher risk of anastomotic leak [4].

The key to a successful procedure is correct preparation of the duodenal stump and a tension-free anastomosis. The duodenal stump should be well-vascularized, with careful attention paid to avoid injury to the common bile duct. Kocker's maneuver may be useful for gaining distance between the duodenal stump and gastric remnant. However, gastro-duodenostomy reconstruction is rarely performed after gastrectomy for cancer in Western countries because the required gastric resection (with a proximal margin ≥ 5 cm from the tumor) and lymphatic dissection are usually too extensive, thus compromising the possibility to achieve a well-vascularized, tension-free anastomosis [5]. Notably, the 5-year survival rates is 50% in patients with negative margins (R0 resection), but only 22% in those with involved margins (R1 resection) [6]. Also, the risk is higher in patients with signet-ring cell carcinoma [6, 7]. An additional problem arises from the fact that Billroth I intervention exposes the patient to a higher risk of biliary reflux than is the case with a Roux-en-Y reconstruction [8].

In studies aimed at identifying the technique of choice, there has been only one randomized trial since the year 2000 comparing mechanical with manual gastro-duodenostomy [9]. The study consisted of 374 patients and showed a significant statistical difference only for the duration of the anastomosis procedure (14 vs. 25 min, $p = 0.02$), while there were no differences in the rates of anastomotic fistulas and strictures. Post-operative mortality and morbidity were also similar. No data are available regarding the recurrence rate, and incurred costs have yet to be analyzed. In our institution, the procedure of choice is manual reconstruction.

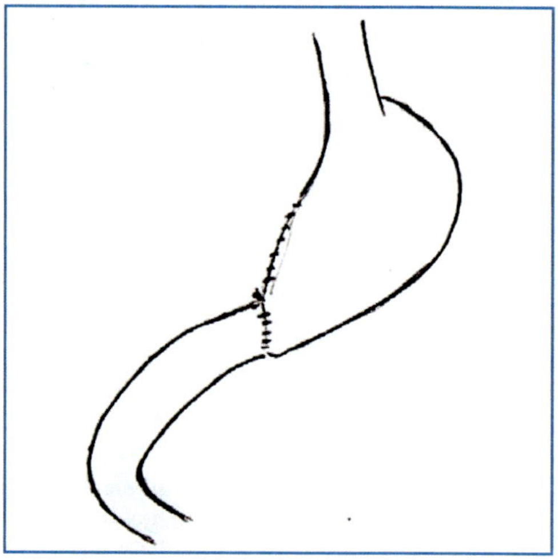

Fig. 10.1 Gastro-duodenal anastomosis: the Billroth I or Péan procedure

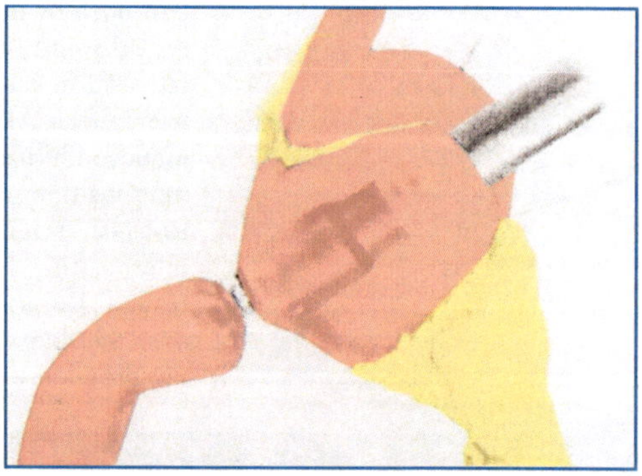

Fig. 10.2 Mechanical gastro-duodenostomy

10.1.2 Gastro-jejunostomy with the First Jejunal Loop (Billroth II Procedure)

A side-to-side anastomosis is made between the gastric remnant and the first jejunal loop. The anastomosis involves either the entire gastric division edge, according to Polya's technique, or a part of the gastric division edge, as described by Finsterer (Fig. 10.3) [10, 11]. In both cases, this reconstruction provides a tension-free anastomosis but there is the likelihood of biliary reflux into the stomach [8]. Also, in both procedures the jejunal loop is placed anisoperistaltically, at 20–30 cm from the angle of Treitz, through the transverse mesocolon, with the afferent loop on the side of the lesser curvature in order to facilitate gastric emptying. With the aim of avoiding biliary reflux, Finsterer recommended performing the anastomosis on the greater curvature side of the gastric remnant, with the jejunal loop placed side-to-side to the closure edge (racket handle), essentially creating a flap. Nevertheless, the advantages of this modification remain theoretical. Conventionally, the anastomosis is hand sewn but mechanical reconstruction using a linear stapler is possible (Fig. 10.4). In this case, careful attention is needed to prevent bleeding. We prefer a double-layer trans-mesocolic gastro-jejunostomy anastomosis according to the Finsterer technique in patients requiring a Billroth II reconstruction. No studies have demonstrated a higher incidence of intestinal obstruction for recurrence after retro-colic reconstruction, while gastric emptying seems to be improved [12].

During the 1970s, the Billroth II rather than the Roux-en-Y reconstruction was the procedure of choice because of the association of the latter with marginal ulcer and emptying problems. Although beginning as early as the 1950s reports suggested a correlation between partial resection for ulcer and gastric stump cancer [13, 14], the surgical approach radically changed only at the end of the 1970s, when more consistent studies were published [15, 16]. Those results showed an association between gastric stump cancer and chronic (20–30 years) biliary reflux. Due to its low rate of complications, Billroth II remains an alternative to Roux-en-Y reconstruction, notably in patients with advanced cancer.

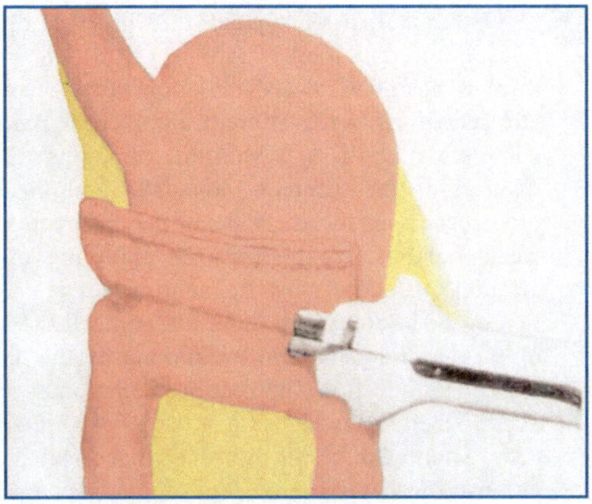

Fig. 10.4 Mechanical gastro-jejunostomy

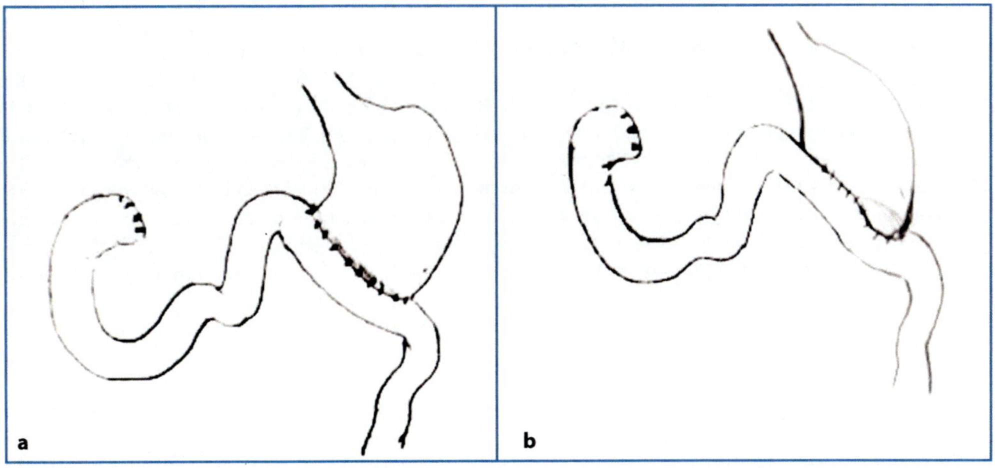

Fig. 10.3 **a** Gastro-jejunostomy or Billroth II reconstruction (Polya's technique); **b** Finsterer modified

One complication typical of Billroth II operations is afferent loop syndrome (ALS), in which there is postprandial accumulation of biliopancreatic secretions in the afferent loop. These patients complain of pain and vomiting. Imaging shows dilation of the afferent loop. The complication often occurs in the early post-operative period (3 weeks) and is due to impaired emptying of the afferent loop. The most frequent causes are: rotation of the afferent loop, internal hernia at the level of the anastomosis, and or kinking at the Treitz angle. In addition, mesocolic hematomas may occur, albeit rarely. Tension at the level of the duodenal stump can result in a duodenal fistula, with potentially catastrophic consequences for the patient. Re-operation is often needed for the treatment of the ALS. The procedure consists of a jejuno-jejunal anastomosis between the afferent and efferent loops (Braun's anastomosis); alternatively, reduction and fixation of the incarcerated loop is possible. ALS can also be a late complication but such cases are difficult to diagnose because the symptomatology is in most cases intermittent. The causes are adhesions, angulations, or torsion involving the afferent loop related to the lenth of it, local recurrence, or weight loss. Surgical treatment consists of conversion to a Roux-en-Y reconstruction. In order to avoid this complication, the surgeon should carefully evaluate the length of the afferent loop, which should typically be 20–30 cm.

10.1.3 Gastro-jejunostomy with Roux-en-Y

After jejunal section at 30–40 cm from the Treitz angle, a side-to-side anastomosis between the distal jejunal stump and the gastric remnant is performed in isoperistaltic position (cul de sac on the greater curvature) through a trans-mesocolic opening. A second jejuno-jejunostomy is realized with the proximal jejunal stump at 60 cm from the gastro-jejunostomy in order to assure bilio-pancreatic transit (Fig. 10.5). The Roux-en-Y prevents biliary reflux. Anastomosis is usually performed manually, but mechanical reconstruction is also possible, either with a circular or a linear stapler. This reconstruction is the same as that performed after total gastrectomy. The results after manual or mechanical anastomosis are similar.

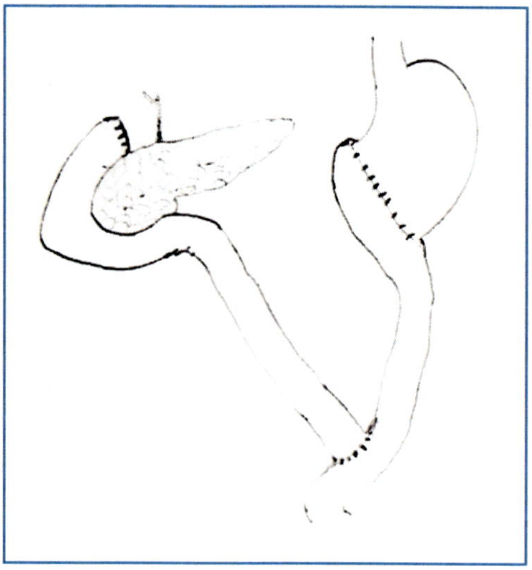

Fig. 10.5 Gastro-jejunal Roux-en-Y reconstruction

Gastric-emptying disorders can occur subsequent to a Roux-en-Y reconstruction (Roux syndrome) [17]. They are usually characterized by gastroparesis and stasis of the alimentary tract in the alimentary limb of the Roux-en-Y [18]. Physiopathological aspects of this disorder include interruption of the pacemaker effect of the duodenum following the jejunal section. Some studies have advocated an ectopic pacemaker in the alimentary limb, with the consequence of reversed motility [19, 20]. Roux syndrome is estimated to occur in 0–10% of patients [21, 22]. Clinically, they complain of post-operative vomiting that in case of a syndrome of old onset is intermittent. Endoscopy usually shows a normal aspect of both the gastric remnant and the anastomosis whereas conventional radiological exams show a dilation of the gastric remnant. The correct diagnosis can often be made by a technetium-labeled-meal scintigram. Treatment is medical, including prokinetics (erythromycin, domperidone, or metoclopramide) but in case of failure surgery is required, specifically, total gastrectomy [23, 24].

There have been many randomized studies comparing gastric reconstruction techniques (Table 10.1), usually Roux-en-Y vs. Billroth I or II reconstruction. Only one study reported a higher morbidity after Roux-en-Y, due to Roux syndrome, while long-term outcome showed better functional and endoscopic results in terms of biliary reflux [21, 22, 25]. No others studies found a statistical difference in post-operative morbidity.

10.2 Total Gastrectomy

After total gastrectomy, three reconstruction techniques are possible: Roux-en-Y with esophago-jejunostomy, jejunal interposition (Longmire's procedure), and reservoir reconstructions.

10.2.1 Roux-en-Y Reconstruction

Described by Roux in 1897, the Roux-en-Y is the simplest and easiest reconstruction after total gastrectomy. The jejunal section, 15–20 cm from the angle of Treitz, is followed by an isoperistaltic end-to-side anastomosis between the esophagus and the distal jejunal stump. A second jejuno-jejunostomy is realized with the proximal jejunal stump, created 60 cm from the esophago-jejunostomy in order to avoid bilio-pancreatic reflux [26] (Fig. 10.6).

The most important technical point is the use of a long and well-vascularized jejunal loop to ensure a tension-free anastomosis. The limb may be brought up through a mesocolic opening or in the pre-colic position. The latter is the preferred solution for preventing early involvement in cases of recurrence. The selected loop should be sectioned close to the angle of Treitz so as to prevent extensive intestinal exclusion, while the marginal arcade should be divided to avoid mesenteric tension.

Esophago-jejunostomy should be end-to-side as this results in a correct calibration of the diameter of the anastomosis, with lower rates of fistulas than end-to-end reconstructions. Anastomosis may be manual or mechanical (Fig. 10.7) but the latter is faster. In manual anastomosis, interrupted sutures are passed through the entire esophageal wall. To assure the success of this important technical aspect, the muscular layer of the esophagus should be sutured separately, 0.5 cm from the muco-submucosal layer, which is usually retracted after the esophageal division. The cul de sac should be as short as possible. Also, single sutures may be passed with a double bite, the first through the entire wall and the second only through the muscular layer (Fig. 10.8) [27]. In mechanical anastomosis, a circular staple (usually 25 mm) is introduced through the jejunal section edge, while the anvil is positioned in the esophagus. The anastomosis is created 6–7 cm from the section edge; after the circular stapler is fired, the jejunal stump is embedded in well-vascularized tissue using a linear stapler.

Roux-en-Y reconstruction coupled with a reservoir improves food intake (Fig. 10.9). An inverted U-shaped pouch about 15 cm in length is fashioned, either manually or mechanically, with the proximal end of the loop. The intestinal loop used to create the reservoir should not be more than 15–20 cm longer than the usual Roux-en-Y limb.

10.2.2 Jejunal Interposition

Also called Longmire's procedure, this intervention aims to create a neo-gastric reservoir while maintaining the physiology of the duodenal transit. The first jejunal loop is divided to obtain a length of 25–30 cm on a good vascular pedicle, as determined using transillumination. The isolated segment is anastomosed, manually or mechanically, in the isoperistaltic position with the esophagus and in the retrocolic position with the duodenum (Fig. 10.10). Anastomosis is followed by a jejuno-jejunostomy. Intestinal interposition also may be performed with a reservoir, as described for Roux-en-Y reconstruction (Fig. 10.11). The selected loop should be 30 cm longer than that used in the standard technique.

10.2.3 Choice of Anastomosis, Reconstruction, and Reservoir

Many studies have sought to identify the optimal reconstruction method after total gastrectomy (Table 10.2). No differences were found in terms of fistula rates after manual or mechanical anastomosis, while the manual technique resulted in fewer strictures. However, mechanical anastomosis may facilitate a transhiatal eso-jejunostomy. Further studies evaluating mechanical reconstruc-

Table 10.1 Randomized studies comparing reconstruction modalities after distal gastrectomy

Author [Reference]	Sample size Indication Operation	Type of reconstructions compared	Postoperative morbidity	Long-term outcome	Conclusion
Chareton et al. [43]	62 Cancer Subtotal gastrectomy	B I vs. B II	n.s. Fistule: 13 vs. 3%	Follow-up: 38 months Survival: n.s. hepatic artery recurrence 23% vs. 3%	Short- and long- term results in favor of B II
Montesani et al. [44]	45 Cancer Subtotal gastrectomy	B I vs. B II vs. Roux-en-Y	n.a.	Follow-up: QoL°: n.s. Reflux (endoscopy and scintigraphy): 33% vs. 47% vs. 13%	Long term results in favor of Roux-en-Y
Ishikawa et al. [21]	50 Cancer Distal gastrectomy	B I vs. Roux-en-Y	8 vs. 29%	Follow-up: 6 months Symptoms: n.s. Gastritis: 62% vs. 30%*	Short-term outcome in favour of B I, long-term results in favor of Roux-en-Y
Haglund et al. [45]	121 Ulcer Antrectomy + selective vagotomy	B I vs. Roux-en-Y	n.s.	Follow-up: 6 months Symptoms: n.s.	
Kojima et al. [22]	133 Cancer Laparoscopic distal gastrectomy	B I vs. Roux-en-Y	n.s.	Follow-up: 1 year Pyrosis: 37 vs. 10%* Eating capacity in favor of Roux-en-Y Gastritis: 34% vs. 12%*	Short- and long-term in favor of Roux-en-Y
Csendes et al. [25]	75 Ulcer Distal gastrectomy + selective vagotomy	B II vs. Roux-en-Y	n.s.	Follow-up: 12-21 years Pyrosis: 33% vs. 3%* Barrett esophagus: 21% vs. 3%* Gastritis: 39% vs. 10%*	Long-term outcome in favour of Roux-en-Y
Rieu et al. [46]	22 Ulcer disease Distal gastrectomy without vagotomy	B II vs. Roux-en-Y	n.s.	Follow-up: 2 years Ulcer disease: 9 vs. 18% Gastritis:* Reflux: n.s.	In favor of Roux-en-Y for gastritis In favor of B II for ulcer disease
Hirao et al. [47]	70 Cancer Distal gastrectomy	Roux-en-Y vs. modified Roux-en-Y	n.s.	Follow-up: 1 year Weight: n.s.	n.s.

(cont.↓)

Noh et al. [20]	90 Cancer Subtotal gastrectomy	Roux-en-Y vs. modified (Noh) B II gastrectomy	n.a.	Follow-up: 2 years Roux syndrome: 30% vs. 12%* Endoscopy: n.s. Weight gain:*	Long term outcome in favour of modified B II Reproducible?
Personal experience	143 Cancer Subtotal gastrectomy	Roux-en Y vs. B II vs. other reconstructions	n.s.	Follow-up: 2 years	n.s.

B, Billroth; *QoL*, quality of life; *n.s.*, not significant; *n.a.*, not available; $*p < 0.05$.

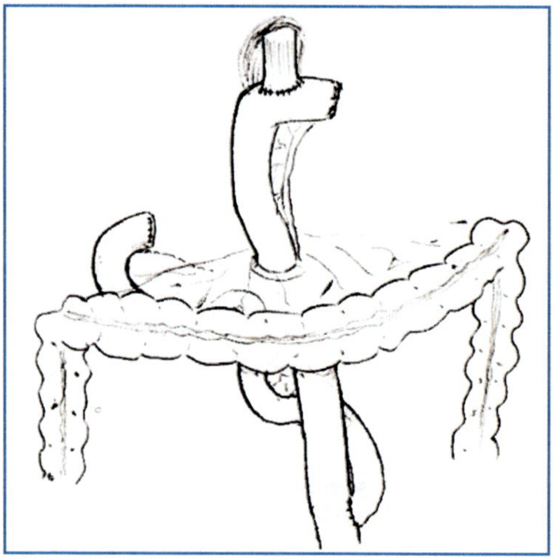

Fig. 10.6 Esophano-jejunal Roux-en-Y reconstruction

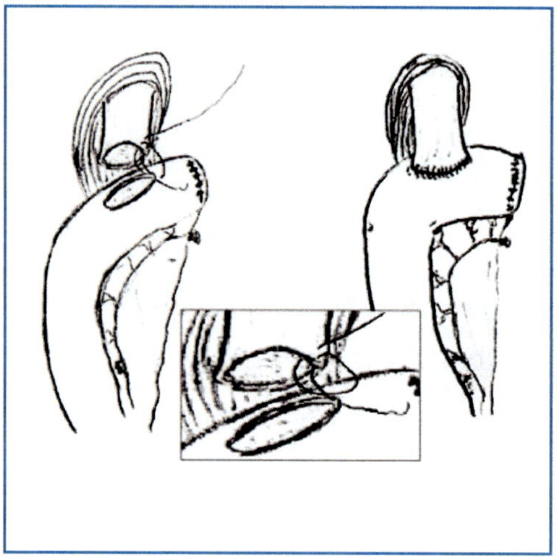

Fig. 10.8 Manual esophago-jejunal double bite suture according to Luigi Tonelli's technique [27]

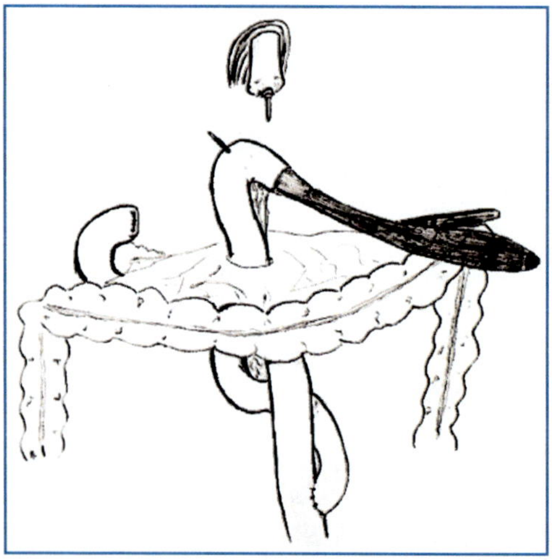

Fig. 10.7 Mechanical Roux-en-Y reconstruction

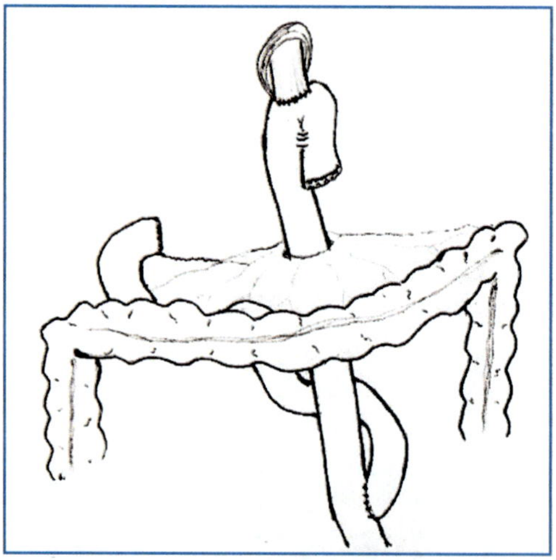

Fig. 10.9 Roux-en-Y reconstruction with reservoir

tion in laparoscopic gastrectomy are required. The advantages of duodenal preservation are the maintenance of physiological transit and the possibility for endoscopic exploration. On the other hand, despite the lack of strong scientific evidence, intestinal interposition seems to expose the patient to a higher risk of biliary reflux and cancer recurrence [28-33]. Mortality and morbidity rates are similar [29, 30, 33], as are weight gain and quality of life. Thus, the theoretical advantages of jejunal interposition have yet to be confirmed by clinical evidence.

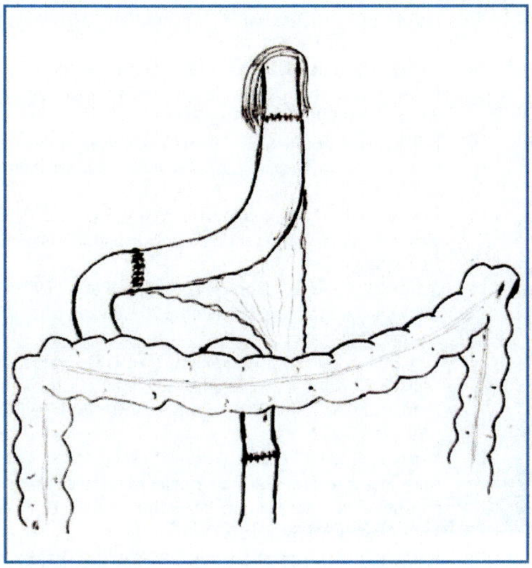

Fig. 10.10 Jejunal interposition (Longmire's procedure)

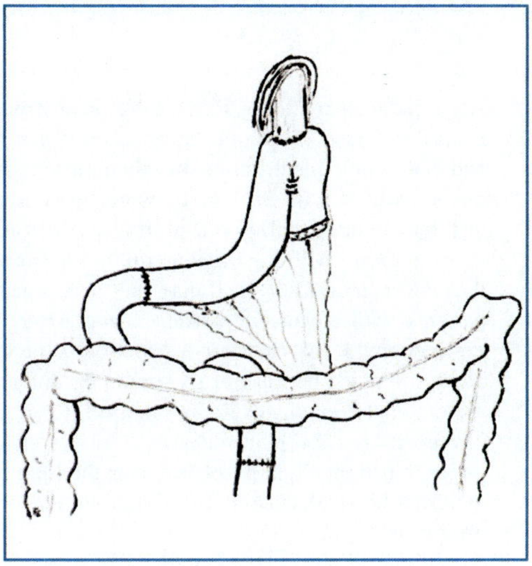

Fig. 10.11 Jejunal interposition with reservoir

Table 10.2 Randomized studies with more than 30 patients per group comparing reconstruction methods after total gastrectomy for cancer

Author [Reference]	Sample size	Reconstructions compared	Postoperative morbidity	Long-term outcome	Conclusion
Fuchs et al. [29]	106	Roux-en-Y + reservoir vs. Interposition + reservoir	n.s.	Follow-up: 36 months Weight gain: n.s.; QoL: n.s.	n.s. between Roux-en-Y + reservoir and Interposition + reservoir
Zhang et al. [48]	149	Roux-en-Y vs. Roux-en-Y + reservoir vs. Interposition + reservoir	n.a.	Follow-up: 6 months Weight gain*; QoV*	In favor of Roux-en-Y with reservoir or interposition vs. Roux-en-Y
Fein et al. [35]	138	Y vs. Y + reservoir	n.s.	Follow-up: 39 months Weight gain: n.s.; QoL:* beginning at 30 months	In favor of reservoir because of long term QoL

n.s., not significant; *QoL*, quality of life; *n.a.*, not available; $*p < 0.05$.

Some surgeons have proposed the creation of a reservoir to increase food intake, thereby improving nutritional status and quality of life; however, the relevant studies have been unable to show differences in morbidity and mortality [30, 31, 33-37]. The data concerning food intake indicate that benefits occur only early on, during the first few years [31, 38-40], but there seem to be improvements in the quality of life of patients in whom a reservoir is placed, notably at 5 years [33, 39, 41, 42].

10.3 Conclusions

After distal gastrectomy, Roux-en-Y reconstruction is the preferred technique because the functional and endoscopic results are better than those accomplished with a Billroth I or II, while there are no differences in mortality and morbidity. Billroth II is preferred to Billroth I reconstruction because of the lower morbidity and may be performed in patients with advanced gastric cancer. After total gastrectomy, Roux-en-Y reconstruction is the technique of choice because of its simplicity and satisfactory nutritional results compared to jejunal interposition. The placement of a reservoir may improve patients' quality of life over the long term and should be discussed for those with a better prognosis.

References

1. Lawrence W Jr (1996) Reconstruction after total gastrectomy: what is preferred technique? J Surg Oncol 63:215-220
2. Lehnert T, Buhl K (2004) Techniques of reconstruction after total gastrectomy for cancer. Br J Surg 91:528-539
3. Piessen G, Triboulet JP, Mariette C (2010) Reconstruction after gastrectomy: which technique is best? J Visc Surg 147:e273-e283
4. Hoya Y, Mitsumori N, Yanaga K (2009) The advantages and disadvantages of a Roux-en-Y reconstruction after a distal gastrectomy for gastric cancer. Surg Today 39:647-651
5. Slim K, Blay JY, Brouquet A et al (2009) Digestive oncology: surgical practices. J Chir (Paris) 146 Suppl 2:S11-S80
6. Piessen G, Messager M, Leteurtre E et al (2009) Signet ring cell histology is an independent predictor of poor prognosis in gastric adenocarcinoma regardless of tumoral clinical presentation. Ann Surg 250:878-887
7. Gouzi JL, Huguier M, Fagniez PL et al (1989)Total versus subtotal gastrectomy for adenocarcinoma of the gastric antrum. A French prospective controlled study. Ann Surg 209:162-166
8. Shinoto K, Ochiai T, Suzuki T et al (2003) Effectiveness of Roux-en-Y reconstruction after distal gastrectomy based on an assessment of biliary kinetics. Surg Today 33:169-177
9. Hori S, Ochiai T, Gunji Y et al (2004) A prospective randomized trial of hand-sutured versus mechanically stapled anastomoses for gastroduodenostomy after distal gastrectomy. Gastric Cancer 7:24-30
10. Pólya E (1911) Zur Stumpfversorgung nach Magenresektion. Zentralblatt für Chirurgie 38:892-894
11. Finsterer H (1918) Ausgedehnte Magenresektion bei Ulcus duodeni statt der einfachen Duodenalresektion bzw. Pylorusausschaltung. Zentralblatt für Chirurgie, Leipzig 45:434-435
12. Lillemoe KD, Sauter PK, Pitt HA et al (1993) Current status of surgical palliation of periampullary carcinoma. Surg Gynecol Obstet 176:1-10
13. Debray C, Roux M, Chevillotte R, Segal S (1950) Cancers of the gastric stump after gastrectomy for ulcer. Arch Mal Appar Dig Mal Nutr 39:702-716
14. Helsingen N, Hillestad L (1956) Cancer development in the gastric stump after partial gastrectomy for ulcer. Ann Surg 143:173-179
15. Kivilaakso E, Hakkiluoto A, Kalima TV, Sipponen P (1977) Relative risk of stump cancer following partial gastrectomy. Br J Surg 64:336-338
16. Schrumpf E, Serck-Hanssen A, Stadaas J et al (1977) Mucosal changes in the gastric stump 20-25 years after partial gastrectomy. Lancet 2:467-469
17. Tonelli F, Corazziari E, Spinelli F (1978) Evaluation of "Alkaline" Reflux Esophagitis after total Gastrectomy in Henley and Roux-en-Y Reconstructive Procedures. World J Surg 2:23-237
18. Van der Mijle HC, Kleibeuker JH, Limburg AJ et al (1993) Manometric and scintigraphic studies of the relation between motility disturbances in the Roux limb and the Roux-en-Y syndrome. Am J Surg 166:11-17
19. Karlstrom LH, Soper NJ, Kelly KA, Phillips SF (1989) Ectopic jejunal pacemakers and enterogastric reflux after Roux gastrectomy: effect of intestinal pacing. Surgery 106:486-495
20. Noh SM, Jeong HY, Cho JS et al (2003) New type of reconstruction method after subtotal gastrectomy (Noh's operation). World J Surg 27:562-566
21. Ishikawa M, Kitayama J, Kaizaki S et al (2005) Prospective randomized trial comparing Billroth I and Roux-en-Y procedures after distal gastrectomy for gastric carcinoma. World J Surg 29:1415-1420
22. Kojima K, Yamada H, Inokuchi M et al (2008) A comparison of Roux-en-Y and Billroth-I reconstruction after laparoscopy-assisted distal gastrectomy. Ann Surg 247:962-967
23. Forstner-Barthell AW, Murr MM, Nitecki S et al (1999) Near-total completion gastrectomy for severe postvagotomy gastric stasis: analysis of early and long-term results in 62 patients. J Gastrointest Surg 3:15-21, discussion
24. Vogel SB, Woodward ER (1989) The surgical treatment of chronic gastric atony following Roux-Y diversion for alkaline reflux gastritis. Ann Surg 209:756-761
25. Csendes A, Burgos AM, Smok G et al (2009) Latest results (12-21 years) of a prospective randomized study comparing Billroth II and Roux-en-Y anastomosis after a partial gastrectomy plus vagotomy in patients with duodenal ulcers. Ann Surg 249:189-194
26. Collard JM, Romagnoli R (2000) Roux-en-Y jejunal loop and bile reflux. Am J Surg 179:298-303
27. Tonelli F, Ficari F. Burci P (1990) Total gastrectomy for gastric carcinoma: which perioperative treatment, surgical technique andt type of digestive reconstruction? Nutrition 6:254-256
28. Adachi S, Inagawa S, Enomoto T et al (2003)Subjective and functional results after total gastrectomy: prospective study for long term comparison of reconstruction procedures. Gastric Cancer 6:24-29
29. Fuchs KH, Thiede A, Engemann R et al (1995) Reconstruction of the food passage after total gastrectomy: randomized trial. World J Surg 19:698-705

30. Iwahashi M, Nakamori M, Nakamura M et al (2009) Evaluation of double tract reconstruction after total gastrectomy in patients with gastric cancer: prospective randomized controlled trial. World J Surg 33:1882-1888
31. Nakane Y, Okumura S, Akehira K et al (1995) Jejunal pouch reconstruction after total gastrectomy for cancer. A randomized controlled trial. Ann Surg 222:27-35
32. Nakane Y, Michiura T, Inoue K et al (2001) A randomized clinical trial of pouch reconstruction after total gastrectomy for cancer: which is the better technique, Roux-en-Y or interposition? Hepatogastroenterology 48:903-907
33. Schwarz A, Buchler M, Usinger K et al (1996) Importance of the duodenal passage and pouch volume after total gastrectomy and reconstruction with the Ulm pouch: prospective randomized clinical study. World J Surg 20:60-66
34. Bozzetti F, Bonfanti G, Castellani R et al (1996) Comparing reconstruction with Roux-en-Y to a pouch following total gastrectomy. J Am Coll Surg 183:243-248
35. Fein M, Fuchs KH, Thalheimer A et al (2008) Long-term benefits of Roux-en-Y pouch reconstruction after total gastrectomy: a randomized trial. Ann Surg 247:759-765
36. Svedlund J, Sullivan M, Liedman B, Lundell L (1999) Long term consequences of gastrectomy for patient's quality of life: the impact of reconstructive techniques. Am J Gastroenterol 94:438-445
37. Tanaka T, Fujiwara Y, Nakagawa K et al (1997) Reflux esophagitis after total gastrectomy with jejunal pouch reconstruction: comparison of long and short pouches. Am J Gastroenterol 92:821-824
38. Iivonen MK, Mattila JJ, Nordback IH, Matikainen MJ (2000) Long-term follow-up of patients with jejunal pouch reconstruction after total gastrectomy. A randomized prospective study. Scand J Gastroenterol 35:679-685
39. Kono K, Iizuka H, Sekikawa T et al (2003) Improved quality of life with jejunal pouch reconstruction after total gastrectomy. Am J Surg 185:150-154
40. Liedman B, Andersson H, Bosaeus I et al (1997) Changes in body composition after gastrectomy: results of a controlled, prospective clinical trial. World J Surg 21:416-420
41. Gioffrè Florio MA, Bartolotta M, Miceli JC et al (2000) Simple versus double jejunal pouch for reconstruction after total gastrectomy. Am J Surg 180:24-28
42. Svedlund J, Sullivan M, Liedman B et al (1997) Quality of life after gastrectomy for gastric carcinoma: controlled study of reconstructive procedures. World J Surg 21:422-433
43. Chareton B, Landen S, Manganas D et al (1996) Prospective randomized trial comparing Billroth I and Billroth II procedures for carcinoma of the gastric antrum. J Am Coll Surg 183:190-194
44. Montesani C, D'Amato A, Santella S et al (2002) Billroth I versus Billroth II versus Roux-en-Y after subtotal gastrectomy. Prospective randomized study. Hepatogastroenterology 49:1469-1473
45. Haglund UH, Jansson RL, Lindhagen JG et al (1990) Primary Roux-Y gastrojejunostomy versus gastroduodenostomy after antrectomy and selective vagotomy. Am J Surg 159:546-549
46. Rieu PN, Jansen JB, Biemond I et al (1992) Short-term results of gastrectomy with Roux-en-Y or Billroth II anastomosis for peptic ulcer. A prospective comparative study. Hepatogastroenterology 39:22-26
47. Hirao M, Kurokawa Y, Fujitani K, Tsujinaka T (2009) Randomized controlled trial of Roux-en-Y versus rho-shaped-Roux-en-Y reconstruction after distal gastrectomy for gastric cancer. World J Surg 33:290-295
48. Zhang JZ, Lu HS, Wu XY et al (2003) Influence of different procedures of alimentary tract reconstruction after total gastrectomy for gastric cancer on the nutrition and metabolism of patients: a prospective clinical study. Zhonghua Yi Xue Za Zhi 83:1475-1478

11 Endoscopic and Surgical Treatment of Early Gastric Cancer

Paolo Morgagni, Luca Saragoni, Filippo Catalano, Alessandro Casadei, and Mario Marini

Abstract

Early gastric cancer (EGC) is defined as a tumor confined to the mucosa/submucosa, irrespective of the presence of lymph node metastases. Only high-quality endoscopic evaluation with chromoendoscopy and biopsy can increase the number of detected EGCs. As the presence of lymph node metastases has a strong adverse influence on patient prognosis, selected criteria must be used to identify the subset of lesions with no risk of lymphatic spread, as these are eligible for endoscopic resection. Conventional endoscopic mucosal resection has gained worldwide consensus for the treatment of selected EGC types but curative resection cannot be always guaranteed for lesions with a diameter > 15 mm. In these patients, a new technique, endoscopic submucosal dissection, allows successful en bloc resection. When conditions for endoscopic treatment cannot be met and lymphatic diffusion cannot be excluded, patients must be treated surgically. Gastrectomy with a clear margin of 2 cm from the lesion and D2 dissection is generally recommended as the treatment of choice. To define radicality and prognosis, the correct application of histological parameters is essential.

Keywords

Early gastric cancer • Chromoendoscopy • Endoscopic mucosal resection • Endoscopic submucosal dissection • D2 gastrectomy • Lymphadenectomy • Pathologic guidelines

11.1 Introduction

One of the reasons for the poor 5-year survival rates in Western patients with gastric cancer (GC) is late diagnosis. The prognosis of these patients could be improved by detecting tumors at an early stage, thus avoiding disease progression to the advanced stage.

Early gastric cancer (EGC) is defined as tumor confined to the mucosa/submucosa, irrespective of the presence of lymph node metastases. Data from Japanese and selected Western centers have shown that the 5-year cancer-specific survival rate of patients with EGC is > 90%. The detection of EGC and thereby better therapeutic results can be achieved using high-quality endoscopic evaluation with chromoendoscopy and biopsy.

P. Morgagni (✉)
Dept. of General Surgery,
"G.B. Morgagni – L. Pierantoni" Hospital,
Forlì, Italy

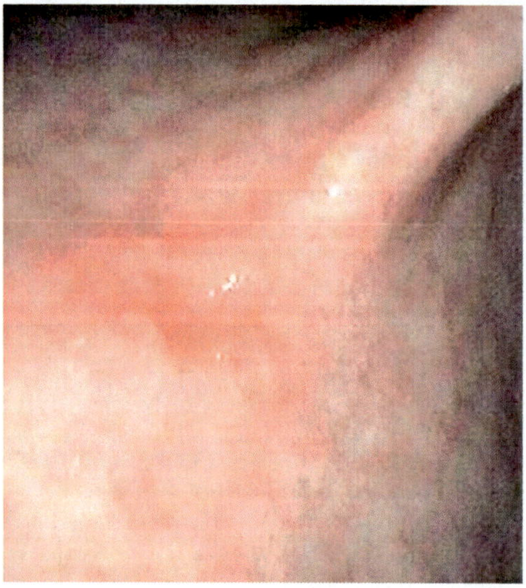

Fig. 11.1 Early gastric cancer: white light aspect

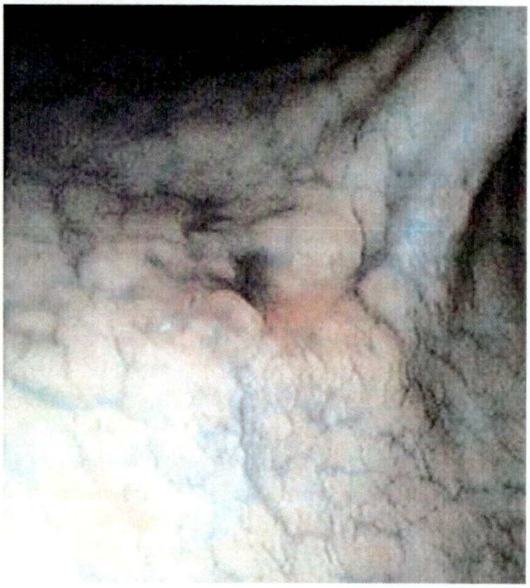

Fig. 11.2 Early gastric cancer after chromoendoscopy

High-quality endoscopy is carried out in the sedated patient, gastric visibility is improved using a mixture of a defoaming and mucolytic agents (dimethylpolysiloxane, pronase, and $NaHCo_3$), which the patient consumes 5 min before the examination. Chromoendoscopy, with indigo carmine, will highlight subtle changes in gastric color, vascularity, and texture, which are the hallmarks of EGC [1] (Figs. 11.1, 11.2).

11.2 Criteria for Endoscopic Mucosal/Submucosal Resection

Lymph node metastases are detected in about 3% of mucosal and 20% of submucosal EGCs and have a strong adverse influence on patients prognosis [2], It is therefore essential to use precise criteria to identify the subset of lesions with no risk of lymphatic spread, as these are eligible for endoscopic resection. Currently, the accepted indications for endoscopic resection of EGC include well-differentiated mucosal cancers < 2 cm in diameter not ulcerated and without lymphatic or vascular involvement [3].

Although Japanese authors have proposed extended criteria for endoscopic resection, in Western countries gastrectomy with radical lymphadenectomy is still recommended for patients not satisfying the standard guideline criteria [4].

Finally, radicality is evaluated on the basis of the histological report, i.e., type of tumor, depth of invasion, lateral and vertical margins status, and lymphovascular invasion.

11.3 Endoscopical Mucosal Resection

Endoscopic mucosal resection (EMR) can be subdivided into three phases: demarcation of the lesion, submucosal injection, and endoscopic resection. During EMR, an endoscope with a 2.8-mm single channel is often used, also in the event of complications [2].

11.3.1 Demarcation

The periphery of the EGC is marked to facilitate recognition of the lesion after submucosal injection and to facilitate resection completeness. The markers are placed 1–3 mm from the margins. Demarcation is performed using the tip of a snare

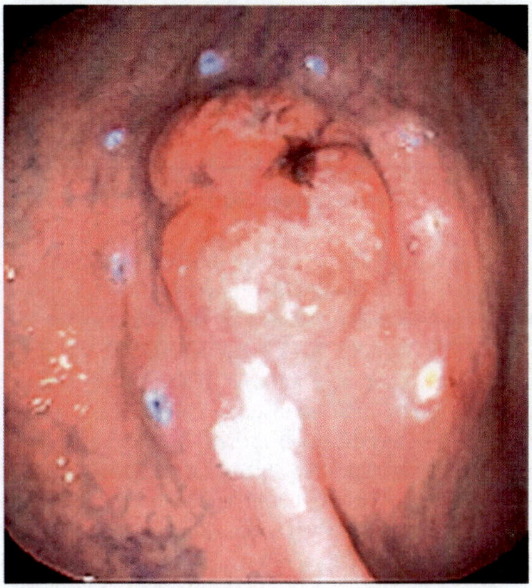

Fig. 11.3 Lesion demarcation with simple needle knife

or a needle knife. Another better method is argon plasma coagulation (APC) (Fig. 11.3).

11.3.2 Submucosal Injection

The lesion is injected submucosally to create a raised bleb, which facilitates its removal, reducing electrocautery and mechanical damage to the deep layers of the gastric wall. The volume of the solution depends on the size and location of the lesion but is usually 5–50 ml; repeated injections are often necessary. The addition of staining dye to the solution aids in the identification of the deep margin during resection. Several different solutions have been developed in an attempt to maintain the submucosal bleb for as long as possible, making the procedure safer and lowering the risk of complications. In Japan, normal saline and glycerol solutions are the most commonly used [5].

11.3.3 Endoscopic Resection

Either the non-suction (lift and cut) or the suction (suck and cut) technique can be used in EMR. In the latter, the lesion is sucked inside a transparent plastic cap placed onto the tip of the endoscope (EMRC) and finally cut. Alternatively, a band ligating device (EMRL) can be employed, usually without submucosal injection. The choice of treatment depends on the experience and preference of the endoscopist and on the size and location of the lesion. In the literature, neither method has been recognized as superior to the other [1, 6, 7] (Table 11.1).

After endoscopic resection, a tattoo may be useful for endoscopic controls. The use of clips for the closure of large mucosal defects after EMR to prevent complications and help healing is not entirely accepted [8].

11.3.4 Injection and Snaring (Lift and Cut)

This is a relatively simple and safe technique for resection of the lesion after submucosal injection.

Table 11.1 Endoscopic mucosal resection methods

Non-suction techniques:
1. Strip off biopsy: injection and snaring
2. Lift and cut biopsy, double snare polypectomy: grasping and snaring
3. Endoscopic resection with hypertonic saline-epinephrine solution: injection, pre-cutting, and snaring
4. Endoscopic mucosal resection using a transparent overtube: grasping and snaring using an overtube
Suction techniques:
1. Endoscopic mucosal resection using a transparent plastic cap: injection and snaring using a cap)
2. Endoscopic mucosal resection using a ligating device: endoscopic variceal ligation and snaring
3. Simple suction technique: snaring using stiff snare

It is based on the use of a snare, which is inserted through a single-channel endoscope. The main problem with this method is the difficulty in treating lesion types IIb and IIc because the snare often slides over the surface of the EGC, making cutting impossible. In these cases, it may be preferable to use snares with a single filament or multiple teeth or, better, to choose another technique [2, 6, 7].

11.3.5 Grasping and Snaring (Strip Biopsy)

A double-channel endoscope can be used to facilitate the lift and cut technique. After submucosal injection, grasping forceps are used to pull the lesion into an opened electrocautery snare that has been introduced through the second channel of the endoscope. The snare is then closed and the lesion resected. This technique is particularly useful for the resection of type IIb and IIc lesions, but the risk of perforation is higher than that of the lift and cut method such that a greater volume of injection solution is therefore necessary [2, 6, 7].

11.3.6 Injection and Snaring Using a Cap (EMRC)

Cylindrical clear plastic caps, straight or oblique, soft or hard, with an outer diameter of 12.9–18 mm, are fixed to the tip of the endoscope. After submucosal injection, a specific crescent-shaped electrocautery snare is opened and positioned on the internal ridge at the tip of the cap. The endoscope is positioned over the EGC and the lesion sucked into the cap; the snare is closed and the lesion resected [1].

11.3.7 Endoscopic Variceal Ligation and Snaring (EMRL)

In this technique, performed with or without submucosal injection, a standard variceal band ligation device captures the lesion such that it is converted into a polypoid lesion. The lesion above or below the band, which is not strong enough to capture the muscularis propria, is then resected with a monofilament snare. EMRL has the advantage of being relatively simple, but en-bloc resection is possible only for lesions < 10–15 mm [2, 6, 7].

11.4 Endoscopic Submucosal Dissection

Conventional endoscopic mucosal resection (EMR) has gained worldwide consensus for the treatment of selected EGC types [2]. Nonetheless, for lesions with a diameter > 15 mm, piecemeal EMR does not always guarantee curative resection [8]. Instead, a new technique, endoscopic submucosal dissection (ESD), has been proposed to guarantee en bloc resection. The feasibility of ESD is still under debate in Western countries due to the lower detection rate of early lesions, the lack of well-established endoscopic criteria for its implementation, and the difficult learning curve. ESD is usually performed and completed with the insulated-tip (IT) knife (Olympus, Tokyo, Japan) technique, first proposed by Hosokawa [9].

11.4.1 Technique

Accurate estimation of the lesion is achieved by spraying 5–10 ml of 0.2% indigo carmine solution directly through the biopsy channel onto the gastric mucosa. Normal mucosa surrounding the lesion is marked at least 5 mm away from the tumor using a standard needle knife (Olympus, Tokyo, Japan) with a forced 20W coagulation current (ICC 200 ERBE Tubingen, Germany). After injection of a saline solution containing epinephrine (0.025 mg/ml) into the submucosa, an initial cut, also called a pre-cut, is made with a needle knife outside the marks in the 60W end-cut mode effect 3. The IT knife is inserted into the pre-cut incision and an electrosurgical current is applied in the 60–80W end-cut mode effect 3 (ICC 200 ERBE, Tubingen, Germany) to complete circumferential mucosal cutting. Epinephrine-containing saline solution is again injected and the IT knife is then used to dissect the submucosa underneath the lesion (Figs. 11.4, 11.5).

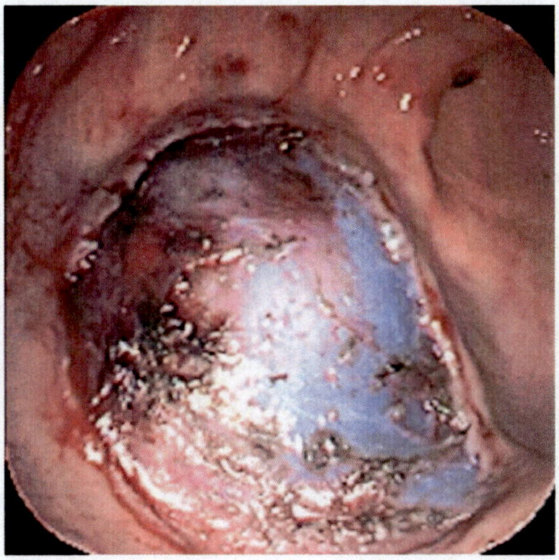

Fig. 11.4 Muscular layer after endoscopic submucosal dissection

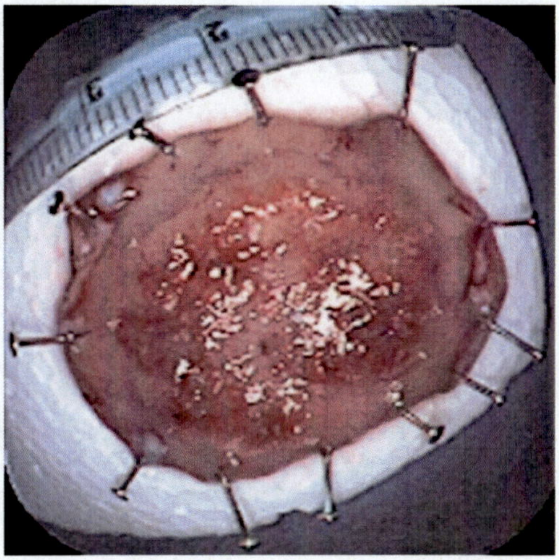

Fig. 11.5 Endoscopic specimen

11.4.2 Complications

The complications of endoscopic resection include pain (typically mild), bleeding, and perforation [10]. Bleeding is the most common complication, occurring in up to 7% of patients. Immediate minor bleeding is not unusual and can be successfully treated by grasping and coagulation using hot biopsy forceps. Delayed bleeding is strongly related to tumor location and size. The risk of perforation during ESD is about 4%; perforations are typically closed using endoclips.

There are only a few studies of ESD treatment in Western patients. One such study, in a GIRCG cohort [11], was limited to a few cases and requires confirmation in a larger trial. Nonetheless, it reported that the achievement of good results for the treatment of EGC depend on the experience of the endoscopist and on all criteria being met for the procedure.

11.5 Pathologic Guidelines for the Assessment of Endoscopic Resections

After EMR or ESD, the specimen must be mounted on a support (e.g., a cork tablet) with the mucous surface facing upwards. It is strongly advisable to mark the lateral margins with India ink. The pathologist must provide the following information: (a) size of the specimen (length, width, thickness), (b) size of the lesion, (c) distance of the lesion from the margins, and (d) type of tumor, as classified according to the Japanese Society of Gastroenterology and Endoscopy (JSGE).

The specimen must then be sampled in its entirety by 2-mm serial sections along the longitudinal axis. The proximal and distal margins should be marked by the endoscopist according to the anatomical landmarks and included separately by the pathologist.

While EMR and ESD primarily have a diagnostic aim, the pathologist should still carry out a therapeutic evaluation derived directly from the complete and correct application of histological parameters, which are essential to this end. These parameters are: (a) macroscopic size, (b) microscopic ulceration, (c) histotype, (d) histological grade, (e) maximum depth of invasion, (f) presence/absence of lymphatic vascular invasion, (g) state of the lateral margins, and (h) state of the deep margin. All of these parameters must be noted in the histological report. A correct histological assessment is possible only if the pathologist strictly adheres to the guidelines on macroscopic samplings [12].

11.6 Surgical Treatment

Patients operated on for EGC in Asian countries typically have a very good prognosis, with low morbidity and mortality rates. Recently, Western institutions have adopted the same techniques, in particular D2 lymphadenectomy, thereby achieving 5- to 10-year patient survival rates of > 90%, morbidity rates of 14.4%, and a mortality rate of 2.2% [13, 14]. Given these results, EGC can be considered as a curable disease.

Lymphatic involvement is the most important and independent prognostic factor. When conditions for endoscopic treatment cannot be met and lymphatic diffusion cannot be excluded, patients must be treated surgically, with accurate lymph node dissection.

Although numerous surgical options have been described depending on the characteristics of the tumor, gastrectomy with a clear margin of 2 cm from the lesion and D2 dissection is generally recommended as the treatment of choice, especially when the risk of advanced cancer cannot be entirely excluded preoperatively.

Multifocality occurs in about 10% of EGC patients [15]. However, this is not considered as an indication for total gastrectomy if a 2-cm distance from the resection site can be guaranteed with subtotal gastrectomy. Although several authors have reported that multifocal cancer generally occurs in areas lateral or distal to the principal lesion, an accurate endoscopy with chromo or magnified technique must still be performed preoperatively, especially at the upper third of the stomach.

Japanese guidelines for EGC recommend different types of dissection: D1 dissection plus gastric artery lymph nodes for small intramucosal differentiated EGC (modified A) and modified A plus hepatic and celiac dissection for small submucosal differentiated tumors (modified B). All other EGCs must be treated, according to the Japanese criteria, with standard D2 dissection. The sentinel lymph node technique has also been proposed, but a general consensus on its use is lacking because of the relatively high incidence of false-negatives, which can result in inappropriate treatment.

In conclusion, limited lymph node dissection can be proposed only if a correct preoperative diagnosis can be guaranteed. If this is not possible, D2 dissection represents the standard treatment. Laparoscopic or robotic surgery can also be proposed if the above mentioned criteria are satisfied.

11.7 Pathologic Guidelines for the Assessment of Surgical Specimens

Surgical specimens are sent to the pathologist mounted on a tablet, with the mucous surface facing upwards. It is advisable that surgeons send the individual lymph node stations already isolated and stored in containers labeled with their exact topography.

The macroscopic examination must meet the following criteria: (a) type of specimen (total or subtotal gastrectomy), (b) type of lymphadenectomy, (c) tumor location, (d) tumor size, (e) macroscopic tumor type (JSGE classification) and Kodama type [16] (Table 11.2), and (f) distance of the tumor from the margins. The lesion must be sampled in its entirety and the histological report must provide all the information listed in Table 11.3.

Table 11.2 Kodama's classification of early gastric cancer

Kodama type	
Small mucosal m	Intramucosal EGC measuring < 4 cm
Small mucosal sm	EGC minimally invading the submucosa and measuring < 4 cm
Super mucosal m	Intramucosal EGC measuring > 4 cm
Super mucosal sm	EGC minimally invading the submucosa and measuring > 4 cm
Penetrating A (PenA)	EGC massively invading the submucosa, with a nodular pattern, and measuring < 4 cm
Penetrating B (PenB)	EGC massively invading the submucosa, with a sawtooth pattern, and measuring < 4 cm
Mixed	Penetrating types A and B and measuring > 4 cm

Table 11.3 Information to be entered in the histological report

Histological type of tumor based on Lauren's classification (or, optionally, WHO classification)
Histological grade (WHO classification)
Maximum depth of invasion of wall
Invasion pattern based on Kodama's classification (see Table 11.2)
Presence /absence of lymphatic vascular and/or venous invasion
State of margins
Total number of lymph nodes examined
Ratio of metastatic lymph nodes out of the total of lymph nodes examined
Staging according to pTNM (7th edition)

References

1. Dinis-Ribeiro M (2006) Chromoendoscopy for early diagnosis of gastric cancer. Eur J Gastroenterol Hepatol 18:831-838
2. Gotoda T(2007) Endoscopic resection of early gastric cancer. Gastric Cancer 10:1-11
3. Japanese Gastric Cancer Association (2004) Gastric cancer treatment guideline (in Japanese). 2nd edn. Kanehara-Shuppan, Tokyo
4. Gotoda T, Yanagisawa A, Sasako M et al (2000) Incidence of lymph node metastasis from early gastric cancer: estimation with a large number of cases at two large centers. Gastric Cancer 3:219-225
5. Gotoda T, Yamamoto H, Soetikno R (2006) Endoscopic submucosal dissection of early gastric cancer. J Gastroentero l41:929-942
6. ASGE Technology Committee (2008) Endoscopic mucosal resection and endoscopic submucosal dissection. Gastrointest Endosc 68:11-18
7. Giovannini M, Cesar Vivian L (2008) Endoscopic resection of superficial gastrointestinal tumors. World J Gastroenterol 14:4600-4606
8. Educhi T, Gotoda T, Oda I et al (2003) Is endoscopic one piece mucosal resection essential for early gastric cancer? Dig Endosc15:113-116
9. Ohkuwa M, Hosokawa K, Boku N et al (2001) New endoscopic treatment for intramucosal gastric tumors using an insulated-tip diathermic knife. Endoscopy 33:221-226
10. Gotoda T (2006) Endoscopic resection of early gastric cancer: the Japanese perspective. Curr Op Gastroent 22:561-569
11. Catalano F, Trecca A, Rodella L et al (2009) The modern treatment of early gastric cancer: our experience in an Italian cohort. Surg Endosc 23:1581-1586
12. Ishikawa S, Togashi A, Inoue M et al (2007) Indications for EMR/ESD in cases of early gastric cancer: relationship between histological type, depth of wall invasion, and lymph node metastasis. Gastric Cancer 10(1):35-38
13. Folli S, Morgagni P, Roviello F et al (2001) Risk factor for lymph node metastases and their prognostic significance in EGC for the Italian Research Group for Gastric Cancer. Jpn J Clin Oncol 3:495-499
14. Roviello F, Rossi S, Marrelli D et al (2006) Number of lymph node metastases and its prognostic significance in EGC: a multicenter Italian study. J Surg Oncol 94:275-280
15. Morgagni P, Marfisi C, Gardini A, Marrelli D (2009) Subtotal gastrectomy as treatment for multifocal EGC. J Gastroint Surg 13:2239-2244
16. Saragoni L, Gaudio M, Morgagni P et al (2000) The role of growth patterns, according to Kodama's classification and lymph node status, as important prognostic factors in early gastric cancer : analysisis of 412 cases. Gastric Cancer 3:134-140

Treatment of Resectable Advanced Gastric Cancer

12

Alberto Marchet, Gian Maria Rossi, Simone Mocellin, and Donato Nitti

Abstract

In Western countries, gastric cancer is still most frequently diagnosed in the advanced stage, with surgery the main treatment modality for advanced gastric carcinoma (T2-T4a). The goal of a potentially curative operation is to remove all visible disease (R0) while achieving adequate resection margins. Splenectomy has not been shown to confer a real beneficial effect on survival rates and is performed only in selected cases. Lymphadenectomy D2, with the removal of at least 16 lymph nodes, is considered the standard treatment for patients with advanced gastric cancer. Laparoscopic distal gastrectomy is a feasible and safe procedure when the principles of radical surgery are met.

Keywords

Advanced gastric cancer • Gastric cancer surgery • Lymphadenectomy • Splenectomy • Gastric cancer epidemiology • Mini-invasive surgery • TNM • Prognosis of gastric cancer • Gastric cancer staging

12.1 Incidence and Prognosis of Advanced Gastric Cancer

Unlike in Japan, where early gastric cancer (T1) is currently the most common type of gastric neoplasm, in Western countries gastric cancer is still most frequently diagnosed in the advanced stage (T2–T4) [1].

The new TNM classification has changed the T subcategories, assigning an independent prognostic value to neoplasms involving the muscularis mucosa (T2; previously classified as T2a) vs. those invading the subserosa (T3; previously classified as T2b), whereas neoplasms with serosal involvement are now classified as T4a and those extending to the adjacent organs as T4b [2].

As the previous TNM classification did not differentiate T2a from T2b tumors, the real incidence of tumors in the new T2 and T3 subcategories reported in the different published series is difficult to define. In an Italian Research Group Gastric Cancer (GIRCG) study, among 1853 patients who underwent radical gastric cancer resection, T2/T3 neoplasms were determined in 29.3% of cases and T4a tumors in 37.1% [3]. In a recent study completed by Nitti et al. on 373 patients who underwent radical resection, the occurrence of T2, T3, and T4a tumors was 13.1, 38.3, and 12.3%, respectively [4]. In the study published by Fotia et al., among the 624 patients with gastric cancer treated by radical resection, the incidence of T2/T3 neo-

A. Marchet (✉)
Dept. of Oncological and Surgical Sciences,
Surgery Section,
University of Padova,
Padova, Italy

plasms was 29% [5]. Likewise, Sarela et al. reported a 30.5% incidence of T2/T3 tumors [6]. In some Japanese series, the incidence of T2/T3 neoplasms ranges from 10% to 38% [7-9]. The different proportions of T2 vs. T3 tumors and T3 vs. T4a tumors reported in the literature [10, 11] may reflect differences in the accuracy of pathological evaluation and the pathologist's ability to differentiate true serosal involvement (T4a) from cases in which infiltration is limited to the subserosa (T3).

Different results have been reported regarding the correlation between the T2, T3, and T4a gastric wall involvement and N categories. In particular, Nitti et al. observed that the number of metastatic lymph nodes increased with the number of examined nodes for T3 and T4a tumors, whereas this was not the case for T1 and T2 tumors. These authors also reported a statistically significant association between T and N categories, with lymph node involvement significantly lower in T2 than in T3 and T4a disease (55 vs. 79 vs. 91%). The incidence of N1 cases was similar for T2 and T3 patients but higher for T4a patients whereas N2 and N3a cases occurred significantly more frequently among T3 and T4a patients than in those with T2 disease [4]. Similar results were reported by Sarela and coworkers [6].

The depth of tumor invasion and the degree of lymph node involvement are considered the main prognostic factors for resectable gastric cancer. Whereas the survival rates of patients with early gastric cancer are high (independent of lymph node status) and those of patients with T4a disease are low, in T2 and T3 gastric cancer the survival rates vary significantly in different series. In the study by Sarela et al., a significantly better 5-year survival was reported for T2 than for T3 patients (64.1 vs. 45.9%, p = 0.005). However, in a subgroup analysis considering only patients with "adequately staged" disease (> 15 lymph node examined), the same authors reported different results: 5-year survival rates of patients with N0 disease were similar among T2 and T3 patients (90 vs. 86%, p = 0.8) and did not significantly differ for N1 disease (56 vs. 44% for T2 vs. T3, p = 0.3). Finally, in a multivariate analysis, Sarela et al. found that N category and site of the primary tumor but not depth of mural invasion were independent factors predictive of death caused by recurrent disease [6]. Similar conclusions were drawn by Fotia et al. in a study comprising 182 patients with radically resected T2/T3 gastric cancer [5].

In a recent study by Nitti et al., the prognosis of patients with T2 disease was reported to be significantly better than that of patients with T3 disease; the 5-year overall survival rate was 73 vs. 31% (p < 0.001). At multivariate analysis, T stage (including the T2/T3 subcategories) was retained as an independent prognostic factor. Furthermore, compared with T1, the risk of death associated was statistically greater with T3 than with T2 tumors (hazard ratio: 1.81 vs. 0.97) and was similar to that of T4a patients (hazard ratio: 1.89) [4]. These results were in line with those reported by Park and coworkers: in a large study (1,118 patients) that included patients with > 15 lymph nodes removed and examined. The authors found a statistically significant 5-year survival advantage for T2 vs. T3 patients (85.5 vs. 55.7%, p < 0.001). In addition, significant differences in the survival rates between T2 and T3 patients were observed when cases were stratified according to N stage. The same investigators found that the TNM classification including the T2/T3 subcategories was significantly associated with prognosis at multivariate analysis [12].

12.2 Type of Resection

Surgery is still considered the main treatment modality for advanced gastric carcinoma. The principles underlying radical surgery for carcinoma of the stomach without macroscopic or microscopic residual disease (R0) are: (a) total or subtotal gastrectomy with disease-free resection margins, (b) en bloc resection of the greater and lesser omentum, (c) removal of loco-regional lymph nodes, and (d) en bloc resection of organs adhering to the tumor.

In the 1970s, many authors considered total gastrectomy the treatment of choice for gastric carcinoma. The reasons supporting this choice were:

1. Hypothetical multicentric lesions. Several studies demonstrated that the percentage of multifocal lesions in gastric cancer ranges from 4.8 to 8.3% and that these lesions involve only the mucosa and submucosa in 80% of cases. Moreover, when multifocal lower-third lesions are detected, a secondary lesion in the upper

third of the stomach is rarely observed. In a recent study on 98 patients with multifocal early gastric cancer, when the principal lesion was situated in the lower third of the stomach, no secondary lesions were detected in the upper third. Thus, the authors concluded that when a chromoendoscopy examination excludes upper-third involvement, subtotal gastrectomy can be considered adequate surgical treatment also for multifocal lower-third gastric carcinoma [13]. Finally, different studies demonstrated that the incidence of gastric cancer recurrence in the gastric stump is not significantly different for multifocal lesions vs. single lesions and the survival rates between the two do not differ.

2. Inadequate resection margins in subtotal gastrectomy. A proximal resection margin of 5 cm (2 cm for early gastric cancer) is considered adequate by Japanese and by Western surgeons. This safe margin of resection can be achieved for lower-third neoplasms and for small neoplasms located in the middle third of the stomach, also when subtotal gastric resection is performed. If subtotal gastrectomy cannot achieve adequate resection margins, total gastrectomy is considered mandatory.
3. Inadequate lymphadenectomy when subtotal gastrectomy is performed. When a distal subtotal gastrectomy is performed, surgeons usually do not remove the left paracardial lymph nodes, the lymph nodes of the splenic hilum and those of the upper greater curvature. However, in lower-third gastric tumors, these lymph nodes are involved in a low percentage of cases.
4. Better survival outcome after total gastrectomy. Several clinical studies demonstrated that the survival of patients with tumors localized in the distal third of the stomach who underwent total gastrectomy was not different from that of patients who underwent gastric resection, which also guaranteed a better functional outcome [14].

12.2.1 Conclusions

As widely accepted, the extent of gastric resection depends on the site of the disease [15]. For tumors of the gastric antrum and pylorus, distal subtotal gastric resection is considered the procedure of choice and is indicated also for middle-third tumors with adequate disease-free resection margins. Total gastrectomy should be performed for middle-third tumors with inadequate resection margins, for upper-third tumors, and for multifocal tumors when there is upper-third involvement. All methods now available for reconstruction and suture are acceptable.

To achieve curative treatment, determination of resection margins is considered one of the key aspects of the surgical procedure [16]. For subtotal gastric resection, a distal resection margin of 2 cm and a proximal resection margin of 5 cm (2 cm in cases of early gastric cancer) are considered adequate. When total gastrectomy is performed, the recommended distal and proximal resection margins are both 2 cm. However, intra-operative examination of frozen sections of the esophageal resection margin is indicated in cases of total gastrectomy. This procedure is also recommended whenever there is any doubt at macroscopic evaluation of resection margin involvement (see chap. 8).

12.3 Splenectomy

The role of splenectomy in the surgical treatment of gastric cancer has changed over the last years based on the availability of new evidence: (1) splenectomy is not necessary to obtain radical resection [17]; (2) the survival of patients who undergo splenectomy is not significantly different from that of patients with spleen preservation, also in cases of upper-third or cardia tumor sites [18]; (3) patients undergoing splenectomy have a longer hospital stay and a significantly higher incidence of post-operative complications than patients who do not undergo splenectomy. For instance, in a Dutch study, the relative risk ratio for morbidity and mortality after resection with curative intent was 3.03 and 2.67, respectively, in 165 patients with splenectomy compared to 546 patients without splenectomy [19] (Fig. 12.1).

12.3.1 Conclusions

Splenectomy should be performed only in patients with gastric cancer involving or adhering to the

Study name	Odds ratio	Lower limit	Upper limit	Z-value	P-value
Bonenkamp et al. [30]	2.680	1.870	3.840	5.371	0.000
Cuschieri et al. [31]	4.450	2.868	6.905	6.660	0.000
Ichikawa et al. [32]	24.000	19.931	28.900	33.528	0.000
Weitz et al. [33]	2.070	1.260	3.400	2.873	0.004
Katai et al. [34]	6.600	1.504	28.970	2.500	0.012
Wu et al. [35]	5.840	1.932	17.656	3.126	0.002
Yu et al. [18]	1.899	0.798	4.519	1.450	0.147
Zhang et al. [36]	1.355	0.469	3.911	0.562	0.574
Nobuoka et al. [37]	3.741	1.838	7.614	3.638	0.000
Marchet et al. [3]	4.660	2.230	9.739	4.092	0.000
Overall effect (meta-risk) *	**4.019**	1.758	9.190	3.297	**0.001**

Statistics for each study

Odds ratio and 95% CI

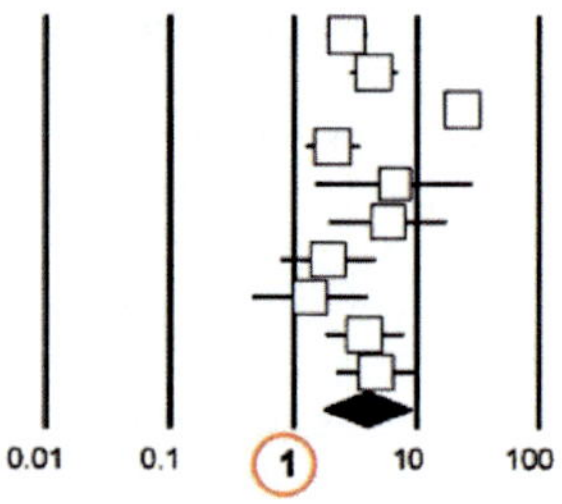

* random effects model

Fig. 12.1 Risk of postoperative complications after gastrectomy: splenectomy versus spleen preservation (preliminary meta-analysis)

spleen and in those with macroscopic intra-operative involvement of the lymph nodes of the splenic hilum or the distal splenic artery. In T4 tumors of the greater curvature, splenectomy can be considered an option. In all other cases, splenectomy should be avoided.

12.4 Lymphadenectomy

The number of metastatic lymph nodes and the ratio between the number of metastatic lymph nodes and the number of lymph nodes examined are among the most important prognostic factors for patients with gastric cancer who undergo radical surgery [3, 20, 21]. The real benefit of extended lymphadenectomy in the treatment of advanced gastric cancer radically resected is still debated in Western countries.

In the Dutch trial published in 1999, the authors concluded that their results did not support the routine use of D2 lymphadenectomy in patients with gastric cancer. Instead, they considered D1 as the standard treatment. The same authors, in a study published in 2004 after a longer follow-up, showed a statistically significant survival advantage for D2 vs. D1 lymphadenectomy only in some patients subgroups (N2 involvement), but noted that it was difficult to identify patients with N2 disease. Therefore, considering the high morbidity and mortality of D2 lymphadenectomy, it was concluded that extended lymph node dissection may be of benefit if morbidity and mortality can be avoided. Recently, the Dutch study results were reviewed. After a 15-year follow-up, the rates of both locoregional recurrence and gastric-cancer-related death were lower after D2 lymphadenectomy than after D1 surgery. Since a technique preserving the spleen and pancreas can be used to reduce surgical morbidity, the authors supported D2 lymphadenectomy as the surgical approach recommended for patients with resectable gastric cancer. In Western countries, these results should definitively answer any questions regarding the extent of lymphadenectomy [20-22].

On the other hand, several studies reported that the total number of removed lymph nodes directly correlates with the survival of patients treated by radical resection. It was also demonstrated that the morbidity and mortality of D2 lymphadenectomy are similar to that of D1 lymphadenectomy in high-volume hospitals, when the procedure is performed by dedicated surgeons [23]. In addition, the results of more recent Western studies on adjuvant chemotherapy showed that when D2 lymphadenectomy is routinely performed, the 5-year survival rate of control arm patients is very high, ranging from 43 to 50% [24]. In the MAGIC and SWOG trials, in which D2 lymphadenectomy was performed in 40 and 10% of patients, respectively, the 5-year survival rates for the treatment arms ranged from 36 to 40% [25, 26]. According to these findings, one can hypothesize that in the UK and USA studies potentially inadequate surgery might have been counterbalanced by chemotherapy/radiotherapy.

12.4.1 Conclusions

In the light of these results, we consider D2 dissection with the removal of at least 16 lymph nodes as the optimal treatment and staging for patients with T2–T4a gastric cancer. A more extensive lymphadenectomy (D3) is not recommended as it is associated with a high incidence of complications and provides no survival advantage [27].

12.5 Mini-invasive Surgery

In recent years, laparoscopy-assisted distal gastrectomy (LADG) has been introduced into clinical practice in the treatment of gastric cancer patients. The results reported in the literature demonstrate that this surgical approach, if performed by "expert hands," can be considered as feasible and safe when the principles of radical surgery are met. Compared to conventional open distal gastrectomy (CODG), LADG is associated with significantly lower blood loss and generally with lower complication rates, shorter time to resumption of oral intake, and an earlier discharge from the hospital; however, during LADG, significantly fewer lymph nodes are removed [28]. A recent meta-analysis demonstrated a similar time to disease recurrence for CODG and LADG, whereas the survival results of LADG vs. CODG cannot be currently determined due to the scarcity of studies published so far on this subject.

References

1. Axon A (2006) Symptoms and diagnosis of gastric cancer at early curable stage. Best Pract Res Clin Gastroenterol 20:697-708
2. Gospodarowicz M, Wittekind C, Sobin L (2009) UICC TNM classification of malignant tumours. 7th edition
3. Marchet A, Mocellin S, Ambrosi A et al (2007) The ratio between metastatic and examined lymph nodes (N ratio) is an independent prognostic factor in gastric cancer regardless of the type of lymphadenectomy: results from an Italian multicentric study in 1853 patients. Ann Surg 245:543-552
4. D. Nitti, A. Marchet, S. Mocellin et al (2009) Prognostic value of subclassification of T2 tumours in patients with gastric cancer. Br J Surg 96: 398-404
5. Fotia G, Marrelli D, De Stefano A et al (2004) Factors influencing outcome in gastric cancer involving muscularis and subserosal layer. Eur J Surg Oncol 30:930-934
6. Sarela AI, Turnbull AD, Coit DG et al (2003) Accurate lymph node staging is of greater prognostic importance than subclassification of the T2 ategory for gastric adenocarcinoma. Ann Surg Oncol 10:783-791
7. Komatsu S, Ichikawa D, Kurioka H et al (2005) Prognostic and clinical evaluation of patients with T2 gastric cancer. Hepatogastroenterology 52:965-968
8. Abe S, Yoshimura H, Nagoaka S et al (1995) Long-term results of operation for carcinoma of the stomach in T1/T2 stages: critical evaluation of the concept of Early Gastric Carcinoma of the stomach. J Am Coll Surg 181:389-396
9. Isozaki H, Fujii K, Nomura E et al (1999) Prognostic factors of advanced gastric carcinoma without serosal invasion (pT2 gastric carcinoma). Hepatogastroenterology 46:2669-2672
10. Hohenberger P, Gretschel S (2003) Gastric Cancer. Lancet 362:305-315
11. Siewert JR, Bittcher K, Stein HJ, Roder JD (1998) Relevant prognostic factors in gastric cancer. Ten-year results of the German Gastric cancer Study. Ann Surg 228:449-461
12. Park do J, Kong SH, Lee HJ et al (2007) Subclassification of pT2 gastric adenocarcinoma according to depth of invasion (pT2a vs pT2b) and lymph node status (pN). Surgery 141(6):757-63
13. Morgagni P, Marfisi C, Gardini A et al (2009) Subtotal gastrectomy as treatment for distal multifocal early gastric cancer. J Gastrointest Surg 13:2239-44
14. Bozzetti F, Marubini E, Bonfanti G et al (1999) Subtotal versus total gastrectomy for gastric cancer: five-year survival rates in a multicenter randomized Italian trial. Italian Gastrointestinal Tumor Study Group. Ann Surg 230:170-178
15. Songun I, Bonenkamp JJ, Hermans J et al (1996) Prognostic value of resection-line involvement in patients undergoing curative resections for gastric cancer. Eur J Cancer 32:433-437
16. Morgagni P, Garcea D, Marrelli D et al (2006) Does resection line involvement affect prognosis in early gastric cancer patients? An Italian multicentric study. World J Surg 30:585-589
17. Maruyama K, Sasako M, Kinoshita T et al (1995) Pancreas-preserving total gastrectomy for proximal gastric cancer. World J Surg19:532-536
18. Yu W, Choi GS, Chung HY (2006) Randomized clinical trial of splenectomy versus splenic preservation in patients with proximal gastric cancer. Br J Surg 93:559-563
19. Bonenkamp JJ, Hermans J, Sasako M et al (1999) Extended lymph-node dissection for gastric cancer. N Engl J Med 340:908-914
20. Dicken BJ, Bigam DL, Cass C et al (2005) Gastric adenocarcinoma: review and considerations for future directions. Ann Surg 241:27-39
21. Nitti D, Marchet A, Olivieri M et al (2003) Ratio between metastatic and examined lymph nodes is an independent prognostic factor after D2 resection for gastric cancer:

analysis of a large European monoinstitutional experience. Ann Surg Oncol 10:1077-1085
22. Songun I, Putter H, Kranenbarg EM et al (2010) Surgical treatment of gastric cancer: 15-year follow-up results of the randomised nationwide Dutch D1D2 trial. Lancet Oncol 11:439-449
23. Birkmeyer JD, Stukel TA, Siewers AE et al (2003) Surgeon volume and operative mortality in the United States. N Engl J Med 349:2117-2127
24. Nitti D, Wils J, Dos Santos JG et al (2006) Randomized phase III trials of adjuvant FAMTX or FEMTX compared with surgery alone in resected gastric cancer. A combined analysis of the EORTC GI Group and the ICCG. Ann Oncol 17:262-269
25. Cunningham D, Allum WH, Stenning SP et al (2006) Perioperative chemotherapy versus surgery alone for resectable gastroesophageal cancer. N Engl J Med 355:11-20
26. Macdonald JS, Smalley SR, Benedetti J et al (2001) Chemoradiotherapy after surgery compared with surgery alone for adenocarcinoma of the stomach or gastroesophageal junction. N Engl J Med 345:725-730
27. Kodera Y, Sasako M, Yamamoto S et al (2005) Identification of risk factors for the development of complications following extended and superextended lymphadenectomies for gastric cancer. Br J Surg 92:1103-1109
28. Shunsuke H, Yuichi A, Hiroshi O et al (2006) Meta-analysis of short-term outcomes after laparoscopy-assisted distal gastrectomy. World J Gastroenterol 12:7676-7683
29. Kun Yang, Xin-Zu Chen, Jian-Kun Hu et al (2009) Effectiveness and safety of splenectomy for gastric carcinoma: A meta-analysis. World J Gastroenterol 15:5352-5359
30. Bonenkamp JJ, Songun I, Hermans J et al (1995) Randomised comparison of morbidity after D1 and D2 dissection for gastric cancer in 996 Dutch patients. Lancet 345:745-748
31. Cuschieri A, Fayers P, Fielding J et al (1996) Postoperative morbidity and mortality after D1 and D2 resections for gastric cancer: preliminary results of the MRC randomised controlled surgical trial. The Surgical Cooperative Group. Lancet 347:995-999
32. Ichikawa D, Kurioka H, Yamaguchi T et al (2004) Postoperative complications following gastrectomy for gastric cancer during the last decade. Hepatogastroenterology 51:613-617
33. Weitz J, Jaques DP, Brennan M et al (2004) Association of splenectomy with postoperative complications in patients with proximal gastric and gastroesophageal junction cancer. Ann Surg Oncol 11:682-689
34. Katai H, Yoshimura K, Fukagawa T et al (2005) Risk factors for pancreas-related abscess after total gastrectomy. Gastric Cancer 8:137-141
35. Wu CW, Chang IS, Lo SS et al (2006) Complications following D3 gastrectomy: post hoc analysis of a randomized trial. World J Surg 30:12-16
36. Zhang CH, Zhan WH, He YL et al (2007) Spleen preservation in radical surgery for gastric cardia cancer. Ann Surg Oncol 14:1312-1319
37. Nobuoka D, Gotohda N, Konishi M et al (2008) Prevention of postoperative pancreatic fistula after total gastrectomy. World J Surg 32:2261-2266

13 Multivisceral Resection for Locally Advanced Gastric Cancer

Fabio Pacelli, Giacomo Cusumano, Fausto Rosa, and Giovan Battista Doglietto

Abstract

The role of multivisceral resection in the setting of locally advanced gastric cancer is still unclear. Previous study studies have reported a higher risk of perioperative morbidity and mortality, with little objective benefit in survival. Accordingly, this approach has been recommended only for selected cases. By contrast, recent studies have shown the feasibility of enlarged resections and the potential advantage of extended resection for clinical T4bN0 gastric adenocarcinoma, with good long-term results. In this chapter, we analyze the state of the art of multivisceral resection for locally advanced gastric cancer, paying particular attention to the short- and long-term outcomes and to the prognostic value of many clinicopathological factors.

Keywords

T4 gastric cancer • Combined organ resection • Prognostic factors • Extended surgery • Survival

13.1 Introduction

Patients with locally advanced gastric cancer have a poor prognosis, especially when compared to patients with early gastric cancer. Globally, extensive radical surgery, aiming at R0 resection, seems to be the most important indicator of long-term survival [1-3]. In the setting of locally advanced gastric cancer, some studies have shown the feasibility of enlarged resections and the potential advantage of extended resection for clinical T4bN0 gastric adenocarcinoma to improve the R0 resection rate of these lesions [4, 5]. Conversely, other studies have reported a higher risk of perioperative morbidity and mortality, with little objective benefit in survival, suggesting this approach only for selected cases [6, 7]. Many potential clinicopathological factors, such as age, tumor size, macroscopic type, depth of invasion, nodal status, distant metastasis, number of resections, and type of resection, have been examined [8-12], but the prognostic value of multivisceral resections in this subset of patients remains controversial.

13.2 Definitions and Indications

The term "locally advanced gastric cancer" refers to tumors infiltrating or adherent to adjacent organs and/or structures with or without lymph node involvement in patients without distant

F. Pacelli (✉)
Digestive Surgery Unit,
Dept. of Surgical Sciences,
Catholic University of Rome, "A. Gemelli" Hospital,
Rome, Italy

G. de Manzoni, F. Roviello, W. Siquini (eds.), *Surgery in the Multimodal Management of Gastric Cancer*,

metastases. With respect to radiation- and chemotherapy-based protocols, gastric carcinomas are considered non-resectable if there is evidence of peritoneal involvement, distant metastases, or locally advanced disease, such as invasion or encasement of major blood vessels [13].

Considering R0 resection as the best therapeutic result and that microscopic infiltration of adjacent organs cannot be confirmed preoperatively or even intraoperatively, the rationale for multivisceral resections is that dissection between the gastric tumor and the adjacent structures should be avoided because of the risk of neoplastic seeding or persistent microscopic residual disease. In addition, when there is suspicion of tumor invasion of a nearby organ, the resection must involve the tumor en bloc with the surrounding tissues.

Even if this concept is well established for many tumors, gastric cancer with T4b invasion represents a particular challenge. In fact, extirpation of the tumor, in some cases, can increase surgical difficulties and increase the likelihood of post-surgical complications. This is particularly true when we consider organs such as the pancreas, esophagus, duodenum, and liver. In addition, T4b invasion is associated with a major tendency of lymph node and peritoneal diffusion, with a lower rate of survival of these patients. Finally, preoperative evaluation to confirm T4a and T4b disease is still inaccurate. Nevertheless, this is a crucial point to minimize unnecessary organ resections in patients with earlier stage disease. Based on all these considerations, the indications for surgery are not completely defined with respect to the number of organs to be resected and the type of resection. Instead, further investigations are needed.

13.3 Postoperative Outcomes

Patients undergoing extended resections experience considerable postoperative morbidity and mortality. In fact, postoperative complications rates in patients undergoing additional organ resection with gastrectomy are reportedly higher than in patients undergoing gastrectomy alone [14, 15]. This increase in overall complications has been implicated in the reduced overall survival associated with multivisceral resections and the skepticism regarding these procedures in patients with T4b disease.

A large retrospective study by Kasakura et al. [15] found that there was no difference in survival between patients undergoing gastrectomy alone and patients with additional organ resection, but there was a higher complication rate. Some retrospective studies evaluating outcomes of patients undergoing total gastrectomy alone, with splenectomy, pancreaticosplenectomy, or esophagectomy showed a survival disadvantage for gastrectomy with additional organ resection [16-19]. This was supported by other studies [4, 6, 10] reporting lower survival in patients undergoing organ resection involving more than one organ.

As shown in Table 13.1, while taking into account the poor homogeneity of studies in the literature, more recent series have shown that gastrectomy with additional organ resection for gastric cancer can be performed with acceptable perioperative morbidity and mortality. Indeed, some authors [5] recommend resection in patients with T4b gastric carcinoma regardless of curability.

13.4 Long-term Results and Prognostic Factors

The main bias of the retrospective studies that have examined multivisceral resection is patient selection, since the patient population in many of them consisted of patients with advanced-stage disease, including peritoneal or metastatic diffusion. This aspect can explain the large differences in long-term results among the different reports. However, the majority still showed an advantage, in terms of 5-year survival, in patients who underwent gastrectomy with multivisceral resections when compared with patients undergoing gastrectomy alone or palliative surgery [4, 8, 20]. Extended surgeries are recommended because better local control of gastric cancer can be achieved with not negligible 5-year survival rates (19.9–38% in different series), as shown in Table 13.1.

Prognostic factors for patients with T4b gastric cancer after multiorgan resection were also investigated but among the features considered in those studies remain a source of great variability. Nevertheless, the features most often identified as

Table 13.1 Main series and results

Series	Year	Cases (*N.*)	PO morbidity	PO mortality	5-year survival	Negative prognostic factors
Isozaki [22]	2000	86	n.r.	n.r.	35%	Tumor location, N+, depth of invasion, extent of lymph node dissection
Saito [12]	2001	156	n.r.	n.r.	38%	R+ resection; peritoneal and liver metastasis
Dhar]19]	2001	150	31.3%	2.6%	25.1%[b]	Splenectomy; esophageal invasion
Piso [24]	2004	33[a]	36%	9%	24%	R+ resection
Carboni [8]	2005	65	27.7%	12.3%	21.8%	R+ resection
Martin [4]	2002	268	n.r.	3.7%	32%	Depth of invasion; nodal status
Kim [5]	2006	95	n.r.	n.r.	19.9%	N+ status
Oñate-Ocaña [11]	2008	74	39%	10.7%	35%	M+ status, Albumin levels, presence of ascites
Kim [20]	2009	34	11,7%	0%	37.8%	R+ resection
Ozer [10]	2009	56	37.5%	12.5%	28.1% [b]	Advanced age, N+ status; resection >1 additional organ
Jeong [7]	2009	47	31.7%	3.3%	31.5%	R+ resection; N3 status
Our series*	2011	112	33.9%	3.6%	27.2%	R+ resection; N status

n.r., not reported; [a]only pancreatic resections; [b]3-year survival.
*Series from the Italian Research Group for Gastric Cancer Study (GIRCG): Digestive Surgery Unit, Catholic University of Rome; Surgical Oncology Unit, University of Siena; Surgery Unit, University of Padova; Upper G.I. Surgery Division, University of Verona.

independent prognostic factors are: completeness of resection, number and type of resected organs, lymph node metastasis, depth of invasion, and peritoneal spreading. These are addressed individually below.

13.5 Completeness of Resection

The main prognostic factor, confirmed in almost every study, is completeness of resection. The 5-year survival rate in patients with T4b gastric cancer undergoing curative resection (R0 resection) ranges from 23 to 46% (Table 13.1). This rate decreases to 17.5–0% in patients undergoing R+ resection [5-8]. Although the study of Kim DY et al. [5] recommended resection in patients with locally advanced gastric carcinoma, regardless of curability, the power of completeness of resection has been globally demonstrated whereas the costs-benefits balance, considering the higher perioperative risks of morbidity and mortality, remains to be evaluated in further studies.

13.6 Number of Resected Organs

According to some studies, the number of resected organs is associated with a poor prognosis [4, 6, 10]. However, the majority of recent reports found that the number of resected organs was not an independent predictor of survival. In addition, there was no statistically significant difference in survival between patients undergoing en bloc resection of one organ and those who had two or five resected organs. As in other series, those reports concluded that the involvement of several organs should not be a contraindication for surgery [5, 7, 20].

13.7 Type of Resected Organs

The most common combination of resected organs is the stomach and the spleen, pancreas, or transverse colon. Many studies have investigated the influence of the additionally resected organ but the data are conflicting. In some studies [18, 19], patients with colon or mesocolon invasion had a significant survival advantage over those with other organ invasions. As for splenectomy, some studies have shown that it is a negative predictor of survival in the treatment of gastric cancer [19, 21], while others found no differences in survival or concluded that the results depended on disease stage [4, 7, 22, 23]. The data regarding pancreatic resections are similar and are often reported together with those for splenectomy [18, 24].

Finally, even in the case of esophageal involvement there are contrasting findings, with several authors suggesting that esophageal invasion does not adversely influence long-term results while, for example in the study of Dhar et al. [19], esophageal invasion was an independent negative prognostic factor in patients with T4b gastric carcinoma, with a relative risk of 2.11.

However, beyond the differences between studies, most of the more recent reports affirm that, on multivariate analysis, splenectomy, pancreatico-splenectomy, colectomy, or the resection of any other organ is not a predictor of poor survival [5, 7, 16].

13.8 Lymph Node Involvement and Depth of Invasion

The depth of invasion and the presence and extent of lymph node metastasis are the most powerful determinants of survival following R0 resection. The study of Martin et al. [4], in which only patients who underwent complete resection were considered, showed that nodal status and T status were independent prognostic factors at multivariate analysis while the T dimension was confirmed only in univariate analysis. Along the same lines, other authors [9, 12] confirmed the prognostic power of lymph node metastatic involvement and added roles for tumor diameter and infiltration pattern.

Finally, the importance of lymph node involvement has been reported in almost all studies, demonstrating the negative power of the presence of lymph node involvement (N+) [4, 5, 22], or only in the case of extensive lymph node metastatic diffusion (N3+) [7], or depending on the number of lymph nodes involved [9].

13.9 Conclusions

In summary, even though patients undergoing extended resections experience considerable post-operative morbidity and mortality, en bloc multi-visceral resection should be the therapeutic choice in patients: (a) with good clinical performance, (b) who have locally advanced gastric cancer without distant metastasis or peritoneal spreading, and (c) in whom complete resection can be realistically obtained. Therefore, in gastrectomy with additional organ resection careful patient selection is mandatory and the procedure should be limited to patients with T4b tumors. Improvements in preoperative assessment to confirm T4a and T4b disease are needed to reduce unnecessary organ resections in patients with earlier stage disease.

References

1. Desai AM, Pareek M, Nightingale PG, Fielding JW (2004) Improving outcomes in gastric cancer over 20 years. Gastric Cancer 7:196-201
2. Michelassi F, Takanishi DM Jr, Pantalone D et al (1994) Analysis of clinicopathologic prognostic features in patients with gastric adenocarcinoma. Surgery 116:804-809
3. Yu CC, Levison DA, Dunn JA et al (1995) Pathological prognostic factors in the second British stomach cancer group trial of adjuvant therapy in resectable gastric cancer. Br J Cancer 71:1106–1110
4. Martin RC 2nd, Jaques DP, Brennan MF, Karpeh M (2002) Extended local resection for advanced gastric cancer: increased survival versus increased morbidity. Ann Surg 236:159-65
5. Kim DY, Joo JK, Seo KW et al (2006) T4 gastric carcinoma: the benefit of non-curative resection. ANZ J Surg 76:453-457
6. Kodama I, Takamiya H, Mizutani K et al (1997) Gastrectomy with combined resection of other organs for carcinoma of the stomach with invasion to adjacent organs: clinical efficacy in a retrospective study. J Am Coll Surg 184:16-22
7. Jeong O, Choi WY, Park YK (2009) Appropriate selection of patients for combined organ resection in cases of gastric carcinoma invading adjacent organs. J Surg Oncol 100:115-120
8. Carboni F, Lepiane P, Santoro R et al (2005) Extended multiorgan resection for T4 gastric carcinoma: 25-year experience. J Surg Oncol 90:95-100
9. Kunisaki C, Akiyama H, Nomura M et al (2006) Surgical outcomes in patients with T4 gastric carcinoma. J Am Coll Surg 202:223-230
10. Ozer I, Bostanci EB, Orug T et al (2009) Surgical outcomes and survival after multiorgan resection for locally advanced gastric cancer. Am J Surg 198:25-30

11. Oñate-Ocaña LF, Becker M, Carrillo JF et al (2008) Selection of best candidates for multiorgan resection among patients with T4 gastric carcinoma. J Surg Oncol 98:336-42
12. Saito H, Tsujitani S, Maeda Y et al (2001) Combined resection of invaded organs in patients with T4 gastric carcinoma. Gastric Cancer 4:206-211
13. National comprehensive cancer network (NCCN) Clinical Practice Guidelines in Oncology (2010) http://www.nccn. org/professionals/physician_gls/PDF/gastric.pdf Accessed 14 August 2010
14. Cuschieri A, Fayers P, Fielding J et al (1996) Postoperative morbidity and mortality after D1 and D2 resections for gastric cancer: preliminary results of the MRC randomised controlled surgical trial. The Surgical Cooperative Group. Lancet 347:995–999
15. Kasakura Y, Fujii M, Mochizuki F et al (2000) Is there a benefit of pancreaticosplenectomy with gastrectomy for advanced gastric cancer? Am J Surg 179:237-242
16. Brady MS, Rogatko A, Dent LL et al (1991) Effect of splenectomy on morbidity and survival following curative gastrectomy for carcinoma. Arch Surg 126:359-364
17. Otsuji E, Yamaguchi T, Sawai K et al (1999) Total gastrectomy with simultaneous pancreaticosplenectomy or splenectomy in patients with advanced gastric carcinoma. Br J Cancer 79:1789-1793
18. Korenaga D, Okamura T, Baba H et al (1988) Results of resection of gastric cancer extending to adjacent organs. Br J Surg. 75:12-15
19. Dhar DK, Kubota H, Tachibana M et al (2001) Prognosis of T4 gastric carcinoma patients: an appraisal of aggressive surgical treatment. J Surg Oncol 76:278-282
20. Kim JH, Jang YJ, Park SS et al (2009) Surgical outcomes and prognostic factors for T4 gastric cancers. Asian J Surg 32:198-204
21. Suehiro S, Nagasue N, Ogawa Y et al (1984) The negative effect of sple- nectomy on the prognosis of gastric cancer. Am J Surg 148:645-648
22. Isozaki H, Tanaka N, Tanigawa N, Okajima K (2000) Prognostic factors in patients with advanced gastric cancer with macroscopic invasion to adjacent organs treated with radical surgery. Gastric Cancer 3:202-210
23. Koga S, Kaibara N, Kimura O et al (1981) Prognostic significance of combined splenectomy or pancreaticosplenectomy in total and proximal gastrectomy for gastric cancer. Am J Surg 142:546-550
24. Piso P, Bellin T, Aselmann H et al (2002) Results of combined gastrectomy and pancreatic resection in patients with advanced primary gastric carcinoma. Dig Surg19:281-285

Surgical Treatment of Liver Metastases from Gastric Cancer

14

Guido A.M. Tiberio, Arianna Coniglio, Gian Luca Baiocchi, and Stefano M. Giulini

Abstract

After a brief description of the clinical characteristics of hepatic metastases from gastric cancer and their different clinical settings, we discuss the natural evolution of the disease, focusing on the extremely poor prognosis of these patients. Through a complete review of the literature, the chapter provides detailed insight into the different therapeutic options, discussing their indications, patient selection criteria, and results. We argue that a correct therapeutic approach can offer to a relatively large percentage of patients (~ 40%) an unexpected 20–40% 5-year survival rate. Our main purpose is to convey the cultural basis that will induce the reader to reconsider the largely predominating passive attitude toward these patients by acknowledging the opportunity to offer better and longer survival to a selected subgroup.

Keywords

Gastric cancer • Hepatic metastases • Synchronous liver metastases • Metachronous liver metastases • Curative intent • Prognostic factor • Treatment • Hepatic resection • Chemotherapy • Best supportive treatment • Radiofrequency ablation • Prognosis

14.1 Clinical Setting

The liver is the most frequent site of hematogenous metastases from gastric cancer, due to the convergence of the gastric venous and lymphatic drainage into the portal bloodstream. Although the real incidence is difficult to assess, hepatic metastases are believed to appear in about 40% of patients with gastric cancer during the course of the disease. At diagnosis, synchronous metastases are detected in 5–20% of patients; among patients submitted to curative gastric resection, 25–30% are eventually diagnosed with metachronous metastases. In both cases, there is an equal distribution between patients with exclusive hepatic involvement and those with concurrent extrahepatic disease, such as peritoneal dissemination, extensive lymph node metastases, or direct neoplastic infiltration of adjacent organs [1, 2].

Synchronous metastases are discovered at the same time as the gastric primary and must be differentiated from direct infiltration of the liver parenchyma by gastric tumors. They can originate from locally advanced, unresectable gastric cancers but also from resectable primaries. More than

G.A.M. Tiberio (✉)
Surgical Clinic,
Dept. of Medical and Surgical Sciences,
University of Brescia,
Brescia, Italy

G. de Manzoni, F. Roviello, W. Siquini (eds.), *Surgery in the Multimodal Management of Gastric Cancer*,

80% of metachronous metastases are detected during early postoperative follow-up (24 months) [3] but there is a general consensus that lesions diagnosed during the very first postoperative period (~ 6 months) are considered as synchronous.

Liver metastases are typically encountered in four clinical conditions: (a) detection of metastatic liver disease leading to diagnosis of gastric cancer; (b) routine work-up of gastric cancer, during which hepatic metastases are detected; (c) intraoperative detection of initially unrecognized hepatic metastases; and (d) detection of hepatic metastases during post-gastrectomy follow-up. Only in the first setting it is possible to recognize metastases-related symptoms; in the other cases, patients are asymptomatic or may display signs and symptoms of gastric tumor.

Clinical examination searches for epigastric or hypochondriac masses and hepatomegaly while signs of peritoneal carcinosis may be detected at rectal examination. Tumor markers are CA 19-9, CEA and CA 72-4. When simultaneously positive, they are strongly suggestive of liver involvement [4].

Metastases from gastric cancer display hypodense and hypo-vascularized patterns at ultrasound and computed tomography imaging and are similar to hepatic metastases from other gastro-enteric primaries. The number, size measurements and location of hepatic metastases, the latter in reference to Couinaud's segmentation, should be described in any radiological report.

Metastatic liver involvement is generally staged according to the system of the Japanese Gastric Cancer Association [5], a simple yet practical classification with direct therapeutic implications (Table 14.1).

Table 14.1 Classification of hepatic metastases from gastric cancer as proposed by the Japanese Gastric Cancer Association [5]

H0	No liver metastases
H1	Liver metastases limited to one lobe of the liver
H2	Isolated diverse metastases in both lobes of the liver
H3	Multiple distributed metastases in both lobes of the liver

14.2 Management of Hepatic Metastases from Gastric Cancer

The positive results achieved by an aggressive multidisciplinary approach to liver metastases from colorectal cancer have not been reproduced in gastric cancer, seemingly due to the biological aggressiveness of the disease. In fact, in the majority of cases, liver metastases are multiple and show a bilobar distribution; when a favorable hepatic involvement exists, it is often associated with extrahepatic disease. Under these conditions, surgery is contraindicated and patients are generally addressed to palliative or, more often, supportive treatments, albeit without appreciable long-term benefit. The standard protocols of chemotherapy offer a certain amelioration of the results compared to supportive treatments. Median survival ranges from 7 to 15 months but long-term survival remains anecdotal [6-8]. In particular, considering the few trials evaluating systemic chemotherapy in the subset of patients with liver-only metastatic involvement, 5-years survival rates do not reach 2% [9].

The recent literature shows that a selected subgroup of patients, accounting for 10–35% of all cases with liver metastases, are candidates for hepatic resection, associated with curative gastrectomy in the presence of synchronous lesions. Resection of liver metastases from gastric cancer is indicated in the absence of extrahepatic disease when complete resection of the metastases can be achieved while preserving postoperative liver function [10, 11]. If these requirements are met, then hepatectomy is a low-risk procedure, with negligible mortality and morbidity rates. The prognosis after hepatectomy remains severe, as intrahepatic recurrence is observed in about two-thirds of patients, but 5-year survival rates of 10–40% have consistently been reported. Notwithstanding, surgery is rarely performed. A recent literature review reported only 436 cases [12], and a French survey recruited only 101 patients from 41 centers [13]. At least in Western countries, a passive attitude toward these patients prevails, as shown by a GIRCG survey reporting that over 60% of patients do not receive specific treatments, including 30% of those with one or two small metastases, and that therapeutic indications are influenced by the patients'

Table 14.2 Series of selected populations submitted to surgical treatment of hepatic metastases

Author [Reference]	N.	T	N	G	H	Ø metastasis	Timing	Margin	MST (months)	N. survivors > 5 years (%)
Ochiai [14]	21	√	√	–	–	n.a.	n.a.	n.a.	18	2 (19)
Miyazaki [15]	21	–	–	–	√	n.a.	–	√	n.a.	2 (9.5)
Fuji [16]	10	–	–	–	–	√	√	n.a.	16	1 (10)
Ambiru [11]	40	–	–	–	–	–	–	√	12	6 (15)
Imamura [17]	17	–	√	√	–	n.a	√	√	12	0
Okano [10]	19	–	–	√	√	–	√	n.a.	21	4 (21)
Zacherl [18]	15	–	–	–	√	–	√	–	8.8	2 (13)[a]
Saiura [19]	10	–	–	–	–	–	–	n.a.	25	2 (20)
Shirabe [20]	36	–	ly	–	√	–	–	–	n.a.	4 (11)
Roh [21]	11	n.a.	–	–	n.a.	–	–	–	19	2 (18)
Chiche [13]	101	–	–	–	√	√	–	√	14,5	11 (10)
Sakamoto [22]	37	√	–	–	√	√	–	–	31	2 (5.4)
Koga [23]	42	√	–	–	√	–	–	–	34	8 (19)
Tsujimoto [24]	17	√	ly	n.a.	–	–	–	n.a.	34	5 (29)

MST, Median survival time; √, prognostic factor; *n.a*, not available; *ly*, lymphatic invasion; [a] alive after 3 years.

determination [3].

In order to promote a pragmatic approach to these patients, recognition of cases that may benefit from surgical treatment can be critical. Various series [10, 11, 13-24] have demonstrated that several clinical and pathological parameters correlate with survival; among these, staging factors of the primary tumor as well as metastases-related and surgery-related variables have been reported more often than others (Table 14.2). Interestingly, however, literature-reported analyses of long-term survivors also show that, if patients presenting with bilobar spread of metastases (H3) are excluded, none of the reported predictive factors, either alone or in combination, are sufficient grounds to deprive a patient of the possibility of long-term survival after hepatic resection. This, in turn, raises concern about the clinical value of prognostic factors emerging from small and super-selected populations submitted to liver resection.

Recently, four papers addressed this topic, analyzing relatively unselected populations of gastric cancer patients who presented with hepatic metastases as the sole site of extrahepatic disease (Table 14.3). In Korea, Cheon et al. [25] studied a cohort of 58 patients and did not find any primary-tumor-related or metastases-related factor of prognostic significance. In Japan, Makino et al. reached similar conclusions in an analysis of 63 cases [26].

Ueda et al., also from Japan [27], studied a cohort of 73 patients who presented with synchronous metastases. Their analysis demonstrated that factors influencing survival were the extent of hepatic involvement (H1/H2 vs. H3) and the presence of macroscopic peritoneal dissemination (P0 vs. P1) at surgical exploration. Focusing on the subgroup of H1/H2 and P0 patients, they showed that the number (1 vs. >1) and size of the hepatic metastases and the N status of the gastric cancer (N0/N1 vs. N2/N3) influenced survival. An Italian survey performed under the auspices of the Italian Research Group on Gastric Cancer [3] studied an unselected cohort of 73 patients who presented with metachronous metastases after curative $D \geq 2$ gastrectomy. The T, N, and G of the gastric primary, when rated T3/T4, N+ and G3, were found to independently display a clear negative prognostic value with cumulative effect.

French authors [28] have stressed that prognostic factors can be helpful in appropriately selecting patients for surgical intervention or, at least, for multidisciplinary evaluation, bearing in mind that the prognosis of these patients is decidedly influenced by therapeutic choices. In fact, all four of the above-mentioned studies strongly highlighted that the main factor influencing long-term survival (p = 0.01–0.001) was the therapeutic approach to liver metastases, in particular when hepatectomy was

Table 14.3 Series considering unselected populations

Author [Reference]	N.	Timing	Prognostic factors	MST (months)	1-; 3-; 5- year survival rates
Cheon [25]	58	Synchronous + metachronous	R0 resection of hepatic metastases	Overall: 16	No hepatic resection: 29.4%; 0%; 0% Hepatic resection ± RFA: 75,3%; 31.7%; 20.8%
Makino [26]	63	Synchronous + metachronous	Resection of hepatic metastases	Overall: 16 Hepatic resection: 31.2	No hepatic resection: 53.2%; 4.2%; 0% Hepatic resection: 82,3%; 46,4%;37.1%
Ueda [27]	72	Synchronous	H; P; R0 Resection of hepatic metastases	n.a.	No hepatic resection: 36.4%; 0%; 0% Hepatic resection ± HAI: 80%; 60%; 60%
Tiberio [3]	73	Metachronous	T; N; G of gastric primary; Resection of hepatic metastases	Overall: 7 BST: 5 Chemotherapy: 12 Hepatic resection: 23	BST: 22%; 2%; 0% Chemotherapy: 45%; 6%; 0% Hepatic resection: 81%; 20%; 20%
Hwang [29]	73	Metachronous	Stage of gastric primary Extrahepatic metastases; H Treatment of hepatic metastases	BST[a]: 3 TACE[a]: 8 Chemotherapy[a]: 15 RFA[a]: 27	BST[a]: 5%; 0%; 0% TACE[a]: 38%; 0%; 0% Chemotherapy[a]: 100%; 0%; 0% RFA[a]: 8%; 50%; 40%

TNGHP, staging designations of gastric cancer and metastatic involvement; *MST*, median survival time; *n.a.*, not available; *BST*, best supportive treatment; *TACE*, trans-arterial chemoembolization; *RFA*, radiofrequency ablation; [a]patients without extrahepatic metastases.

performed. In the GIRCG study, hepatectomy was associated with a five-fold increase in the survival of patients with a less favorable prognosis (>1 negative prognostic factor), with the 5-year survival rate of that series reaching 20%. Furthermore, both Cheon et al. and Ueda et al. provided evidence that the possibility to perform a radical operation (R0 vs. R1) was a significant factor influencing long-term survival; they reported 5-year survival rates of 20 and 60%, respectively. It is worth noting that in synchronous cases radical surgery was intended to address not only the hepatic lesions, with resection as prescribed by good surgical practice, but also the gastric tumor, to be treated by standard curative D ≥ 2 gastrectomy [24, 25].

Published series report survival achieved by surgery alone, with only a few series that included postoperative adjuvant chemotherapy. Better results would therefore be possible through the systematic adoption of modern, state-of-the-art chemotherapy protocols, as suggested by Ueda, who reported an outstanding 80% 5-year survival rate in a subgroup of eight patients submitted to radical surgery followed by hepatic artery infusion chemotherapy.

Nonetheless, despite all efforts, these patients generally die of cancer progression. Hepatic recurrence is observed in about 70% of cases and in about half of them is associated to extrahepatic relapse [3, 12, 13]. This observation raises concern about the timing of treatment, in order to avoid inappropriate surgery. A simple "wait and see" strategy may be acceptable once a potential candidate for curative surgery is encountered. It can be easily suggested in patients with favourably located metachronous lesions but contraindicated in case of critically located liver metastases and, in general, in case of synchronous metastases, especially those associated with symptomatic gastric cancer. Adam et al. [28] envisaged a multidisciplinary approach to these patients and, in particular, suggested that systemic chemotherapy be started at diagnosis whenever possible, in order to offer its advantages to a greater number of patients and to effectively select cases for surgery.

The literature does not offer an adequate insight into re-do hepatectomy in case of exclusive hepatic recurrence; such reports are exceedingly rare and do not allow any conclusions to be drawn.

Some series in the literature advocate the use of radiofrequency ablation (RFA) in the treatment of metastases from gastric cancer. This ablative technique is employed either as an alternative to or in association with hepatectomy, following the therapeutic guidelines for hepatocellular carcinoma or for metastases from colo-rectal cancer. It is difficult to evaluate the exact role of this treatment as the number of reported procedures is very low and their data cannot be effectively extrapolated from the context. However, a paper by Hwang et al. [29] considered 72 patients with metachronous metastases submitted to different treatments but not to hepatectomy. The 15 patients without extrahepatic disease treated by RFA ± chemotherapy had a median survival of 22 months, with 3- and 5-year survival rates of 50 and 40%, respectively, similar to those reported in the best surgical series. These data are consistent with those of Cheon et al. [25]: in their experience, a subgroup of nine patients submitted to RFA compared favorably with 22 patients submitted to radical surgery, with a 4-year survival of 40 and 20%, respectively. These results need further confirmation but highlight the potential of RFA in the management of these particular cases. In fact, for these patients, whose general condition often contraindicates surgery, a less invasive, and less expensive, ablative technique may represent an interesting opportunity.

14.3 Conclusions

An unexpected 20–40% 5-year survival rate can be achieved in a subgroup of gastric cancer patients presenting with hepatic metastases, if adequate treatment is provided. Both the gastric primary and hepatic involvement display simple clinical and biological characteristics that are of prognostic value and may be helpful in selecting therapeutic strategy–bearing in mind that the best results are achieved by surgical treatment, which should be proposed whenever possible.

References

1. Dicken BJ, Bigam DL, Cass C et al (2005) Gastric adenocarcinoma. Review and considerations for future directions. Ann Surg 241:27-39
2. D'Angelica M, Gonen M, Brennan MF et al (2004) Patterns of initial recurrence in completely resected gastric adenocarcinoma. Ann Surg 240:808-816
3. Tiberio GAM, Coniglio A, Marchet A et al (2009) Metachronous hepatic metastases from gastric carcinoma: a multicentric survey. EJSO 35:486-491
4. Marrelli D, Roviello F, De Stefano A et al (2004) Risk factors for liver metastases after curative surgical procedures for gastric cancer: a prospective study of 208 patients treated with surgical resection. J Am Coll Surg 198:51-58
5. Japanese Gastric Cancer association (1998) Japanese classification of gastric carcinoma. 2nd English edition. Gastric Cancer 1:10-24
6. Cocconi G, Carlini P, Gamboni A et al (2003) Cisplatin, epirubicin, leucovorin and 5-fluorourail (PELF) is more active than 5-fluorouracil, doxorubicin and methotrexate (FAMTX) in advanced gastric carcinoma. Ann Oncol 14:1258-1263
7. Lee J, Kang WK, Kwon JM et al (2007) Phase II trial of irinotecan plus oxaliplatin and 5-fluorouracil/leucovorin in patients with untreated metastatic gastric adenocarcinoma. Ann Oncol 18:88-92
8. Cao W, Yang W, Lou G et al (2009) Phase II trial of infusional fluorouracil, leucovorin, oxaliplatin and irinotecan (FOLFOXIRI) as first-line treatment for advanced gastric cancer. Anticancer Drugs 20:287-293
9. Yoshida M, Ohtsu A, Boku N et al (2004) Long-term survival and prognostic factors in patients with metastatic gastric cancers treated with chemotherapy in the Japan Clinical Oncology Group (JCOG) study. JJCO 34:654-659
10. Okano K, Maeba T, Ishimura K et al (2002) Hepatic resection for metastatic tumors from gastric cancer. Ann Surg 235:86-91
11. Ambiru S, Miyazaki M, Ito H et al (2001) Benefits and limits of hepatic resection for gastric metastases. Am J Surg 181:279-283
12. Kerkar SP, Kemp CD, Avital I (2010) Liver resections in metastatic gastric cancer. HPB 12:589-596
13. Chiche L, Ducreux M, Lebreton G et al (2005) Métastases hépatiques des cancers de l'estomac. In : Adam R, Chiche L, eds. Chirurgie des métastases hépatiques de cancers non colorectaux non endocrine. Monographies de l'association Française de Chirurgie. Arnette, Paris pp 45-59
14. Ochiai T, Sasako M, Mizuno S et al (1994) Hepatic resection for metastatic tumours from gastric cancer: analysis of prognostic factors. Br J Surg 81:1175-1178
15. Miyazaki M, Itoh H, Nakagawa K et al (1997) Hepatic resection of liver metastases from gastric carcinoma. Am J Gastroenterol 92:490-493
16. Fujii K, Fujioka S, Kato K et al (2001) Resection of liver metastasis from gastric adenocarcinoma. Hepatogastroenterology 48:368-371
17. Imamura H, Matsuyama Y, Shimada R et al (2001) A study of factors influencing prognosis after resection of hepatic

metastases from colorectal and gastric carcinoma. Am J Gastroenterol 96:3178-3184
18. Zacherl J, Zacherl M, Scheuba C et al (2002) Analysis of hepatic resection of metastasis originating from gastric adenocarcinoma. J Gastrointest Surg 6:682-689
19. Saiura A, Umekita N, Inoue S et al (2002) Clinicopathological features and outcome of hepatic resection for liver metastasis from gastric cancer. Hepatogastroenterology 49:1062-1065
20. Shirabe K, Shimada M, Matsumata T et al (2003) Analysis of the prognostic factors for liver metastasis of gastric cancer after hepatic resection: a multi-institutional study of the indications for resection. Hepatogastroenterology 50:1560-1563
21. Roh HR, Suh KS, Lee HJ et al (2005) Outcome of hepatic resection for metastatic gastric cancer. Am Surg 71:95-99
22. Sakamoto Y, Sano T, Shimada K et al (2007) Favorable indications for hepatectomy in patients with liver metastasis from gastric cancer. J Surg Oncol 95:534-539
23. Koga R, Junji Y, Shigekazu O et al (2007) Liver resection for metastatic gastric cancer: experience with 42 patients including eight long-term survivors. JJCO 37:836-842
24. Tsujimoto H, Ichikura T, Ono S et al (2010) Outcomes for patients following hepatic resection of metastatic tumors from gastric cancer. Hepatol Int 4:406-413
25. Cheon SH, Rha SY, Jeung H-C et al (2008) Survival benefit of combined curative resection of the stomach (D2 resection) and liver in gastric cancer patients with liver metastases. Ann Onc 19:1146-1153
26. Makino H, Kunisaki C, Izumisawa Y et al (2010) Indication for hepatic resection in the treatment of liver metastasis from gastric cancer. Anticanc Res 30:2367-2376
27. Ueda K, Iwahashi M, Nakamori M et al (2009) Analysis of the prognostic factors and evaluation of surgical treatment for synchronous liver metastases from gastric cancer. Langenbecks Arch Surg 394:647-653
28. Adam R, Chiche L, Aloia T et al (2006) Hepatic resection for noncolorectal nonendocrine liver metastases. Ann Surg 244:524-535
29. Hwang S-E, Yang D-H, Kim C-Y (2009) Prognostic factors for survival in patients with hepatic recurrence after curative resection of gastric cancer. World J Surg 33:1468-1472

Hyperthermic Intraperitoneal Chemotherapy in Gastric Cancer: Indications and Technical Notes

15

Gianni Mura, Orietta Federici, and Alfredo Garofalo

Abstract

Synchronous and metachronous peritoneal carcinomatosis (PC) is the most important issue in gastric cancer (GC) recurrence. Progress in the therapeutic challenge posed by PC has been made through a new treatment consisting of cytoreductive surgery (CRS) and hyperthermic intraperitoneal chemotherapy (HIPEC), developed over the last two decades. This chapter provides a review of the literature and recent results. Current indications for HIPEC in GC are: for curative purposes in addition to CRS in the treatment of PC; as palliative treatment for otherwise untreatable ascites; and as adjuvant treatment in the absence of PC for tumors infiltrating the serosal layer. There is abundant evidence that a multimodality approach offers survival benefits over surgery alone. In selected patients and in experienced centers, HIPEC after radical CRS can prolong survival and reduce peritoneal recurrences. The early identification of GC patients at high risk for peritoneal disease is a task for the future.

Keywords

Gastric cancer • Peritoneal carcinomatosis • Cytoreductive surgery • Hyperthermic intraperitoneal chemotherapy • HIPEC • Surgical resection • Surgical cytoreduction • Hyperthermia, induced • Micrometastasis • Molecular biology • RT-PCR • Randomized controlled trials

15.1 Rationale

The loco-regional progression of gastric cancer (GC) frequently results in peritoneal carcinomatosis (PC), with random distribution on the peritoneal surface. The molecular mechanisms by which GC gives rise to PC remain to be clarified but may include chemokines. These small secretory proteins control the migration and activation of leukocytes and other cell types through interactions with a group of transmembrane receptors. Expression of the chemokine receptors CXCR4/CXCL12 has been shown to play a role in the development of PC from GC, as evidenced in a xenograft animal model in which treatment with a CXCR4 antagonist suppressed the PC development. Moreover, CXCR4 expression on the primary tumors of patients with advanced GC was shown to significantly correlate with the occur-

G. Mura (✉)
Dept. of Surgery,
Valdarno Hospital,
Arezzo, Italy

G. de Manzoni, F. Roviello, W. Siquini (eds.), *Surgery in the Multimodal Management of Gastric Cancer*,

rence of PC, strongly suggesting that CXCR4-expressing GC cells are preferentially attracted to the peritoneum, where the receptor's ligand, CXCL12, is abundantly produced. Growth factors such as vascular endothelial growth factor (VEGF) and VEGF-C are thought to be associated with the development of peritoneal metastasis. Furthermore, the relevance of interactions between VEGF, CXCR4, and CXCL12 in the development of peritoneal metastasis was recently demonstrated [1]. These results provide very interesting diagnostic and therapeutic perspectives for GC-related PC.

At surgical exploration, from 15 to ≥ 50% of patients present with PC, especially when there is serosal involvement by the tumor [2, 3]. The prognosis of these patients is very poor, as median survival is less than 6 months [4, 5]. PC developing from GC is likewise associated with a poor prognosis, with median survival ranging from 1–1.6 to 3.1–9 months [6]. The risk of peritoneal recurrence is particularly high in patients with diffuse Lauren's type tumors and serosal infiltration [7].

Even after curative resection of GC, there is a major problem with PC recurrence. Two Italian studies, with 441 and 200 GC patients, showed peritoneal recurrence in 17 and 32.9% at the median follow-up of 48 and 42.3 months, respectively [7, 8]. A Korean study of 500 GC patients who underwent standardized radical surgery found that, within 5 years after gastrectomy, PC is the most frequent form (51.7%) of recurrence [9]. A prospective randomized controlled trial (RCT) in Japan involving 530 patients treated with curative gastrectomy also found peritoneal recurrence as the most frequent event (15.8%) at 3 years follow-up [10].

Conventional surgery is not adequate for PC; instead, current treatments are systemic chemotherapy and palliative therapy, albeit with no hope of cure. Synchronous and metachronous PC is therefore the most important issue in GC recurrence and metastasis. Over the last two decades, a new therapeutic strategy, consisting of cytoreductive surgery (CRS) and hyperthermic intraperitoneal chemotherapy (HIPEC), has been developed. This multimodal approach takes advantage of surgery to reduce the visible tumor burden and of regional hyperthermic chemotherapy to eradicate microscopic peritoneal implants.

The well-codified surgical procedures that comprise CRS depend on the extent of peritoneal disease [2, 11]. The aim of CRS is complete macroscopic cytoreduction as a pre-condition for HIPEC. Residual disease is classified intraoperatively using the completeness of cytoreduction (CC) score. The efficacy of intraperitoneal chemotherapy reaches its highest degree in the absence of visible residual disease (CC-0) or in the presence of neoplastic residuals ≤ 2.5 mm (CC-1). The main theoretical advantage of intraperitoneal chemotherapy is that it allows the direct administration of a high local concentration of potentially effective drugs while incurring minimal systemic exposure and toxicity. Experimental studies have demonstrated that hyperthermia (42–43°C) may have an important therapeutic effect on tumor tissue when applied alone [12]; moreover, hyperthermia synergistically enhances the chemosensitivity of neoplastic cells to antimitotic agents and allows deeper penetration of drugs into tumor tissue [13].

Nowadays, HIPEC can be considered the standard treatment for peritoneal mesothelioma, pseudomyxoma peritonei, and—when a complete CRS is possible—for PC arising from colorectal cancer [5, 14]. For GC, the results are more controversial and HIPEC has yet to be adopted as standard therapy.

15.2 Indications

Current indications for HIPEC in GC patients are the following: (1) for curative purposes in addition to CRS in the treatment of PC; (2) as palliative treatment for otherwise untreatable ascites; and (3) in the absence of PC, as adjuvant treatment for tumors infiltrating the serosal layer.

15.2.1 HIPEC in the Treatment of PC

Since the first report concerning the possibility of treating PC with HIPEC and the following papers from Sugarbaker et al in the 1980s [15,16] many studies have been carried out examining cytoreduction associated with HIPEC in the treatment of PC. Series of CRS and HIPEC for GC-related PC evaluated in the late 1990s [17] reported overall median survivals between 6.6 and 27.7 months, with great improvement (up to 43 months) in patients treated by radical CRS.

In 49 consecutive patients with PC from advanced GC submitted to CRS and HIPEC, Glehen reported an overall median survival of 10.3 months; median survival was of 21.3 months for 25 of the 49 patients who received CC-0 and CC-1 surgery vs. 6.1 months for patients with residual nodules > 5 mm in diameter ($p < 0.001$) [18].

Very interesting results were recently obtained in a multi-institutional study [14] consisting of 159 patients with PC from GC (44% synchronous) among 1290 patients treated by CRS plus HIPEC for PC of nongynecologic malignancies. The overall median survival was 9.2 months and the 1-, 3-, and 5-year survival rates were 43, 18, and 13%, respectively. Median survival for the 85 CC-0 patients was 15 months with 1-, 3-, and 5-year survival rates of 61, 30, and 23%, respectively. The 37 CC-1 patients and 30 CC-2 patients had a median survival of 4 months and none of them was alive at 2 years [14]. The only independent prognostic indicator at multivariate analysis was the completeness of CRS, as confirmed by Yonemura et al. [19]. In a recent study, median survival was 43.4 months for CC-0/CC-1 patients vs. 9.5 and 7.5 months in CC-2 and CC-3 patients, respectively [20]. These results emphasize the fact that HIPEC, for this indication, should not be recommended in patients in whom complete CRS cannot be achieved.

In conclusion, CRS + HIPEC in the treatment of PC arising from GC is an aggressive combined therapy still under investigation. Notwithstanding, several studies carried out in Europe and Asia show the possibility of 5-year survival rates of ~25% until recently, an unexpected outcome.

15.2.2 HIPEC as Palliative Treatment for Neoplastic Ascites

For patients who are not candidates for CRS and who present with neoplastic therapy-resistant ascites, HIPEC is indicated as a palliative treatment. The clinical management of malignant ascites using a myriad of conventional treatment modalities has been inconsistent, temporary at best, and generally unsatisfactory. Palliative HIPEC provides definitive treatment of neoplastic ascites with resulting improvements in the quality of life of these patients. Abdominal sclerosis and the induction of dense adhesions are probably the major factor influencing the technique's efficacy. The use of video laparoscopic surgery approaches has resulted in low morbidity and mortality and limited surgical trauma, allowing possible treatment of the entire peritoneal surface. In addition, laparoscopic viscerolysis is a low-risk procedure. A complete and definitive disappearance of the ascites was observed in 94% of these patients [21, 22].

15.2.3 HIPEC in the Adjuvant Setting for Advanced GC without PC

Perhaps the most promising indication for HIPEC is as adjuvant treatment. Peritoneal recurrence develops in 60% of patients with pT4a or pT4b tumors after curative resection [23]. In serosa-invading tumors, invisible implants are already present in the peritoneal cavity at the time of curative surgery, and the peritoneum is the only site of first recurrence in 40–60% of patients [5]. Therefore, peritoneal dissemination alone usually results in the death of 20–40% of patients with GC [24].

Cytological examination of peritoneal washings at the time of primary tumor resection is frequently positive. Free peritoneal cells are associated with an average survival of 4 months vs. 21 months for patients with negative cytology [23, 25]. The majority of patients with positive cytology on peritoneal lavage develop PC, although it also occurs in patients with negative cytological results. These observations indicate that conventional cytology lacks sensitivity for the detection of residual cancer cells and the prediction of peritoneal spread. Many recent reports have emphasized the clinical significance of molecular diagnosis using reverse transcriptase-polymerase chain reaction (RT-PCR) analysis for more sensitive detection of GC cells in peritoneal lavage. Fujiwara analyzed the survival of 123 patients with serosa-invading GC. The prognosis of the 29 patients with positive cytology in the peritoneal lavage was very poor, and most of them died within 1 year after surgery. Among the 93 patients with negative cytology (CY0), 49 had a positive genetic diagnosis and a significantly poorer prognosis than those with negative genetic results. More than half of the patients with positive PCR and CY0 developed peritoneal recurrence after surgery, while almost all patients with negative PCR and CY0 had no peritoneal recurrence after surgery [26]. These results have been confirmed by many authors (e.g., [24]), who concluded that molecular diagnosis based on peritoneal lavage fluid is useful to predict peritoneal recurrence for patients with serosal invasion of GC [27].

Four prospective RCTs from Japan and Korea evaluated adjuvant HIPEC after potentially curative GC resection. The first found no significant difference between the two groups of patients, presumedly because of the small number enrolled [28], but the other three studies reported positive responses: In Fujimoto's 141 patients, HIPEC significantly reduced the incidence of peritoneal recurrence ($p < 0.001$) and improved the survival rate ($p = 0.03$) without adverse postoperative events [29]. Yonemura randomized 139 patients in three arms, surgery alone, surgery plus HIPEC, and intraperitoneal chemotherapy without hyperthermia. The 5-year survival was 61% in the HIPEC group compared to 43 and 42% in the other two groups [30]. Zhang confirmed a reduction in recurrence and an improvement in survival, both statistically significant, for patients treated with surgery plus HIPEC [31].

In 2001, the results of a controlled study of 103 patients with serosal-involving GC who underwent surgical resection alone or surgical resection plus HIPEC were published. The 5-year survival rate was significantly higher in the experimental group when patients with distant metastases were excluded ($p = 0.0379$). The most common recurrence pattern was loco-regional in the HIPEC group and peritoneal in the control group [32].

Yan systematically reviewed 13 RCTs and the ten of acceptable quality were subsequently meta-analyzed. Overall, 1648 patients with resectable advanced GC, with macroscopic serosal invasion but without distant metastases or PC, were randomly assigned to receive surgery combined with intraperitoneal chemotherapy or surgery without intraperitoneal chemotherapy. Meta-analysis established that, compared with current standard treatments, HIPEC is associated with significant improvement in the survival of patients with advanced GC ($p = 0.002$). However, the authors pointed out the need for a well-designed prospective multi-institutional RCT [33].

On the basis of the reported results and rationale, a cooperative European multicentric randomized study to determine the role of HIPEC in the prevention of peritoneal dissemination after curative GC resection in patients at high risk for peritoneal recurrence has been proposed. Its aim is to evaluate the added value of HIPEC to D2 gastric resection plus systemic therapy with respect to the survival of patients with serosal-infiltrating GC or/and free cancer cells in peritoneal washing [34].

15.3.3 Principles of Technique and Complications

HIPEC associated with surgery can be performed using either the closed or the open technique. In the closed version, after cytoreduction, gastrectomy, and anastomoses are completed, the drains are positioned and the abdominal wall is closed. HIPEC is thus initiated with the abdominal cavity closed. The position of the operating bed is changed every 15 min to facilitate circulation of the perfusate into the abdomen. In the open version, at the end of the CRS, the abdominal wall is suspended by a retractor, such as the Thompson (Thompson Surgical Instruments, Traverse City, MI, USA) or the Flexitrac (Medicon Instrumente, Tuttlingen, Germany), with stitches or clamps on the skin. The abdominal cavity is covered by a plastic sheet, thereby creating an artificially closed area. The surgeon inserts his or her hand through an incision in the sheet, and mixes the solution in order to obtain more homogeneous spreading of the perfusate in the abdomen.

With both techniques, in-flow and out-flow abdominal drains are inserted and connected to an external circuit including the pumping system and the heat exchanger. Performer-LRT (Rand, Mirandola, Italy) and Exiper (Menfis bioMedica, Bologna, Italy) are examples of modern HIPEC-dedicated devices providing an integrated system that monitors temperature, pressure, and flow. The chemotherapeutic agents are added into the circuit as soon as the abdominal temperature reaches 41.5–42.5°C. Lavage with 5% dextrose through the drains during the early postoperative period is suggested. The purpose is to prevent free cells from embedding in the fibrin, the so-called cathedrals of cancer, resulting in disease recurrence. Postoperative lavage must be performed every hour until a clear liquid is obtained and then continued every 2 h thereafter for the first 12 h postoperatively [11].

Postoperative mortality after CRS and HIPEC is 2–4%; morbidity is relatively high (25–41%) but comparable to that following major gastrointestinal surgery. The morbidity rates seem to be related to the extension of CRS rather than to the HIPEC itself. The anastomosis following total or subtotal gastrectomy in combination with CRS and HIPEC is relatively safe. In a series of 49 patients submitted to HIPEC for PC of gastric origin, 13 underwent subtotal and 26 total gastrectomy. Major complications occurred in 13 patients but no leakage at the esophago- or gastro-jejunostomy was observed [18]. Piso analyzed 37 patients who underwent gastric resection with curative intent for PC. No leakages occurred at the site of the esophageal or gastric anastomosis/suture [35].

15.4 Conclusions and Perspectives

Neither surgery alone nor systemic chemotherapy is adequate treatment for PC whereas a multimodality approach clearly offers survival benefits over the former. In selected patients and in experienced centers, HIPEC after radical CRS can prolong survival and reduce peritoneal recurrences. The surgical technique of peritonectomy is complex and has a long learning curve. To date, complete cytoreduction and HIPEC has yielded unexpected results, with 5-year survival rates of 19–25% [14, 20]. The use of HIPEC in the adjuvant setting in patients with GC infiltrating the serosal layer looks very promising, but needs to be confirmed, perhaps by the forthcoming European trial [34]. Pre-operative laparoscopy with cytology is mandatory for peritoneal staging and further therapeutic choices. The introduction into clinical practice of genetic diagnostic techniques for peritoneal lavage from patients with GC will soon increase the number of candidates for more aggressive treatments, including HIPEC [26]. In the near future, CXCR4 expression in biopsy specimens and CXCL12 levels in peritoneal washing may serve as useful molecular markers, identifying a subset of GC patients at very high risk of peritoneal recurrence. Furthermore, by targeting CXCL12, a therapy including CXCR4 antagonists may become part of the multi-modal treatment of PC [1].

References

1. Yasumoto K, Koizumi K, Kawashima A et al (2006) Role of the CXCL12/CXCR4 axis in peritoneal carcinomatosis of gastric cancer. Cancer Res 66:2181-2187
2. Sugarbaker PH, Yonemura Y (2000) Clinical pathway for the management of respectable gastric cancer with peritoneal seeding: Best palliation with a ray of hope for cure. Oncology 58:96-107
3. Bozzetti F, Yu W, Baratti D et al (2008) Locoregional treatment of peritoneal carcinomatosis from gastric cancer. J Surg Oncol 98:273-276
4. Sadeghi B, Arvieux C, Glehen O et al (2000) Peritoneal carcinomatosis from non-gynecologic malignancies: results of the EVOCAPE 1 multicentric prospective study. Cancer 88:358-363
5. al-Shammaa HAH, Li Y, Yonemura Y (2008) Current status and future strategies of cytoreductive surgery plus intraperitoneal hyperthermic chemotherapy for peritoneal carcinomatosis. World J Gastroenterol 14:1159-1166
6. Chu DZ, Lang NP, Thompson C et al (1989) Peritoneal carcinomatosis in nongynecologic malignancy. A prospective study of prognostic factors. Cancer 63:364-367
7. Roviello F, Marrelli D, de Manzoni G et al (2003) Prospective study of peritoneal recurrence after curative surgery for gastric cancer. Br J Surg 90:1113-1119
8. Muratore A, Zimmitti G, Lo Tesoriere R et al (2009) Low rates of loco-regional recurrence following extended lymph node dissection for gastric cancer. Eur J Surg Oncol 35:588-592
9. Moon YW, Jeung HC, Rha SY et al (2007) Changing patterns of prognosticators during 15-year follow-up of advanced gastric cancer after radical gastrectomy and adjuvant chemotherapy: a 15-year follow-up study at a single Korean institute. Ann Surg Oncol 14:2730-2737
10. Sakuramoto S, Sasako M, Yamaguchi T et al (2007) Adjuvant chemotherapy for gastric cancer with S-1, an oral fluoropyrimidine. N Engl J Med 357:1810-1820
11. Garofalo A, Corona F, Valle M et al (2008) The role of hyperthermic Intraperitoneal chemotherapy. In De Giuli M (ed) Management of gastric cancer. Recent advances. Minerva Medica, Turin
12. Giovanella BC, Stehlin JS, Morgan AC et al (1976) Selective lethal effect of sopranormal temperature on human neoplastic cells. Cancer Res 36:3944-3950
13. Wallner K, Li G (1987) Effect of drug exposure duration and sequencing on hyperthermic potentiation of mitomycin C and cisplatin. Cancer Res 47:493-495
14. Glehen O, Gilly FN, Arvieux C et al (2010) Peritoneal car-

cinomatosis from gastric cancer: a multi-institutional study of 159 patients treated by cytoreductive surgery combined with perioperative intraperitoneal chemotherapy. Ann Surg Oncol 17:2370-2377
15. Spratt J, Adcock M, Muskovin M et al (1980) Clinical delivery system for intraperitoneal hyperthermic chemotherapy. Cancer Res 40:256-60
16. Sugarbaker PH (1989) Surgical treatment of peritoneal carcinomatosis: 1988 Du Pont lecture. Can J Surg 32:164-170
17. Sayag-Beaujard AC, Francois Y, Glehen O et al (1999) Intraperitoneal chemo-hyperthermia with mitomycin C for gastric cancer patients with peritoneal carcinomatosis. Anticancer Res 19:1375-1382
18. Glehen O, Schreiber V, Cotte E et al (2004) Cytoreductive surgery and intraperitoneal chemohyperthermia for peritoneal carcinomatosis arising from gastric cancer. Arch Surg 139:20-26
19. Yonemura Y, Kawamura T, Bando E et al (2005) Treatment of peritoneal dissemination from gastric cancer by peritonectomy and chemohyperthermic peritoneal perfusion. Br J Surg 92:370-375
20. Yang XJ, Li Y, Yonemura Y (2010) Cytoreductive surgery plus hyperthermic intraperitoneal chemotherapy to treat gastric cancer with ascites and/or peritoneal carcinomatosis: Results from a Chinese center. J Surg Oncol 101:457-464
21. Valle M, Van der Speeten K, Garofalo A (2009) Laparoscopic hyperthermic intraperitoneal peroperative chemotherapy (HIPEC) in the management of refractory malignant ascites: A multi-institutional retrospective analysis in 52 patients. J Surg Oncol 100:331-334
22. Ba MC, Cui SZ, Lin SQ et al (2010) Chemotherapy with laparoscope-assisted continuous circulatory hyperthermic intraperitoneal perfusion for malignant ascites. World J Gastroenterol 16:1901-1907
23. Bando E, Yonemura Y, Takeshita Y et al (1999) Intraoperative lavage for cytological examination in 1297 patients with gastric carcinoma. Am J Surg 178:256-262
24. Yonemura Y, Bando E, Kinoshita K et al (2003) Effective therapy for peritoneal dissemination in gastric cancer. Surg Oncol Clin N Am 12:635-648
25. Bonenkamp JJ, Songun I, Hermans J et al (1996) Prognostic value of positive cytology findings from abdominal washings in patients with gastric cancer. Br J Surg 83:672-674
26. Fujiwara Y, Doki Y, Taniguchi H et al (2007) Genetic detection of free cancer cells in the peritoneal cavity of the patient with gastric cancer: present status and future perspectives. Gastric Cancer 10:197-204
27. Katsuragi K, Yashiro M, Sawada T et al (2007) Prognostic impact of PCR-based identification of isolated tumor cells in the peritoneal lavage fluid of gastric cancer patients who underwent a curative R0 resection. Br J Cancer 97:550-556
28. Hamazoe R, Maeta M, Kaibara N (1994) Intraperitoneal thermochemotherapy for prevention of peritoneal recurrence of gastric cancer - final results of a randomized controlled study. Cancer 73:2048-2052
29. Fujimoto S, Takahashi M, Mutou T et al (1999) Successful intraperitoneal hyperthermic chemoperfusion for the prevention of postoperative peritoneal recurrence in patients with advanced gastric carcinoma. Cancer 85:529-534
30. Yonemura Y, de Aretxabala X, Fujimura T et al (2001) Intraoperative chemohyperthermic peritoneal perfusion as an adjuvant to gastric cancer: final results of a randomized controlled study. Hepatogastroenterol 48:1776-1782
31. Zhang W, Su D, Wang K et al (1998) Clinical study in prophylactic use of intraperitoneal hyperthermic chemoperfusion for the prevention of peritoneal metastasis in patients with advanced gastric carcinoma. Shanxi Yiyao Zazhi 27:67-69
32. Kim JY, Bae HS (2001) A controlled clinical study of serosa-invasive gastric carcinoma patients who underwent surgery plus intraperitoneal hyperthermo-chemo-perfusion (IHCP). Gastric Cancer 4:27-33
33. Yan TD, Black D, Sugarbaker PH et al (2007) A systematic review and meta-analysis of the randomized controlled trials on adjuvant intraperitoneal chemotherapy for resectable gastric cancer. Ann Surg Oncol 14:2702-2713
34. Nissan A, Garofalo A, Esquivel J (2010) Cytoreductive surgery and hyperthermic intra-peritoneal chemotherapy (HIPEC) for gastric adenocarcinoma: why haven't we reached the promised land? J Surg Oncol 102:359-360
35. Piso P, Slowik P, Popp F et al (2009) Safety of gastric resections during cytoreductive surgery and hyperthermic intraperitoneal chemotherapy for peritoneal carcinomatosis. Ann Surg Oncol 16:2188-194

Postoperative Course: Morbidity, Mortality, and Treatment of Complications

16

Giovanni de Manzoni, Luca Cozzaglio, Simone Giacopuzzi, and Antonella Ardito

Abstract

Over the last two decades, better assessment of operative risk as well as better surgical technique and perioperative management have led to a large reduction in postoperative mortality in Western countries. At present, in Western specialized centers postoperative mortality ranges from 2% to 5% with 3.9% reported by the GIRCG (Italian Research Group for Gastric Cancer) network. These figures, although representing a noteworthy surgical achievement, still lag behind values reported by Japanese series (0.8–2.7%) probably because in Western countries the patients are older and have more advanced cancer as well as a higher number of associated diseases. Postoperative complications are usually directly related to the type of surgery: total or subtotal gastrectomy, combined resection of neighboring organs, and type of node dissection (D1, D2, D3). This chapter analyzes the incidence, etiopathogenesis, diagnosis, treatment, and prognosis of the most frequent complications in gastric cancer surgery.

Keywords

Gastric cancer surgery • Morbidity • Mortality • Anastomotic leakage • Duodenal stump leakage • Pancreatic fistula • Total gastrectomy • Subtotal gastrectomy • Splenectomy • Pancreatectomy • Lymphadenectomy • Endoscopy • Esophageal stent

16.1 Postoperative Morbidity and Mortality

Over the last two decades, the outcomes of gastric cancer surgery have greatly improved in Western countries, as better assessment of operative risk, better surgical technique, and advances in perioperative management have led to a large reduction in postoperative mortality. At present, in Western specialized centers postoperative mortality ranges from 2% to 5%, [1-5] with 3.9% reported by the GIRCG (Italian Research Group for Gastric Cancer) network. These figures, although representing a noteworthy surgical achievement, still lag behind those reported by Japanese series (0.8–2.7%) [6, 7], probably because in Western countries the patients are older and have more advanced cancer as well as a higher number of associated diseases.

Postoperative complications are usually directly related to the type of surgery: total or subtotal gastrectomy, combined resection of neighboring

G. de Manzoni (✉)
Dept. of Surgery,
Upper G.I. Surgery Division,
University of Verona,
Verona, Italy

G. de Manzoni, F. Roviello, W. Siquini (eds.), *Surgery in the Multimodal Management of Gastric Cancer*,

Table 16.1 Morbidity and mortality after splenectomy and splenopancreasectomy in the most recent literature

Author [Reference]	Morbidity		
	Splenectomy Yes	Splenopancreatectomy Yes	No
Verlato [20]**	29.6	39.5	17.4
Danielson [98]		40.9	22.8
Yu [102]	15.4		8.7
Lo [103]		42,5	32.3
Yamamoto [104]**	24.1	41,9	9.1
Yang [105][a]	15.3		8.7
Sasako [106]**	32.7	39.8	11.6
	Mortality		
	Splenectomy/Pancreatectomy		
	Yes	No	
Csendes [4]	4.0	3,0	
Ozer [8]	7.3	3,3	
Verlato [20]	5.0	3,7	
Yu [102]	1.9	1,0	
Lo [103]	6.3	4,8	
Yamamoto [104]	1.4	0	
Yang [105][a]	3,0	2.0	
Sasako [106]**	12.6	5.6	

[a]Meta-analysis.
**Statistically significant.

Table 16.2 Morbidity and mortality after different extension of lymphadenectomy in the most recent literature

Author [Reference]	Lymphadenectomy		
	D1	D2 D3 Morbidity	
Wu [5]**	7.3	17.1	
Lewis [9]	36	28	
Cuschieri [16]**	28	46	
Verlato [20]	18.4	19.2	21.4
Danielson [98]**	16.8	33	33
Hartgrink [99]**	25	43	
Dicken [101]**	25	43	
Sano [25]		20,9	28.1
Yang [100]**	25.5	44.3	
	Mortality		
Lewis [9]		12	8.3
Cuschieri [16]**	6.5	13	
Verlato [20]	3.6	2.9	3.0
Danielson [98]	1.8	3.7	3.7
Hartgrink [99]**	4	10	
Dicken [101]**	6.5	13	
Sano [25]		0.8	0.8
Yang [100]	3.6	7.1	

**Statistically significant.

organs, and type of lymph node dissection (D1, D2, D3). Total gastrectomy is still associated with greater morbidity than subtotal gastrectomy (12.9–37.5 vs. 8.9–14%) [8-11] and, according to some authors, a higher mortality (2–12.5 vs. 0.9%–1.6) [1, 8–11]. In the GIRCG experience, while surgical morbidity was significantly greater after total gastrectomy (23% vs. 17%; $p < 0.032$), postoperative mortality did not change as a function of the surgical procedure, suggesting that surgical complications were adequately managed.

Over the years, the incidence of pancreatectomy during gastric cancer surgery has been reduced to about 4%, a value confirmed both in the GIRCG experience and in the recent JCOG randomized trial on para-aortic lymphadenectomy. By contrast, the incidence of splenectomy is highly variable: < 10% in the GIRCG experience and around 36% in Japan, as it is still routinely performed in total gastrectomy. Splenectomy and splenopancreatectomy are associated with a higher incidence of surgical complications and thus in some but not in all series with a higher mortality (Table 16.1).

The majority of authors report that extended lymph node dissection (D2 or D3) entails a higher risk of complication than is the case with D1 (Table 16.2). However, in the GIRCG experience, the extent of lymphadenectomy had no impact on postoperative mortality. Similar results have been reported by other European observational studies (in selected patients centers) and by Far East randomized trials [12, 13]. Also, the large increase in postoperative morbidity and mortality observed in European randomized trials has been attributed to the limited pre-trial experience of the participating surgeons (Table 16.2) [14].

16.2 Anastomotic Leakage

The reported incidence of esophagojejunal anastomotic leaks after gastric cancer surgery varies widely in the literature, ranging from 4 to 27% in European multicenter studies [15-18] with an average of 5–8% [19, 20] in major recent series. A lower leakage rate is recorded after gastrojejunal anastomosis (1.9–2.2%) [1, 22, 23]. It should be noted that the mortality rate associated with anastomotic dehiscence is still very high, up to 50%, even with gastrojejunal anastomosis [1, 15, 19,24].

16.2.1 Etiology and Risk Factors

Both systemic and local factors are believed to influence the incidence of leakage. Systemic factors include advanced cancer stage and poor performance status, with impaired cardiovascular and respiratory function potentially compromising blood supply, tissue oxygenation, and healing at the anastomotic site [25]. A recent study failed to support the negative effects of malnutrition or obesity on anastomotic failure [26]. Local factors include localized infections, impaired vascularization of the lower esophagus or graft end, and mechanical traction on the sutures.

16.2.2 Diagnosis

A widely accepted classification of leakage is still lacking in the current literature. Some authors base the definition on radiographic findings whereas others refer to the clinical impact (minor or major). We have adopted the classification proposed by Schuchert et al., [27] which relies on objective endoscopic (degree of anastomotic dehiscence) as well as clinical (degree of intervention required) parameters.

The clinical presentation of an anastomotic leak ranges from trivial to severe. Abdominal pain, pyrexia, tachycardia, abscess, gastrointestinal contents within the abdominal drain, and a high white blood cell count are frequent findings while in the most severe cases there is systemic sepsis. Early diagnosis and a proper assessment of disease severity are crucial since treatment aggressiveness and invasiveness should be proportional to leakage severity and potential lethality.

Routine contrast radiology is still performed by most centers before the patient is allowed to start oral intake, even though there is no consensus on the timing, which currently varies from postoperative day 3 to day 14. It should be noted that the sensitivity of this examination is quite low (66% in the Lamb experience) [24, 28, 29] so that a normal contrast study may not exclude a leak. For this reason, routine postoperative studies to identify a leak are no longer warranted; however, patients with clinical suspicion or subtle clinical signs of septic illness must be radiologically examined as soon as possible, using oral contrast administration as the first step.

Recently, endoscopy with minimal air insufflation has been proposed to diagnose a suspected leak, as this approach allows direct visualization of the anastomotic site, determination of the percent disruption of the anastomotic circumference, and even the placement of a transanastomotic nasojejunal tube. This procedure seems to have a very high sensitivity in leakage detection, around 95–100% [30-32].

The diagnostic work up of a patient with a suspected leak also includes a CT scan. While this is definitely a second-line test in leak assessment, it will reveal whether the leak is contained, with only a small perianastomotic fluid collection, or whether there is an undrained abscess or signs of mediastinitis.

16.2.3 Treatment and Prognosis

Given the spectrum of severity, there is no standard management. Nevertheless, coordinated and aggressive interventions by surgical and intensive care units allow the vast majority of patients to be successfully treated. Initial medical treatment consists of elimination of oral intake and decompression of the anastomotic area with a nasogastric tube, together with broad-spectrum antibiotics. Parenteral nutrition or, preferentially, enteral nutrition via an endoscopically placed fine-bore nasojejunal tube could be important. The infected perianastomotic fluid collections must be adequately drained, with percutaneous drainage under computed tomography or ultrasonographic guidance effective for most patients.

Surgical intervention is indicated whenever the patient's clinical condition deteriorates despite medical treatment. This can arise in the setting of sepsis, due to mediastinitis or peritonitis, and is often predictive of subsequent death, probably because it is a marker of disease severity. Indeed, secondary surgical repair is usually not effective but instead typically serves as an adjunctive strategy if surgical drainage of widespread peritoneal or mediastinal soilage is requested.

Recently, endoscopic minimally invasive treatment has taken on an important role in the management of anastomotic leaks [33-35]. The different techniques range from the application of fibrin glue or a metallic clip to the use of self-expanding covered stents. However, prior to endoscopic treatment it is necessary to adequately drain the external peri-anastomotic collections and to perform internal endoscopic lavage and debridment until the anastomotic fistula is sufficiently cleaned. Hence, when the leak is small, i.e., involving < 30% of the anastomotic circumference and/or the diameter of the hole is < 1.5 cm, endoscopic clipping is indicated even if multiple endoscopic sessions are usually needed. For larger dehiscences, temporary placement of a silicon-covered self-expanding stent is an effective option for cure. Stent placement has the advantage of immediate leak occlusion in a single endoscopic session.

A stent has to be removed within 3 months to avoid long-term complications, such as fistulization or upper-gastrointestinal hemorrhage. In this respect, self-expanding plastic stents are probably much easier to remove than metal stents such as the Ultraflex, which often becomes strongly embedded in the esophageal wall.

16.3 Fistula of Duodenal Stump

16.3.1 Introduction

Duodenal fistula (DF) after gastrectomy is relatively rare, with an incidence of about 3%, but is a life-threatening problem with a high rate of complications, an overall mortality of 7–67% [36-38], and a very long period of hospitalization. Nonetheless, spontaneous closure occurs in 28–92% of patients [37, 39, 40]. In 1944, Christopher, in his textbook of surgery, said, "There is not a more serious complication in abdominal surgery, except for massive hemorrhages, than an external duodenal fistula [41].

Many published studies dealing with postoperative DF were based on small series of patients and in many case [36-40] surgery had been performed not only after gastric surgery but also after operations on the biliary tract, duodenum, pancreas, and kidney. Moreover, many series also considered DF following duodenal trauma, duodenal ulcer perforation, Crohn's disease, and pancreatitis. Consequently, an accurate description of the natural history and management of this complication is still lacking. The most recent and largest published series comprised 3785 gastrectomies for malignant diseases in a retrospective multicenter study at eleven Italian centers. There were 68 DF, corresponding to a frequency of 1.8% (range 0.3–6.3) [42].

16.3.2 Etiology

Possible causes of postoperative DF include inadequate closure of the duodenal stump, devascularization, inflamed duodenal wall, local hematoma, incorrect drain position or migration of the drain into the duodenum [43], duodenal resection line involvement [42], and postoperative distension of the duodenum. Among the technical causes, some authors have suggested that DF is more frequently associated with Billroth II reconstructions, due to the difficult emptying of the afferent jejunal loop [44]. However, these data have not been confirmed by other authors [42]. Surprisingly, improved surgical techniques and the use of staplers have not decreased the frequency of DF [42].

16.3.3 Presentation

The most common sign of DF is the presence of duodenal fluid in the surgical drainage or its leakage through the abdominal wall, as confirmed by CT scan, fistulography, or exploratory surgery. The onset of DF varies greatly in terms of timing, output, and clinical presentation. Two types of DF, early and late, are recognized. Early DF is uncommon; it typically occurs during the first few postoperative days, usually without sepsis, and is in most cases related to technical problems involving the sutures. Late DF is more common; it usually develops at about postoperative day seven, but the variability is very large and it may first present 20 days postoperatively [42]. Therefore, this complication must be suspected also in outpatients who have recently undergone gastrectomy.

The daily output of DF can be as little as 40 mL and as much as 3300 mL [36, 42]. Symptoms associated with leakage of duodenal fluid are fever and right abdominal pain followed by skin irritation or excoriation around the site of leakage. Patients with a DF very often develop other complications, such as intra-abdominal abscess, wound infection, necrosis or dehiscence, diffuse peritonitis, sepsis, malnutrition, fluid and electrolyte disturbances, acute cholecystitis, pancreatitis, abdominal bleeding and the formation of new fistulas in neighboring abdominal organs, and pneumonia [36, 42].

The symptoms associated with DF have partially changed with respect to the data reported in the oldest literature, which date back about 30 years. Some new features have been acquired and others have been lost, such as fluid, electrolyte and acid/base imbalances, and dermatitis. The incidence of cholecystitis has decreased, probably because patients are encouraged to eat or are provided with enteral nutrition. However, we have observed an approximately 20% frequency of new fistulas in neighboring abdominal organs, such as jejunum, colon, pancreas, and gastric stump [42], perhaps related to a the recovery time; in other words, while the DF heals, patients may be at risk of developing new fistulas.

16.3.4 Prognosis

Recent advances in medical therapy have dramatically reduced the mortality of DF, from 40% to 16% since 1980. Mortality is due to sepsis followed by multiple organ failure and is highest in the first weeks after onset [42] despite the very long healing time, thus necessitating the maximum medical effort at the early stage. The healing rate of DF is about 80%, with healing occurring any time between a few days to a few years later [42]. Recurrences are very common, even after several months since the apparent healing, but they usually are not severe and do not compromise the prognosis.

Higher mortality rates are associated with the presence of other complications, the need for multiple reoperations, age > 65 years, and serum albumin < 25 g/L [36–38, 40, 42]. Additional factors, according to some authors [36], are fistula output > 200 mL/day, anemia with serum hemoglobin < 10 g/100 mL, weight loss > 15% of usual weight [45], delay in DF diagnosis, and previous radiotherapy.

Levy et al. [46] proposed a severity score of DF based on nine risk factors: abdominal wall necrosis, previous radiotherapy, multiple laparotomy, shock, respiratory insufficiency, septicemia, renal failure, upper gastrointestinal hemorrhage, and pulmonary embolism. However, the usefulness of this score has not been confirmed by other authors [39].

16.3.5 Therapy

The management of DF remains controversial but medical therapy is preferred to surgery. The latter is indicated only for complications not treatable by other means, such as in the case of abdominal sepsis, bleeding, or fistulas in neighboring organs [42].

Medical therapy is mainly based on prevention or early detection and includes treatment of infections, adequate external drainage of the fistula, protection of skin excoriations, maintenance of fluid and electrolyte balance, and nutritional support by enteral or parenteral nutrition.

The use of somatostatin and its analogue octreotide in the management of DF is based on inhibition of gastrointestinal hormone secretion or exocrine secretory responses. The available information suggests a benefit in terms of fistula output only in some patients, but without any significant increase in spontaneous closure rates [47].

In many cases DF is treated percutaneously, with the main procedures being abscess drainage, transhepatic biliary drainage by placing the catheter tip into the duodenum thereby draining the bile, intestinal, and pancreatic secretions [48], or transhepatic biliary drainage coupled with an occlusion balloon to stop biliary flow [49] followed by fistula obliteration using cyanoacrylate or prolamine [50].

Surgical procedures proposed for the treatment of DF include closure of the fistula, placement of a tube into the abdomen to drain the duodenal fluid, abscess drainage, tube duodenostomy (either alone or coupled with continuous intraluminal infusion and aspiration) [46], fistula repair with a rectus abdominis muscle flap [51], serosal patch repair using the jejunum or omentum, and feeding-tube jejunostomy. Simple closure or repair of an established DF is associated with a high recurrence rate. A large duodenal defect not controlled by tube duodenostomy or draining abundant amounts of fluid for > 6 weeks can be closed by a Roux-en-Y duodenojejunostomy [52]; occasionally, pancreatoduodenectomy is necessary and can be lifesaving [53]. Surgery is always mandatory in cases of diffuse peritonitis and severe sepsis, but nowadays surgical closure of DF is indicated only for a select group of patients in whom medical therapy has failed.

Fasting and nasogastric suction are not necessary and an oral diet should always be encouraged as it improves outcome [42].

16.4 Pancreatic Fistula

16.4.1 Introduction

Although gastric surgery has achieved a low rate of morbidity and mortality [54], pancreatic fistula (PF) remains a serious complication after extended gastrectomy associated with pancreaticosplenectomy [21, 55, 56]. In a Japanese major clinical trial enrolling 523 patients with advanced gastric cancer, PF was the most common complication after extended gastrectomy [7].

The incidence of PF after gastrectomy reportedly ranges from 0 to 22%, specifically [21, 55-58], between 0% and 2% [21, 56] in the absence of associated pancreatic resection and between 7% and 22% after distal pancreatosplenectomy [21]. This large variability in incidence is partly explained by the different definitions of PF adopted by different studies. Thus, in July 2005, the International Study Group on Pancreatic Fistula (ISGPF) developed and published a definition and clinical grading for postoperative PF [59]. Despite differences in the criteria used to define a PF [21, 59, 60], most investigations report a considerable percentage of subclinical cases in the absence of pancreatic resection.

Once PF develops, it can lead to other major complications, such as intra-abdominal abscess, bleeding, anastomotic leakage, fistula to neighboring organs, and pleural effusion. Moreover, in many series PF is one of the complications most predictive of death [61, 62].

16.4.2 Definition

Postoperative PF is generally defined as a leak from the pancreatic ductal system around the pancreas and containing pancreas-derived, enzyme-rich fluid originating from the raw pancreatic surface. A broad definition begins with the following criteria: output, either through a drain or the abdominal wall, of any measurable volume of fluid after postoperative day 3, with an amylase concentration greater than three-fold higher than the upper normal serum value [16, 59].

The ISGP recognizes three grades of PF [59]. Grade A postoperative PF, also called "transient fistula," is the most common and has no clinical impact. It requires little change in management or deviation from the normal clinical pathway. The patient is fed orally and remains clinically well; the use of nutritional support, antibiotics, or somatostatin analogues is not indicated. A grade B fistula requires a change in management or adjustment in the clinical pathway. The patient is often not fed orally but instead supported with parenteral or enteral nutrition. The peripancreatic drains are usually maintained in place; however, if the fistula is not fully drained then a CT scan may detect a peripancreatic collection requiring repositioning of the drains. When associated with abdominal pain, fever, and/or leukocytosis, antibiotics are usually required and somatostatin analogues may be administered. Grade C PF demands a major change in clinical management. Clinical stability may be borderline and clinical intervention is aggressive: the patient is fed only with total parenteral nutrition and treated intravenously with antibiotics and somatostatin analogues, often in an intensive care unit setting. A CT scan usually reveals a worrisome, peripancreatic fluid collection requiring percutaneous drainage.

16.4.3 Etiology

Pancreatic fistula is the main complication of extended (D2) or superextended (D3) lymphadenectomy [63, 64] associated with pancreaticosplenectomy or splenectomy. The development of postoperative PF is related to an operative trauma with an associated injury to pancreatic tissue.

Both the Medical Research Council Gastric Cancer Surgical Trial and the Dutch Gastric Cancer Group trial documented an increased postoperative morbidity and mortality related to PF that developed after pancreaticosplenectomy. It has therefore been argued that pancreaticosplenectomy should be performed in D2 gastrectomy only if there is a direct extension of the disease to the pancreas. Indeed Maruyama et al. demonstrated that pancreas-preserving D2 gastrectomy still provided good lymph node clearance [65].

Reported risk factors for PF development are BMI > 25 [66], hyperlipidemia [67], and the presence of comorbidities, such as hypertension, cardiac dysfunction, and diabetes mellitus [34]. Accordingly, the higher incidence of PF after pancreaticosplenectomy reported by Western randomized controlled trials with respect to Japanese studies can likely be attributed to the higher prevalence of obesity in Western countries [68].

16.4.4 Presentation

The presence of PF may be suspected on the basis of both clinical symptoms and biochemical findings.

PF fluid can have a "sinister appearance" that may vary from dark brown to milky to clear and resembling pancreatic fluid. Clinical findings may include nausea, anorexia, abdominal pain, and distension with impaired bowel function, delayed gastric stump emptying, fever (>38° C), serum leukocyte count > 10,000 cells/mm^3, and increased serum C-reactive protein. Patients with PF are also at risk of electrolyte imbalance, particularly related to the loss of sodium and bicarbonate, and malnutrition. PF patients have a greater susceptibility to infection because of the many invasive lines and the fact that they are often immunocompromised secondary to protein losses through the pancreatic fluid.

Imaging documentation is seldom necessary for the diagnosis; nevertheless, CT scan, fistulography, and NMR may be useful to identify the anatomy of the pancreatic duct, the size and location of the PF, intra-abdominally associated abscess, bleeding, erosion, or migration of the drain into a neighboring organ. Endoscopic retrograde pancreatography is the most sensitive and specific modality to identify the pancreatic duct anatomy and the characteristics of PF.

16.4.5 Prognosis

For many years, postoperative PF was the main concern for surgeons performing pancreatic resections because it was responsible for a high mortality and prolonged hospital stay [69]. Although some authors have reported that in recent years mortality due to PF has substantially decreased, the impact on the postoperative complication rate is still significant [70]. The reported PF rate after distal pancreatectomy is 0–60% [71-73] and after central pancreatectomy 0–40% [74].

The occurrence of PF raises two main issues: prevention and treatment. The postoperative management of surgical drains may be one of the key steps in decreasing the rate and severity of PF. Prophylactic drains after pancreatic surgery allow monitoring of the occurrence of intra-abdominal bleeding and the development of pancreatic or other fistulas. However, the surgical placement of drains may result in an increased risk of intra-abdominal infections [75]. Indeed, drains left in place for > 4 days have been reported to significantly increase the rate of both PF and intra-abdominal infections. Moreover, drains left in place for several days may cause additional complications, such as enteric fistula due to decubitus of the surgical drain. One study even suggested that prophylactic drains after pancreatic surgery are useless [76].

The reported success rate of conservatively treated PF is about 80%, but patients with a high-output fistula and signs of severe sepsis or hemorrhage should undergo laparotomy [57]. Both the reoperation rate and the mortality rate vary greatly, ranging from 2.8% to 65.8% and 0% to 22%, respectively [7, 55, 63, 77].

16.4.6 Therapy

Measurement of amylase levels in the drainage fluid is a simple and useful method to monitor PF and to plan appropriate management. Initially, the patient is allowed nothing by mouth and fed with total parenteral nutrition in the attempt to minimize pancreatic exocrine excretion, maintaining a good electrolyte balance and nutritional status. In many patients, this simple approach allows a spontaneous closure, while in others adjunctive measures are needed. Somatostatin and octreotide are potent inhibitors of pancreatic endocrine and exocrine functions, but their administration does not seem to decrease the incidence of PF when given prophylactically; however, they may be useful to decrease the fistula's output, thus limiting protein and electrolytes losses [58, 78].

Pancreatic fluid leakage is often followed by contamination, resulting in a left subphrenic abscess. Contamination does not seem to be caused by retrograde infection through the drainage tubes but by contamination of the pancreas fluid itself. This is presumably due to bacterial translocation from the bowel or to retrograde contamination caused by dysfunction of the duodenal papillae. In such cases, the appearance of an intra-abdominal abscess must be suspected and treatment promptly initiated, with percutaneous drainage performed in the presence of septic signs.

When the amount of PF fluid is relatively small, thick mucinous fluid can block the tube, preventing adequate drainage, in which case continuous drain irrigation or repetitive flushing with saline solution is suggested. In the presence of large amounts of PF fluid, continuous irrigation is recommended to reduce the risk of secondary bleeding from major arteries. If the patient's general condition is good, without signs of sepsis or impaired bowel function, food intake or enteral nutrition does not interfere with healing, but rather maintains enteral mucosal integrity. When drainage is adequate and sepsis is controlled, antibiotics should be stopped. The site around the skin of a PF should be promptly protected because of the erosive action of pancreatic fluid.

If PF fluid persists despite proper drainage, nutritional optimization, pancreatic rest, and octreotide use, the next step is endoscopic therapy. Endoscopic retrograde pancreatography with papillary decompression through sphincterectomy or transampullary stenting allows for the preferential flow of pancreatic fluid into the duodenum by decreasing the differential pressure, thus facilitating closure of the ductal defect [79].

Fibrin glue has been used to attempt PF closure by obliteration of the fistulous track. Although it does not seem to be effective as a sole modality, there are some reports of its successful use in conjunction with endoscopic stenting [80].

While conservative therapies are successful in the management of most cases of PF, those patients with a worsening clinical status, progressive sepsis, impending organ failure, or vascular complications require re-exploration. Secondary surgery consists of the placement of optimized drainages, but postoperative mortality is markedly elevated [81].

In patients with other unfavorable characteristics, such as the inability to cannulate the fistula during endoscopic retrograde pancreatography, a ductal stricture or a large defect not amenable to endoscopic therapy, or a disconnected pancreatic duct, surgery is required.

16.5 Chylous Fistula

16.5.1 Introduction

Chylous fistula (CF) is a complication of many surgical retroperitoneal procedures [82, 83] and it is caused by damage to or interruption of major lymphatic vessels, such as the thoracic duct, cisterna chyli, or one of their major tributaries [84]. Although CF is an unusual complication of gastric surgery [85, 86], its rate is most likely underestimated because only prolonged leakage with serious consequences is usually reported in the literature. CF generally is associated with D3 dissection, in which the incidence is 5–10% [87, 88].

16.5.1 Definition

Chylous fistula is defined as the presence of milky flow in drainage tubes or on aspiration, in excess of 200 ml/day, with a triglyceride ratio of CF vs. serum > 2 [88, 89]. Postoperative CF can lead to the accumulation of lymphatic fluid in the peritoneal cavity, resulting in chyloperitoneum and then chylous ascites.

16.5.2 Etiology

The postoperative development of CF indicates damage to an abdominal lymphatic vessel. In the abdomen, the cisterna chyli primarily drains the intestinal lymphatics; specifically, the efferents from the superior mesenteric and celiac group of lymph nodes. The cisterna chyli lies on the anterior aspect of the first or second lumbar vertebra, on the right side of the aorta, but this classic anatomy is present in only 50% of individuals, whereas in the others a distinct cisterna chyli is replaced by a lymphatic plexus, McVay described 16 different anatomic variants of the abdominal lymphatic plexus and cisterna chyli [90]. During D3 dissection, the retroperitoneal lymphatics and fat are excised, causing a possible severance or interruption of the lymphatic vessels; therefore, surgeons should be aware of the inconsistent anatomy of the abdominal lymphatic system and cisterna chyli, and the variable lymphatic plexus as well [91].

16.5.3 Presentation

Chylous fistula usually becomes apparent with increased oral intake, typically 3–12 days after surgery. Before the patient is allowed oral intake, the drainage fluid is almost always serous, but the presence of fat in the diet leads to an increase in fluid output coupled with a change in its quality. In fact, during fasting, the rate of chyle production is 1 ml/kg/h whereas after a fatty meal it can increase to as much as 220 ml/kg/h. CF can easily be diagnosed by the characteristic milky-beige odorless fluid seen through the surgical drain. Laboratory investigation of the drainage fluid (chylomicrons, triglycerides, lymphocytes count, alkaline pH, positive staining for fat with Sudan red) will confirm the diagnosis (CF output is variable but can reach 2000–3000 ml/day) [92].

In patients without any surgical drain, chylous ascites may be diagnosed after a delay of weeks or months. It is characterized by the presence of progressive abdominal distension, shortness of breath, and dyspnea, resulting from increased abdominal pressure; patients also may complain of weight gain. Other features include abdominal pain, nausea, early satiety, fever, night sweats, diarrhea, and steatorrhea, a shortage of fat-soluble vitamins, and then weight loss and malnutrition. Sometimes patients who have undergone abdominal surgery may present with an acute onset of CF. However, in the majority of cases, the diagnosis requires paracentesis, which is the most important diagnostic tool.

16.5.4 Prognosis

Patients often have a low performance status due to cancer and the effects of the primary operation and thus may be further debilitated by the serious consequences of CF. In fact, CF causes a constant loss of water, electrolytes, proteins, fats, and fat-soluble vitamins, leading to nutritional depletion and therefore a prolonged hospital stay. Persistent CF is mainly associated with an increased risk of local infections, wound complications, immunosuppression, and sepsis; accordingly, CF fluid must be cultured if infective signs appear because the risk of severe infections, in particular by *Candida albicans*, is considerable. The prognosis of patients with CF is usually good; if nutritional or infective complications are prevented, CF spontaneously heals in over 80% of the cases within 10–90 days. The drainage can be removed when there is no fluid in the tube and no ascites in the peritoneal cavity.

16.5.5 Therapy

Therapy of postoperative CF may be a challenging problem. In some cases, CF developing after D3 dissection is a reversible condition, and initial therapy consisting of restricted oral intake and low-fat diet supplementation may be sufficient [88]. Most authors recommend an oral diet with medium-chain triglycerides (MCT) and total parenteral nutrition (TPN). The MCT are bound to albumin and directly absorbed into the portal venous system, which diminishes the lymphatic flow. In addition, several promising new medical therapies have recently been introduced: somatostatin and octreotide decrease intestinal absorption of fats; orlistat is an inhibitor of gastric and pancreatic lipases that blocks the conversion of triglycerides to free fat acids, thus inhibiting bowel fat absorption [93]. Diuretics can be used to reduce the CF volume. Also, many techniques have been proposed, such as low-dose radiotherapy, sclerosing agents, subatmospheric pressure dressings, and percutaneous embolization of the cisterna chyli. These treatments, alone or in combination with other conservative measures, may be able to avoid the need for surgical re-interventions.

Another study suggested the creation of a peritoneal-venous shunt between the abdominal cavity and superior vena cava, in order to minimize fluid loss [94], but the high rate of complications, such as sepsis and shunt blockage, and improvements in TPN techniques have discouraged the use of this therapy.

If alimentary modifications, TPN, and the other conservative therapies fail, relaparotomy with ligature of the lymphatic vessels and/or the placement of fibrin glue on the CF may be proposed [95, 96]. Prior to surgery, lymphangiography or lymphoscintigraphy may be used to investigate the CF [95]; intraoperative administration of an oil solution via a nasogastric tube can be helpful in identifying the location of the leakage. However, surgery may occasionally fail to identify the leak, in which case re-intervention is associated with significant morbidity and mortality.

Jayabose et al. reviewed the literature in 1989 and reported successful surgical exploration only in 37% of CF patients [89]. A more recent paper analyzed 156 patients with postoperative CF. In the 105 who were treated conservatively, closure of the lymphatic fistula required several weeks to 2 months whereas 51 patients were successfully treated surgically [97]. In conclusion, medical therapy is preferred and surgery must be performed only when conservative therapies fail.

References

1. Pedrazzani C, Marrelli D, Rampone B et al (2007) Postoperative complications and functional results after subtotal gastrectomy with Bilroth II reconstruction for primary gastric cancer. Dig Dis Sci 52:1757-1763
2. Gil-Rendo A, Hernández-Lizoain JL, Martínez-Regueira F et al (2006) Risk factors related to operative morbidity in patients undergoing gastrectomy for gastric cancer. Clin Transl Oncol 8:354-361
3. Ibànez Aguirre et al (2006) Laparoscopic gastrectomy for gastric adenocarcinoma. Long- term results. Rev Esp Enferm Dig 98:491-500
4. Csendes A, Burdiles P, Rojas J et al (2002) A prospective randomized study comparing D2 total gastrectomy versus total D2 total gastrectomy plus splenectomy in 187 patients with gastric carcinoma. Surgery 131:401-407
5. Wu CW, Hsiung CA, Lo SS et al (2004) Randomized clinical study of morbidity after D1 and D3 surgery for gastric cancer. Br J Surg 91:283-287
6. Ikeguchi M et al (2001) Postoperative morbidity and mortality after gastrectomy for gastric carcinoma. Hepatogastroenterology 48:1517-1520
7. Sano T, Sasako M, Yamamoto S et al (2004) Gastric Cancer Surgery: Morbidity and mortality results from a prospective randomized controlled trial comparing D2 and extended para-aortic lymphadenectomy – Japan ClinicalOncology Group Study 9501. J Clin Oncol 22:2767-2773
8. Ozer I, Bostanci EB, Orug T et al (2009) Surgical outcomes and survival after multiorgan re-section for locally advanced gastric cancer. Am J Surg 198:25-30
9. Lewis WG, Edwards P, Barry JD et al (2002) D2 or not D2? The gastrectomy question. Gastric Cancer 5(I):29
10. Bozzetti F, Marubini E, Bonfanti G et al (1999) Subtotal versus total gastrectomy for gastric cancer: five-year survival rates in a multicenter randomized Italian trial. Italian Gastroin-testinal Tumor Study Group. Ann Surg 230:170-178
11. Degiuli M, Calvo F (2006) Survival of early gastric cancer in a specialized European center. Which lymphadenectomy is necessary? World J Surg 30:2193-2203
12. Sasako M, Sano T, Yamamoto S et al (2008) D2 lymphadenectomy alone or with para-aortic nodal dissection for gastric cancer. N Eng J Med 359:453-462
13. Wu CW, Hsiung CA, Lo SS et al (2006) Nodal dissection for patients with gastric cancer: a randomised controlled trial. Lancet Oncol 7:309-315
14. McCulloch P, Niita ME, Kazi H et al (2005) Gastrectomy with extended lymphadenectomy for primary treatment of gastric cancer. Br J Surg 92:5-13
15. Bonenkamp JJ, Hermans J, Sasako M et al (1999) Extended lymph-node dissection for gastric cancer. Dutch Gastric Cancer Group. N Engl J Med 340:908-914
16. Cuschieri A, Weeden S, Fielding J et al (1999) Patient survival after D1 and D2 resections for gastric cancer: long-term results of the MRC randomized surgical trial. Surgical Co-operative Group. Br J Cancer 79:1522-1530
17. Roder JD, Bottcher K, Busch R et al (1998) Classification of regional lymphnode metastasis from gastric carcinoma. German Gastric Cancer Study Group. Cancer 82:621-631
18. Fernàndez A et al (2010) Self- expanding plastic stents for the treatment of post- operative esophago- jejuno anastomotic leak. A case series study. Rev Esp Enferm Dig 102:704-710
19. Sierzega M, Kolodziejczyk P, Kulig J (2010) Polish Gastric Cancer Study Group. Impact of anastomotic leakage on long-term survival after total gastrectomy for carcinoma of the stomach. Br J Surg 97:1035-1042
20. Verlato G, Roviello F, Marchet A et al (2009) Indexes of surgical quality in gastric cancer surgery: experience of an Italian network. Ann Surg Oncol 16:594-602
22. Martin RC 2nd, Jaques DP, Brennan MF, Karpeh M (2002) Extended local resection for advanced gastric cancer: increased survival versus increased morbidity. Ann Surg 236:159-165
23. Kowalski C, Kastuar S, Mehta V, Brolin RE (2007) Endoscopic injection of fibrin sealant in repair of gastrojejunostomy leak after laparoscopic Roux-en-Y gastric bypass. Surg Obes Relat Dis 3:438-442
24. Lamb PJ (2004) Prospective study of routine contrast radiology after total gastrectomy British Journal of Surgery 91:1015-1019
25. Sano T, Sasako M, Yamamoto S et al (2004) Gastric cancer surgery: morbidity and mortality results from a prospective randomized controlled trial comparing D2 and extended para-aortic lymphadenectomy. J Clin Oncol 22:2767-2773

26. Pacelli F, Papa V, Rosa F et al (2008) Four hundred consecutive total gastrectomies for gastric cancer: a single-institution experience. Discussion 775 Arch Surg 143:769-775
27. Schuchert MJ, Abbas G, Nason KS et al (2010) Impact of anastomotic leak on outcomes after transhiatal esophagectomy. Surgery 148:831-838
28. Sauvanet A, Baltar J, Le Mee J, Belghiti J (1998) Diagnosis and conservative management of intrathoracic leakage after esophagectomy. Br J Surg 85:1446-1449
29. Tirnakiz MB, Deschamps C, Allen MS et al (2005) Effectiveness of screening acqueous contrast swallow in detecting clinical significant leaks after esophagectomy for cancer. Eur Surg Res 37:123-128
30. Griffin SM, Lamb PJ, Dresner SM et al (2001) Diagnosis and management of a mediastinal leak following radical oesophagectomy. Br J Surg 88:1346-1351
31. Hogan BA, Winter DC, Broe D et al (2008) Prospective trial comparing contrast swallow, computed tomography and endoscopy to identify anastomotic leak following oesophagogastric surgery. Surg Endosc 22:767-771
32. Strauss C, Mal F, Perniceni T et al (2010) Computed tomography versus water-soluble con-trast swallow in the detection of intrathoracic anastomotic leak complicating esophagogas-trectomy (Ivor Lewis): a prospective study in 97 patients. Ann Surg 251:647-651
33. Rodella L, Laterza E, G. de Manzoni et al (1998) Endoscopic clipping of anastomotic leakages in esophagogastric surgery. Endoscopy 30:453-456
34. Salminen P, Gullichsen R, Laine S (2009) Use of self-expandable metal stents for the treatment of esophageal perforations and anastomotic leaks. Epub Surg Endosc 23:1526-1530
35. Schubert D, Scheidbach H, Kuhn R et al (2005) Endoscopic treatment of thoracic esophageal anastomotic leaks by using silicone-covered, self-expanding polyester stents. Gastrointest Endosc 61:891-896
36. Rossi JA, Sollenberger LL, Rege RV et al (1986) External duodenal fistulas. Arch Surg 121:908-912
37. Tarazi R, Coutsofides T, Steiger E, Fazio (1983) VW Gastric and duodenal cutaneous fistulas. World J Surg 7:463-473
38. Edmunds LH jr, Williams GM, Welch CE (1960) External fistulas arising from the gastroin-testinal tract. Ann Surg 152:445-471
39. Garden OJ, Dikes EH, Carter DC (1988) Surgical and nutritional management of postoperative duodenal fistulas. Dig Dis Sci 33:30-35
40. Reber HA, Roberts C, Way LW, Dumphy JE (1978) Management of external gastrointestinal fistulas. Ann Surg 188:460-467
41. Christopher F (1944) Textbook of Surgery, 3rd ed. W.B. Saunders Company Philadelphia
42. Cozzaglio L, Coladonato M, Biffi R et al (2010) Duodenal Fistula after Elective Gastrectomy for malignant Disease. An Italian Retrospective Multicenter Study. Journal of Gastrointestinal Surgery 14:805-811
43. Ravishankar HR, Malik RA, Burnett H, Carlson GL (2001) Migration of abdominal drains into the gastrointestinal tract may prevent spontaneous closure of enterocutaneous fistulas. Ann R Coll Surg Engl 83:337-338
44. de Alves JB (1968) Treatment of the postgastrectomy external duodenal fistula. International Surgery 49:248-251
45. Fazio VW, Coutsoftides T, Steiger E (1983) Factors influencing the outcome of treatment of small bowel cutaneous fistulas. World J Surg 7:481-488
46. Levy E, Cugnenc PH, Frileux P et al (1984) Postoperative peritonitis due to gastric and duodenal fistulas. Operative management by continuous intraluminal infusion and aspiration: report of 23 cases. Br J Surg 7:543-546
47. Hesse U, Ysebaert D, de Hemptinne B (2001) Role of somatostatin-14 and its analogues in the management of gastrointestinal fistulae: clinical data. Gut 49(Suppl 4):iv11-iv21
48. Villar R, Fernàndez R, Gonzàles J et al (1996) High-output external duodenal fistula: treatment with percutaneous transhepatic biliary/duodenal drainage. Cardiovasc Intervent Radiol 19:371-373
49. Ardito A, Cozzaglio L, Cimino M et al (2010) Feasibility and efficacy of percutaneous transhepatic biliary drainage and occlusion balloon (PTBD-OB) in the management of duodenal stump fistola after gastrectomy for cancer".
XXXIII Congresso Nazionale SICO Milano 10-12 Giugno 2010
50. Bianchi A, Solduga C, Ubach M (1988) Percutaneous obliteration of a chronic duodenal fistula. Br J Surg 7:572
51. Chander J, Lal P, Ramteke VK (2004) Rectus abdominis muscle flap for high-output duodenal fistula: novel technique. World J Surg 28:179-182
52. Ujiki GT, Shields TW (1981) Roux-en-Y operation in the management of postoperative fistulas. Arch Surg 116:614-617
53. Musicant ME, Thompson JC (1969) The emergency management of lateral duodenal fistula by pancreatoduodenectomy. Surg Gynecol Obstet 128:108-114
54. McCulloch P (2006) The role of surgery in patients with advanced gastric cancer. Best Pract Res Clin Gastroenterol 20:767-787
55. Okabayashi T, Kobayashi M, Sugimoto T et al (2005) Postoperative pancreatic fistula following surgery for gastric and pancreatic neoplasm: is distal pancreaticosplenectomy truly safe? Hepatogastroenterology 52:233-236
56. D'Amato A, Santella S, Cristaldi M et al (2004) The role of extended total gastrectomy in advanced gastric cancer. Hepatogastroenterology 51:609-612
57. Katai H, Yoshimura K, Fukagawa T et al (2005) Risk factors for pancreatic-related abscess after total gastrectomy. Gastric Cancer 8:137-141
58. Sasako M, Katai H, Sano T et al (2000) Management of complications after gastrectomy with extended lymphadenectomy. Surg Oncol 9:31-34
59. Bassi C, Dervenis C, Butturini G et al (2005) Postoperative pancreatic fistula: an international study group (ISGPF) definition. Surgery 138:8-13
60. Kunisaki C, Makino H, Suwa H et al (2007) Impact of splenectomy in patients with gastric adenocarcinoma of the cardia. J Gastrointest Surg 11:1039-1044
61. Bonenkamp JJ, Songun I, Hermans J et al (1995) Randomized comparison of morbidity after D1 and D2 dissection for gastric cancer in 996 Dutch patients. Lancet 345:745-748
62. Cuschieri A, Fayers P, Fielding J et al (1996) Postoperative morbidity and mortality after D1 and D2 resections for gastric cancer: preliminary results of the MRC randomized controlled surgical trial. The Surgical Cooperative Group. Lancet 347:995-999
63. Lo SS, Wu CW, Shen KH et al (2002) Higher morbidity and mortality after combined total gastrectomy and pancreaticosplenectomy for gastric cancer. World J Surg 26:678-682
64. Yamamoto M, Baba H, Kakeji Y et al (2004) Postoperative morbidity/mortality and survival rates after total gastrectomy with splenectomy/pancreaticosplenectomy for patients with advanced gastric cancer. Hepato-Gastroenterol 51:298-302
65. Maruyama K, Sasako M, Kinoshita T et al (1995) Pancreas preserving total gastrectomy for proximal gastric cancer. World J Surg 19:532-536
66. Chikara Kunisaki et al (2006) Predictive Factors for Pancreatic Fistula After Pancreati-cosplenectomy for Advanced Gastric-Cancer in the Upper Third of the Stomach. J Gastr Surg 10:132-137
67. van der Kallen CJ, Voors-Pette C, de Bruin TW (2004) Abdominal obesity and expression of familial combined hyperlipidemia.

Obes Res 12:2054-2061
68. Keaney JF Jr (2000) Atherosclerosis: From lesion formation to plaque activation and endothe-lial dysfunction. Mol Aspects Med 21:99-166
69. Griffanti Bartoli F, Arnone GB, Ravera G et al (1991) Pancreatic fistula and relative mortality in malignant disease after pancreaticoduodenectomy. Review and statistical meta-analysis regarding 15 years of literature. Anticancer Res 11:1831-1848
70. Buchler MW, Friess H, Wagner M et al (2000) Pancreatic fistula after pancreatic head resection. Br J Surg 87:883-889
71. Rosso E, Bachellier P, Oussoultzoglou E et al (2006) Toward zero pancreatic fistula after pancreaticoduodenectomy with pancreaticogastrostomy. Am J Surg 191:726-732
72. Balzano G, Zerbi A, Cristallo M et al (2005) The unsolved problem of fistula after left pancre-atectomy: the benefit of cautious drain management. J Gastrointest Surg 9:837-842
73. Knaebel HP, Diener MK, Wente MN et al (2005) Systematic review and metaanalysis of tech-nique for closure of the pancreatic remnant after distal pancreatectomy. Br J Surg 92:539-546
74. Roggin KK, Rudloff U, Blumgart LH et al (2006) Central pancreatectomy revisited. J Gastrointest Surg 10:804-812
75. Kawai M, Tani M, Terasawa H et al (2006) Early removal of prophylactic drains reduces the risk of intra-abdominal infections in patients with pancreatic head resection. Prospective study for 104 consecutive patients. Ann Surg 244:1-7
76. Conlon KC, Labow D, Leung D et al (2001) Prospective randomized clinical trial of the value of intraperitoneal drainage after pancreatic resection. Ann Surg 234:487-494
77. Lin JW, Eng M, Cameron JL et al (2004) Risk factors and outcomes in postpancreaticoduodenectomy pancreaticocutaneous fistula. J Gastrointest Surg 8:951-959
78. Torres AJ, Landa JI, Moreno-Azcoita M et al (1992) Somatostatin in the management of gastrointestinal fistula. Arch Surg 127:97-100
79. Halttunen J et al (2005) The endoscopic management of pancreatic fistulas Surg Endosc 19:559-562
80. Fisher A, Baier P et al (2004) Endoscopic management of pancreatic fistulas secondary to intraabdominal operation. Surg Endosc 18:706-708
81. Frymerman AS et al (2010) Impact of Postoperative Pancreatic Fistula on Surgical OutcomeThe Need for a Classification-driven Risk Management. J Gastrointest Surg 14:711-718
82. Ablan CJ, Littooy FN, Freeark RJ (1990) Postoperative chylous ascites: diagnosis and treatment. Arch Surg 125:270-3
83. Kaas R, Rustman LD, Zoetmulder FAN (2001) Chylous ascites after oncological abdominal surgery: incidence and treatment. EJSO 27:187-189
84. Gaglio PJ, Leevy CB, Koneru B (1996) Peri-operative chylous ascites. J Med 27:369-376
85. Rajasekar A, Ravi NR, Diggory RT (2000) Chylous ascites: a rare complication of radical gastrectomy. Int J Clin Pract 54:201-203
86. Halkic N, Adbelmoumene A, Suardet L, Mosimann F (2003) Postoperative chylous ascites after radical gastrectomy. A case report. Minerva Chir 58:389-391
87. Chew-Wun Wu, Mao-Chih Hsieh, Su-Shun Lo et al (1996) Results of curative gastrectomy for carcinoma of the distal third of the stomach. J Am Coll Surg 183: 201-217
88. Yol S, Bostanci EB, Ozogul Y et al (2005) A rare complication of D3 dissection for gastric carcinoma: chyloperitoneum. Gastric Cancer 8:35-38
89. Jayabose S, Kogan S, Berezin S et al (1989) Combined occurrence of chyloperitoneum and chylothorax after surgery and chemotherapy for Wilm's tumor. Cancer 64:1790-1795
90. McVay CB Thoracic cavity and its contents. In: Anson BJ, McVay CB (eds). Surgical anatomy. Philadelphia: WB Saunders, pp. 460-463
91. Pabst TS, McIntyre KE Jr, Schilling JD et al (1993) Management of chyloperitoneum after abdominal aortic surgery. Am J Surg 166:194-198
92. Benedix F, Lippert H, Meyer F (2007) Post surgical lympho cutaneous fistula, chylous ascites and chylothorax-infrequent but serious complications: etiology, diagnosis and therapeutic options. Zentralbl Chir 13:529-538
93. Fairweather M, Santos A P, Ravindra K, Cheadle WG (2010) Chylous ascites Am Surg 76: 442-444
94. Silk YN, Goumas WM, Douglass HO et al (1991) Chylous ascites and lymphocyst management by peritoneovenous shunt. Surgery 110:561-565
95. Cárdenas A, Chopra S (2002) Chylous ascites. Am J Gastroenterol 97:1896-1900
96. Shen WB, Sun YG, Xia S et al (2005) The diagnosis and therapy of chylous ascite. Zhonghua Wai Ke Za Zhi 43:25-28
97. Leibovitch I (2002) Postoperative chylous ascites–the urologist's view. Drugs Today (Barc) 38:687-697
98. Danielson H, Kokkola A, Kiviluoto T et al (2007) Clinical outcome after D1 vs D2-3 gastrec-tomy for treatment of gastric cancer. Scand J Surg 96:35–40
99. Hartgrink HH, van de Velde CJ, Putter H et al (2004) Extended lymph node dissection for gastric cancer: who may benefit? Final results of the randomized Dutch gastric cancer group trial. J Clin Oncol 22(11):2069-2077
100. Yang SH, Zhang YC, Sharma N et al (2009) An evidencebased medicine review of lymphade-nectomy extent for gastric cancer. The American Journal of Surgery 197:246–251
101. Dicken BJ, Bigam DL, Cass C et al (2005) Gastric adenocarcinoma: review and considerations for future directions. Ann Surg 241(1):27-39
102. Yu W, Choi GS, Chung HY (2006) Randomized clinical trial of splenectomy versus splenic preservation in patients with proximal gastric cancer. Br J Surg 93(5):559-563
103. Lo SS,Wu CW, Shen KH et al (2002) Higher morbidity and mortality after combined total gastrectomy and pancreaticosplenectomy for gastric cancer. World J Surg 26(6):678-682
104. Yamamoto M, Baba H, Kakeji Y et al (2004) Postoperative morbidity/mortality and survival rates after total gastrectomy, with splenectomy/pancreaticosplenectomy for patients with advanced gastric cancer. Hepatogastroenterology 51(55):298-302
105. Yang K, Chen XZ, Hu JK et al (2009) Effectiveness and safety of sple-nectomy for gastric carcinoma: a meta-analysis. World J Gastroenterol 15(42):5352-5359
106. Sasako M (1997) Risk factors for surgical treatment in the Dutch gastric cancer trial. Br J Surg 84:1567-1571

Long-term Results after R0 Resection in the Surgical Treatment of Gastric Cancer

17

Franco Roviello, Giovanni Corso, and Daniele Marrelli

Abstract

The International Union against Cancer and the American Joint Committee on Cancer system define residual tumor as R0 when the surgical procedure is concluded without any evidence of macroscopic residual tumor. This index is considered an important factor in terms of the prognosis and long-term survival of gastric carcinoma patients. Our data demonstrate that prognosis and survival differ in high- vs. low-risk areas of gastric cancer; in particular, we determined that prognosis is better in high-risk areas for gastric cancer in patients undergoing R0 surgery. These differences may also take into account the multiple etiologies of gastric tumors. In this chapter, we discuss the R classification in gastric cancer, focusing on long-term survival after radical surgery (R0) and stratifying these data with respect to high- and low-incidence areas for gastric carcinoma development.

Keywords

Gastric cancer • Radical surgery • High- and low-risk areas

17.1 Introduction

Long-term survival in patients with gastric cancer (GC) after curative (R0) resection is strongly influenced by pTNM stage classification, in which lymphatic dissemination is the main predictor of tumor recurrence. Furthermore, it has been demonstrated that extended lymphadenectomy may decrease the risk of tumor relapse after gastric resection, with several other prognostic factors indicative of long-term outcome. Indeed, overall 5-year survival for GC after curative (R0) resection is extremely variable, and significant differences in survival have been reported from institutions throughout the world.

In R1 and R2 cases, prognosis is determined primarily by the absence or presence of distant metastases while the pTNM classification is of minor significance; by contrast, in R0 patients, pTNM is a good predictor of prognosis.

Figure 17.1 provides an overview of gastric carcinoma management with respect to the R0, R1, and R2 classification. In this chapter, we review the overall survival of GC patients who underwent radical (R0) surgery, as reported by several institutions located in different geographic areas.

F. Roviello (✉)
Dept. of Human Pathology and Oncology,
Section of General Surgery and Surgical Oncology,
Translational Research Laboratory,
University of Siena,
Siena, Italy

G. de Manzoni, F. Roviello, W. Siquini (eds.), *Surgery in the Multimodal Management of Gastric Cancer*,

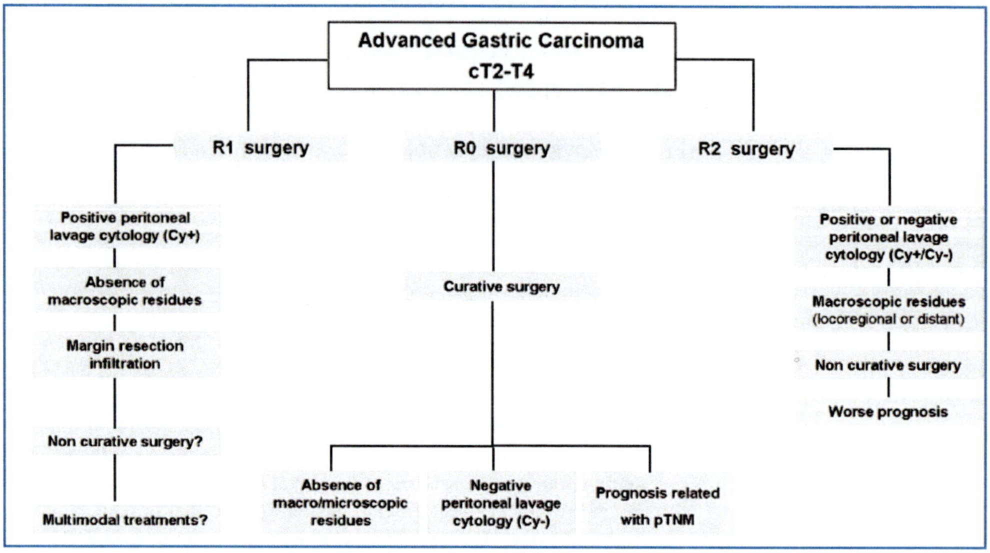

Fig. 17.1 The proposed flow-chart is a model for gastric carcinoma management with respect to the R0, R1, and R2 classification

17.2 Definition of R0 Resection

The residual tumor (R) classification system was defined by Hermanek and Colleagues in 1994 [1, 2]. Surgery is defined as "potentially curative" (R0) when the surgical procedure is concluded without any evidence of macroscopic residual tumor in the tumor bed, lymph nodes, and/or at distant sites. In addition, macroscopic and microscopic examination of resection margins is negative. R1 and R2 indicate, respectively, microscopic and macroscopic residual tumor. According to this definition, the R classification is considered as a predictor of prognosis, in which good long-term survival can be expected only in R0 patients. However, this classification system is currently discussed controversially by different authors because the definitions do not consider the presence of tumor dissemination through the blood stream, peritoneal dissemination, and/or lymphatic involvement. Consequently, the presence of microscopic and distant residual disease could be missed [3]. In this regard, clinical pre-operative staging is fundamental, including the selection of the appropriate modality to determine the extent of tumor spreading: endoscopic ultrasound, computed tomography, positron emission tomography, magnetic resonance imaging, or laparoscopic exploration [4]. More recently, the International Union against Cancer (UICC)/American Joint Committee on Cancer (AJCC) system defined as R0 resection a complete resection of the primary cancer without macroscopic or microscopic residual disease. Patients with intraperitoneal cancer cells, identified by cytology examination after lavage, are classified as having R1 disease. According to the new UICC/AJCC TNM, the number of positive lymph nodes is considered a strong prognostic determinant, and cases with positive peritoneal cytology are considered as M1 and included in stage IV [5, 6].

17.3 Long-term Results after R0 Resection in High-incidence Areas

In this and the following sections, we analyze R0 GC cases and the long-term results, as reported from areas around the world where there is either a high or a low incidence of GC. Among the areas with a high GC incidence are Japan, Korea, China, and Latvia. In Korea and Japan, extended lymph node dissection (D2 or D3) is routinely performed.

Three studies of interest were carried out in Japan. Maruyama et al. [7] analyzed the data of 8851 patients with primary gastric carcinoma (JGCA 2006). The authors identified 4959 GC patients as having R0 disease (namely curability A); the cumulative 5-year survival was 88.5% [7]. A Japanese study based on tumor histology grade was performed on 1119 GC patients, including a subset of R0 cases. The tumors were graded as follows: grade 1, well differentiated; grade 2, moderately differentiated; and grade 3, poorly differentiated [8]. Five-year survival was 71% for patients with grade 1, 65.7% for those with grade 2, and 66.7% for those with grade 3 disease. In the third Japanese study [9], the outcome of 587 GC patients who underwent R0 gastrectomy with D2 lymphadenectomy was analyzed. Five-year survival according to the AJCC/UICC staging system was 94.6% for Ia, 88.4% for Ib, 70.6% for II, 54.1% for IIIa, 35.5% for IIIb, and 25.6% for IV.

A population of 9998 GC patients was analyzed by Ahn et al. [10] from Korea, which has the world's highest incidence of GC. Overall 5-year survival in their R0 resection patients was 66.4%. According to the TNM stage, the 5-year disease-free survival of patients with stages Ia, Ib, IIa, IIb, IIIa, IIIb, and IIIc was 95.1, 88.4, 84, 71.7, 58.4, 41.3, and 26.1%, respectively.

Among Asian countries, a paper described 2159 patients in China who underwent both en bloc resection of primary GC and D2/D3 lymphadenectomy, without microscopic or macroscopic residual disease (R0). The 5-year disease-free survival of patients with stages I, II, III, and IV was 84, 50.8, 29.1, and 12.4%, respectively [11].

The advantage of these Asian studies was that in each one screening programs led to the diagnosis of GC at an early stage of the disease. Furthermore, most patients achieved radical (R0) resection with D2 or D3 lymphadenectomy.

Good results were also reported in a Latvian study of 444 patients with GC who underwent R0 surgery [12]. Five-year survival was 52.5% but considering pTNM stage was 89.7% for stage Ia, 72.6% for stage Ib, 52.9% for stage II, 34.8% for stage IIIa, 27.4% for stage IIIb, and 18.7% for stage IV.

Considered as a whole, the overall 5-year survival of patients from high-incidence areas treated by R0 surgery is approximately 44-88%. The lowest overall survival was registered in China (44%) and the highest in Japan (88.5%).

17.4 Long-term Results after R0 Resection in Low-incidence Areas

Among the countries with a low GC incidence, we consider studies from the USA, Germany, and Norway.

In the USA, the 711 patients analyzed in the study of Strong et al. [13] were treated in a specialized center by R0 resection, with extended lymphadenectomy performed in most cases. The authors reported an overall 5-year survival rate of 58%. The study of Cunningham et al. [14] consisted of 436 patients; overall 5-year survival after R0 resection in this group was 33%. In a trial comparing chemoradiotherapy after surgery vs. surgery alone, Macdonald et al. [15] reported an overall 5-year survival of 44% in 281 patients treated by gastrectomy and chemoradiotherapy vs. 28% in 275 patients treated by surgery alone. Notably, in that trial only 10% of patients were treated by D2 dissection.

A study from Germany analyzed 124 GC patients who underwent curative surgery (R0) with D2 lymphadenectomy [16]; the overall survival rate over a period of 94 months was 51%. A multicentric study was conducted in Germany by Siewert et al. [17], in which 1182 consecutive patients underwent radical surgery with D1 or D2 lymphadenectomy. The 5-year survival rate with respect to stage was: Ia 82.8%, Ib 68.3%, II 42.9%, IIIa 28.2%, IIIb 16.7%, and IV 17.3%. Long-term survival was better in patients receiving R0 surgery and D2 lymphadenectomy at stage II (29% vs. 56.7%). In another Western study, from Norway [18], 97 patients underwent R0 surgery for gastric carcinoma with D1 lymphadenectomy; 5-year survival was 39%.

In low-incidence areas (USA, Norway, Germany), there are more cases of advanced stage disease and thus a lower overall 5-year survival (28-58%) than in high-incidence areas (Korea, Japan, China, Latvia), where survival is 44–88%. Specifically, the American data showed lower overall 5-year survival in GC patients with R0 resection (28-58%), with similar results in the population from Norway (39%). In Germany, the overall survival rate (42–51%) is within the range of that in high-incidence areas. Generally, however, patients with R0 GC in countries with a higher incidence of the disease have a better prognosis than analogous patients in low-incidence countries.

17.5 The Experience of the Italian Research Group for Gastric Cancer

The Italian Research Group for Gastric Cancer (GIRCG) assessed a prognostic score predicting tumor recurrence in GC patients with curative resection (R0) [19] based on 536 patients who underwent UICC R0 resection at three surgical department in Italy (University of Siena, University of Verona, and Morgagni Hospital of Forlì). During the follow-up period, tumor relapse was identified in 50.7% of these patients. The results of this study demonstrated that the predicted and observed risk of recurrence overlapped, with a sensitivity of 83.5% and specificity of 81.1%. The statistical model identified nodal status, pT stage, tumor location, extent of lymphadenectomy, and advanced age as independent predictors of recurrence.

Extended lymphadenectomy (D2) is considered the standard approach for the treatment of advanced GC, with benefits in long-term survival. The GIRCG demonstrated that the 5-year overall survival was 54% in patients with R0 surgery and D2 lymphadenectomy, and with a real survival benefit for patients with locoregional lymph node involvement [20]. Another study [21], conducted on 286 R0 GC patients treated with super-extended (D3) lymphadenectomy, demonstrated a potential benefit of this procedure, especially in patients with pT2 disease and positive nodes (5-year overall survival 60%).

The overall geographic Italian area is considered to be at low-risk for GC, but in some regions of the country the incidence is relatively high [22, 23]. In Tuscany, for example, the estimated incidence of GC is three-fold higher than in Southern Italy. GC patients in Tuscany have a 5-year survival probability of 63.2% compared to 48% in patients in Southern Italy.

Table 17.1 reviews the overall survival rate reported in the literature for GC patients undergoing potentially curative surgery (R0).

Table 17.1 Overall survival rate reported in the literature in patients with gastric cancer who underwent potentially curative surgery (R0)

Author [Reference]	Country	Risk area	N. of patients	UICC	Lymphadenectomy	Follow-up end-time (months)	Overall survival (%)
Inoue et al. [8]	Korea	High	9.998	R0	D2-D3	60	55.6
Maruyama et al. [7]	Japan	High	4.959	R0	D2	60	88.5
Ichikura et al. [9]	Japan	High	1.119	R0	Unknown	60	67.8
Ahn et al. [10]	Japan	High	587	R0	D2	60	61.5
Sun et al. [11]	China	High	2.159	R0	D2-D3	60	44.0
Sivinis et al. [12]	Latvia	High	444	R0	D1	60	52.5
Strong et al. [13]	USA	Low	711	R0	D2	60	58.0
Cunningham et al. [14]	USA	Low	436	R0	Unknown	60	33.0
McDonald et al. [15]	USA	Low	556	R0	D1	60	28-44[a]
Roukos et al. [16]	Germany	Low	124	R0	D2	94	51.0
Siewert et al. [17]	Germany	Low	1.182	R0	D1-D2	60	42.7
Lello et al. [18]	Norway	Low	97	R0	D1	60	39.0
[Present report]	Italy-Tuscany Italy-Southern	High Low	545 89	R0 R0	D2-D3 D2-D3	60 60	63.2 48.0

[a]Surgery alone vs. surgery + radio-/chemotherapy.

17.6 Conclusions

Radical resection (R0) for GC offers the possibility of cure although it requires complete surgical removal of the tumor. The UICC classification for GC considers curative resection (R0) as a good predictive prognostic factor; nevertheless, the limitation of this classification (R0 vs. R1) is the risk of overlooking microscopic tumor diffusion, especially in cases with hematogenous or peritoneal metastasis. Therefore, the R classification may represent a more valid prognostic indicator when associated with pTNM stage.

The overall survival of R0 patients who undergo GC resection is 30-70%, and varies notably in different institutions worldwide. The survival rate of R0 GC patients is better in high-incidence than in low-incidence areas. This difference has been explained by: (a) differences in the disease itself; (b) stage migration; and (c) differences in treatment. These explanations are probably not mutually exclusive. Moreover, environmental factors can interact with and influence molecular pathways, as can single-nucleotide polymorphisms and dietary and life-style habits.

The widespread introduction of screening programs in high-incidence countries has resulted in the detection of early stage GC, which in turn would explain differences in prognosis; in addition, those countries generally have a better diagnostic and therapeutic approach, which is also likely play a prognostic role. This points to the need for a standard surgical approach to the treatment of GC; for example, it has been demonstrated that extended (D2) and superextended (D3) lymphadenectomy are associated with better R0 outcome in advanced cases of GC, also in low-risk areas.

References

1. Hermanek P, Wittekind C (1994) Residual tumor (R) classification and prognosis. Semin Surg Oncol 10:12-20
2. Hermanek P (1995) pTNM and residual tumor classifications: problems of assessment and prognostic significance. World J Surg 19:184-190
3. Biondi A, Persiani R, Cananzi F et al (2010) R0 resection in the treatment of gastric cancer: Room for improvement. World J Gastroenterol 16:3358-3370
4. Kwee RM, Kwee TC (2007) Imaging in local staging of gastric cancer: a systematic review. J Clin Oncol 25:2107-2116
5. Fleming ID, Cooper JS, Henson DE et al (1997) American Joint Committee on Cancer staging manual, 5th edition. Philadelphia: Lippincott-Raven
6. Edge SB, Byrd DR, Compton CC et al (2010) AJCC Cancer Staging Handbook, 7th edn. New York: Springer-Verlag
7. Maruyama K, Kaminishi M, Hayashi K-I et al (2006) Gastric Cancer treated in 1991 in Japan: data analysis of nationwide registry. Gastric Cancer 9:51-66
8. Inoue K, Nakane Y, Michiura T et al (2002) Histopathological grading does not affect survival after R0 surgery for gastric cancer. Eur J Surg Oncol 28:633-636
9. Ichikura T, Tomimatsu S, Uefuji K et al (1999) Evaluation of the new American Joint Committee on Cancer/International Union Against Cancer Classification of lymph node metastasis from gastric carcinoma in comparison with Japanese classification. Cancer 86:553-558
10. Ahn HS, Lee H-J, Hahn S et al (2010) Evaluation of the Seventh American Joint Committee on Cancer/International Union against cancer classification of gastric adenocarcinoma in comparison with the sixth classification. Cancer 116: 5592-5598
11. Sun Z, Li D, Wang Z et al (2009) Prognostic significance of microscopic positive margins for gastric cancer patients with potentially curative resection. Ann Surg Oncol 16:3028-3037
12. Sivins A, Pedrazzani C, Roviello F et al (2009) Surgical treatment of gastric cancer in Latvia: results of centralized experience. Eur J surg Oncol 35:481-485
13. Strong VE, Song KY, Park CH et al (2010) Comparison of gastric cancer survival following R0 resection in the United States and Korea using an internationally validated nomogram. Ann Surg 251:640-646
14. Cunningham SC, Kamangar F, Kim MP et al (2005) Survival after gastric adenocarcinoma resection: eighteen-year experience at a single institution. J Gastrointest Surg 9:718-725
15. Macdonald JS, Smalley SR, Benedetti J et al (2001) Chemoradiotherapy after surgery compared with surgery alone for adenocarcinoma of the stomach or gastroesophageal junction 345:725-730
16. Roukos DH, Lorenz M, Karakostas K et al (2001) Pathological serosa and node-based classification accurately predicts gastric cancer recurrence risk and outcome, and determines potential and limitation of a Japanese-style extensive surgery for Western patients: a prospective with quality control 10-year follow-up study. Br J Cancer 84:1602-1609
17. Siewert JR, Bottcher K, Stein HJ et al (1998) Relevant prognostic factors in gastric cancer. Ann Surg 228: 449-461
18. Lello E, Furnes B, Edna T-H (2007) Short and long-term survival from gastric cancer. A population-based study from a county hospital during 25 years. Acta Oncol 46:308-315
19. Marrelli D, De Stefano A, de Manzoni G et al (2005) Prediction of recurrence after radical surgery for gastric cancer. Ann Surg 241:247-255
20. Roviello F, Marrelli D, Morgagni P et al (2002) Survival benefit of extended D2 lymphadenectomy in gastric cancer with involvement of second level of lymph nodes: a longitudinal multicenter study. Ann Surg Oncol 9:894-900

21. Roviello F, Pedrazzani C, Marrelli D et al (2010) Super-extended (D3) lymphadenectomy in advanced gastric cancer. Eur J Surg Oncol 36:439-446
22. Marrelli D, Pedrazzani C, Corso G et al (2009) Different pathological features and prognosis in gastric cancer patients coming from high-risk and low-risk areas of Italy. Ann Surg 250:43-50
23. Marrelli D, Pedrazzani C, Roviello F (2010) Gastric cancer prognosis: strong correlation between incidence and survival. Ann Surg Oncol 17:340-341

Surgical Treatment of Gastric Cancer Infiltrating the Esophago-gastric Junction

18

Giovanni de Manzoni, Andrea Zanoni, and Corrado Pedrazzani

Abstract

Tumors infiltrating the esophago-gastric junction (EGJ) are characterized by a worse prognosis than cancers of the middle and lower thirds of the stomach. The definition, classification, and treatment of these tumors have yet to be definitively standardized. Complete resection of the tumor is considered the main goal of surgery, although the best approach and the appropriate extent of surgical resection continue to be debated. This chapter discusses the extent of gastric and esophageal resection as well as that of lymph node dissection. Long-term results and the main factors affecting prognosis are presented. The limits of primary surgery are defined and the adoption of pre-operative multimodality treatments in the context of controlled clinical trials encouraged.

Keywords

Esophago-gastric junction • Siewert Classification • TNM Classification • Surgery • Resection margins

18.1 Introduction

The incidence of gastric cancer, especially intestinal-type tumors of the lower third of the stomach, has been decreasing. Conversely, the incidence of diffuse-type tumors involving all parts of the stomach has remained stable whereas tumors located around the esophago-gastric junction (EGJ) have become more common, as reported in studies from the US and Europe [1, 2].

G. de Manzoni (✉)
Dept. of Surgery,
Upper G.I. Surgery Division,
University of Verona,
Verona, Italy

Controversies exist regarding the definition, classification, and staging of tumors arising in proximity to the EGJ, due to the border location of the cardia region, between the esophagus and stomach. The previous version of the TNM staging system (AJCC-UICC, 6th edn.) classified tumors involving the EGJ as esophageal when > 50% of the cancer occupied the esophagus, and as gastric when > 50% of the cancer infiltrated the stomach. For tumors located equally above and below the EGJ, the histology determined the origin, with Barrett's adenocarcinoma most likely to be esophageal in origin [3].

Siewert proposed classifying EGJ tumors into types I, II, and III depending on the relative extent of involvement of either the esophagus or the stomach (Fig. 18.1). Briefly, in type I, the center of the tumor lies 1–5 cm above the anatomic EGJ;

G. de Manzoni, F. Roviello, W. Siquini (eds.), *Surgery in the Multimodal Management of Gastric Cancer*,

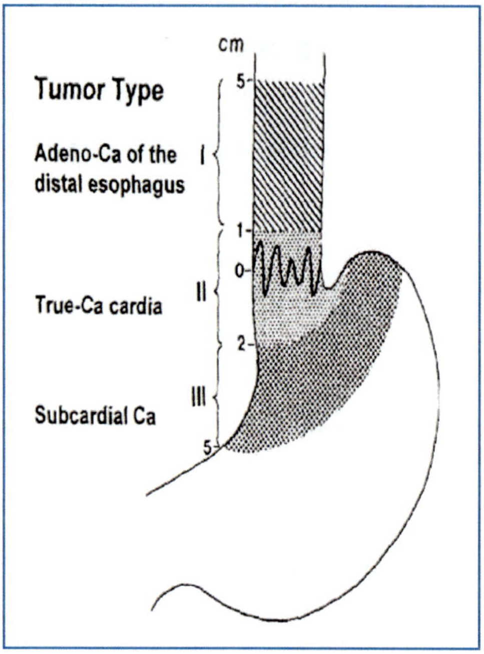

Fig. 18.1 Schematic representation of the Siewert classification

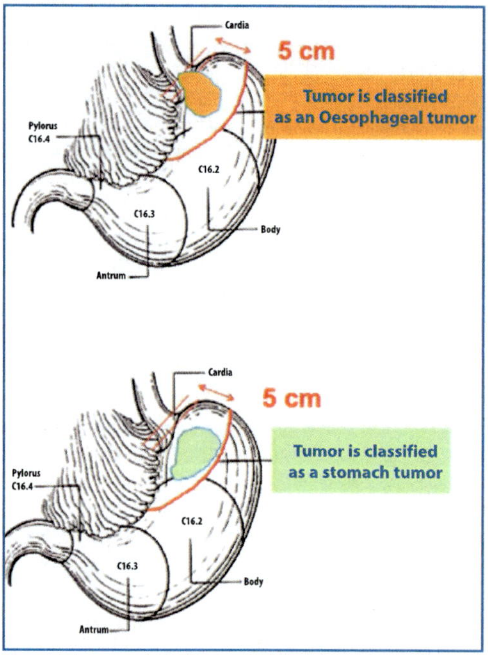

Fig. 18.2 Definition of tumors arising near the esophago-gastric junction (EGJ) according to the new TNM staging system, 7th edn. (Courtesy of Prof. Christian Witteking)

in type II, the tumor lies 1 cm above to 2 cm below the anatomic EGJ; and in type III, the center is 2–5 cm below the anatomic EGJ [4]. Although this classification did not demonstrate a prognostic value per se, it proved to be a useful tool in planning the surgical approach [5, 6]. Furthermore, Siewert's classification has allowed the discrimination of tumors with different etiologies and peculiar clinical and biological characteristics [4, 7]. Its major limit is the characterization of type II tumors, as their etiology, definition, and treatment are still debated. Currently, they are considered and managed as esophageal tumors by some and as gastric tumors by others [8, 9].

The new TNM staging system (AJCC-UICC, 7th edn.) radically changes the categorization of tumors located in this region. All tumors whose centers are located within 5 cm below the anatomic EGJ and which infiltrate the junction are classified as esophageal cancers. Otherwise, those tumors located within 5 cm below but not infiltrating the EGJ are considered gastric cancers [10]. Hence, type III tumors according to the Siewert classification are here considered and staged as esophageal cancers. Differently, if the tumor's center is located > 5 cm away from the EGJ, it is classified as gastric even if it infiltrates the EGJ or the esophagus (Fig. 18.2).

18.2 Surgical Treatment

Radical resection is the mainstay of therapy for tumors infiltrating the EGJ, although survival results after surgery alone are poorer than those following the resection of gastric cancers not infiltrating the junction. Five-year survival rates after R0 resection for tumors whose centers are located within 5 cm above and below the EGJ are 25–40% [5, 6, 8, 11]. The worse prognosis is mainly due to the great propensity of tumors infiltrating the esophagus to lymphatic dissemination, a consequence of the extensive lymphatic system in the submucosa. As soon as the cancer breaches the muscularis mucosae, it invades the associated lymphatics, which drain into regional lymph nodes but also directly into the thoracic duct [12]. Thus, lymphatic dissemination and the ability to completely remove the tumor (R0 resection) are indeed the main factors affecting prognosis [5, 11-14]. Incomplete surgical resection, either macroscopic (R2 resection) or microscopic (R1 resection), implies a very small chance of long-term survival [5, 6, 13].

18.2.1 Extent of Gastric and Esophageal Resection

Positive resection margins are a key factor precluding the success of surgical resection [13, 15, 16]. In the treatment of tumors involving the EGJ, the proximal extent of the tumor into the esophagus as well as its distal infiltration into the stomach should be taken into consideration and evaluated carefully. This means that, depending on the tumor's extent, the option of performing a thoracotomy to achieve adequate proximal resection margins and a gastrectomy to obtain distal clearance should be considered for every patient. The mode of subsequent reconstruction is influenced by the level of gastric resection.

Gastrectomy should be considered mandatory in patients with gastric cancers infiltrating the EGJ and in those with Siewert type III tumors. In such cases, esophageal resection is accomplished through a trans-hiatal or trans-thoracic resection, depending on the extent of esophageal infiltration. In this setting, Sasako and colleagues randomized 167 patients to either a trans-hiatal or a left thoraco-abdominal approach to treat gastric cancer of the cardia or subcardia infiltrating the distal esophagus for ≤ 3 cm. In this trial, there were no differences in the length of esophageal resection, frequency of local recurrence, and overall survival between the two approaches. The authors concluded that a left thoraco-abdominal approach is not justified to treat cardia or subcardia tumors when the extent of esophageal invasion is ≤ 3 cm [15]. Furthermore, a recent analysis on the quality of life of this group of patients demonstrated worse short-term results [17].

Barbour and colleagues specifically analyzed the influence of esophageal resection margins and operative approach on the outcome of patients treated for adenocarcinoma of the EGJ. They concluded that resection margins > 5 cm of the in vivo distal esophagus lead to a better prognosis. Thus, while esophagectomy should be strongly recommended for patients with Siewert type I tumors, the surgical approach may be individualized to achieve this goal for those with Siewert types II and III tumors [16].

In our current practice, all patients with cancers infiltrating the EGJ and with the bulk of the tumor involving the stomach are treated by total gastrectomy with distal esophageal resection. The convenience of adding a thoracotomy is evaluated on a case-by-case basis. The patient's age and fitness together with the tumor's characteristics (esophageal infiltration > 2–3 cm) as well as the possibility of achieving adequate proximal resection margins (R0 resection at frozen section and a clear margin > 5 cm) are the main factors taken into consideration.

18.2.2 Extent of Lymph Node Dissection

Lymph node involvement is a critical determinant of prognosis in tumors involving the EGJ [5, 12, 14, 18]. The peculiar position of the EGJ allows tumors in this region to readily spread, both proximally to the mediastinal lymph nodes and distally to the abdominal nodes [18-20]. In a recent series, we demonstrated that mediastinal lymph nodes are involved in 46% of Siewert type I, 30% of type II, and 9% of type III tumors. Conversely, abdominal nodes are involved in all cases in which lymph node metastases are present. Furthermore, tumors of the three Siewert types often spread to second-tier abdominal nodes. Above all, left gastric artery nodes (station 7) are affected in 14–60% of type I, 18–65% of type II, and 10–42% of type III tumors [18, 19, 21-23]. Likewise, the percentage of metastases to the common hepatic artery (station 8) and celiac trunk (station 9) nodes cannot be considered negligible (10–18%).

Interestingly, metastases to the para-aortic nodes (station 16) are an extremely common event in upper-third gastric cancers and in type III cancers. In our series, nodal involvement of para-aortic stations was determined in about 30% of the patients who underwent D3 lymphadenectomy [19, 24]. A similar rate was reported by authors from Japan [25-27].

The long-term advantage of extended lymphadenectomy has been difficult to prove in gastric and esophageal cancers, due to the paucity of cases and the limitations of randomized controlled trials published to date; nonetheless, recent data seem to establish the superiority of extended lymphadenectomy both in disease control and in long-term survival, with no increase in morbidity and mortality. At present, the adoption of extended lymphadenectomy seems to be justified and advisable, as supported by the Taiwan trial [28] and the final results of the Dutch trial [29].

Regarding para-aortic node dissection in a prophylactic setting, the Japanese trial failed to demonstrate an advantage for tumors involving all regions of the stomach [30]. Conversely, in a clinical setting, we recently determined very high survival rates after D3 lymphadenectomy for patients with tumors not infiltrating the serosa [24]. Our results are consistent with the post-hoc analysis of the Japanese trial, in which potential benefits for pT2 patients and those with tumors located in the upper stomach were reported [30]. These results together with those of Kurokawa et al., which refuted the possibility of a poorer outcome in terms of quality of life for patients undergoing para-aortic node dissection [17], seem to justify the use of this extended procedure in order to obtain R0 resection, when no major increase in morbidity and mortality is expected.

18.2.3 Splenectomy

The side effects of splenectomy and the merits of the procedure with respect to the long-term prognosis in the treatment of gastric cancer is described elsewhere in this volume. Infiltration of the EGJ from proximal gastric cancer does not account for the frequency of metastatic nodes at the splenic hilum [19, 31]. Accordingly, the indications for splenectomy remain unchanged.

18.3 Long-term Results and the Main Factors Affecting Prognosis

Patients with gastric cancers arising close to the cardia and subcardia have a poorer prognosis than those with tumors of the middle and distal parts of the stomach. Survival rates of patients with tumors infiltrating the esophagus or reaching the EGJ are very similar to those determined for patients with primary esophageal cancers. Of note, considering tumors whose centers are located 5 cm above and below the EGJ, no differences in prognosis were observed between the three Siewert types [5, 6, 11].

18.3.1 Type of Resection (R Category)

Complete surgical resection (R0 resection) should be considered the primary aim of surgery, given that there is virtually no chance of cure for patients with residual tumor [5, 6, 13]. Indeed, median survival after macroscopically incomplete surgical resection (R2 resection) is very short, usually well below 12 months [5, 6]. Accordingly, given the complexity of the necessary surgical procedure and the related short-term results in terms of quality of life, surgery should be considered unreasonable in palliative cases.

The presence of microscopic residual tumor (R1 resection) is similarly considered to strongly influence prognosis [13, 15, 16, 32]. No possibility of cure has been reported by the majority of authors in studies of patients with positive peritoneal washing or positive resection margins. Nonetheless, the rare long-term survivor with microscopic involvement of the resection margin has been described in large series [5].

A positive peritoneal washing is more frequently observed in patient whose tumors predominantly extend into the stomach and it is always indicative of a poor prognosis. In the new TNM classification, positive peritoneal cytology is considered as systemic disease; hence, tumors with cancer cells demonstrated in the peritoneal lavage are classified as stage IV [10].

Consistent with the literature results [5, 8, 11], in our experience the median survival time for 113 patients who underwent a potentially curative resection (R0 resection) for type II or III EGJ adenocarcinoma was 26 months with 3- and 5-year survival rates of 44 and 35%, respectively [14].

18.3.2 Depth of Tumor Invasion (pT Category)

As for gastric cancers of the middle and lower third of the stomach, the depth of tumor invasion alters the prognosis. Typically, tumors infiltrating the EGJ show two main peculiarities: (a) the prognosis, as evaluated on a stage by stage basis, is poorer and (b) due to the lack of a serosal layer in the cardia region, the prognosis of tumors with transmural growth and those with serosal invasion is similar [6, 33].

Five-year survival rates for tumors infiltrating the submucosal layer (pT1) are reported to be 50–80% [5, 6, 33]. These poor results are mostly related to the frequent nodal involvement (20%-40%) [6, 12].

For pT2 and pT3 tumors, the new TNM classification does not overcome the limits of the previous edition. In fact, tumors of the EGJ region are now divided into those infiltrating the muscularis propria (pT2) and those infiltrating the adventitia (pT3). However, firstly, the new classification does not consider tumors arising on the anterior aspect of the cardia and in the subcardia region covered by the serosa. Secondly, it does not differentiate between tumors with transmural growth and tumors infiltrating but not penetrating the muscularis propria even though they differ in terms of prognosis. Characteristically, tumors with transmural growth that do not infiltrate the serosa due to their location (pT3) share with pT4a tumors a similarly poor 5-year survival rate (~20%) after surgery alone [6, 33].

When adjacent organ invasion is demonstrated at primary surgery (pT4b), patients with tumors infiltrating the EGJ have a very small chance of long-term survival, with an extremely poor median survival time as well. In view of these results, multimodality treatment should be strongly encouraged in this setting.

18.3.3 Nodal Involvement (pN Category)

In adenocarcinomas infiltrating the EGJ, lymph node involvement is the main predictor of survival [34, 35] and a major determinant of locoregional recurrence [36, 37]. Similar to the previous classification for gastric cancer, the new TNM classification considers different pN classes based on the number of involved regional lymph nodes. The definition of regional nodes varies between esophageal and gastric cancer classifications; hence, regional nodes are considered differently for tumors classified as EGJ and those of the stomach infiltrating the EGJ. For EGJ adenocarcinomas, regional nodes are defined as those in the esophageal drainage area, which includes the para-esophageal nodes of the neck and the celiac axis nodes [10]. For gastric cancers infiltrating the EGJ, regional nodes are considered those in the gastric drainage area, with the retropancreatic, para-aortic, portal, retroperitoneal, and mesenteric nodes considered as non-regional nodes. The lower para-esophageal and mediastinal nodes are classified as non-regional nodes, although no detailed description is provided [10].

In our experience [14, 19] and in that of several other groups [35, 38, 39], the chances of cure after surgery alone are limited to patients with < 4–6 positive lymph nodes. Nonetheless, due to the paucity of cases, no data have been published comparing pN1 (1–2 positive nodes) and pN2 (3–6 positive nodes) cases either for EGJ tumors or for gastric cancers infiltrating the junction.

In contrast to what is reported in the new TNM classification, there seems to be virtually no chance of cure for EGJ adenocarcinomas with second-tier abdominal lymph node metastases, even after extended lymphadenectomy. The same applies to EGJ tumors with mediastinal lymph node involvement, as recently confirmed by Peters et al. [20].

18.4 Multimodality Treatments

An evaluation of the multimodality treatment protocols proposed to date for tumors infiltrating the EGJ is beyond the scope of this chapter. Nonetheless, we would like to highlight the limits of primary surgery as the sole treatment of this type of tumor. It is our opinion that the use of pre-operative multimodality treatments should be strongly encouraged in the context of controlled clinical trials for tumors of the EGJ as well as for gastric cancers infiltrating the EGJ with transmural growth and/or nodal involvement, as determined at staging work-up.

References

1. Wu H, Rusiecki JA, Zhu K et al (2009) Stomach carcinoma incidence patterns in the United States by histologic type and anatomic site. Cancer Epidemiol Biomarkers Prev 18:1945-1952
2. Marrelli D, Pedrazzani C, Morgagni P et al on behalf of the Italian Research Group for Gastric Cancer (2011) Changing clinical and pathological features of gastric cancer in the period 1991-2005. A statistical evaluation of the Italian research group for gastric cancer (IRGCC) database. Br J Surg. Epub ahead of print
3. American Joint Committee on Cancer (2006) AJCC Cancer Staging Atlas. Springer Science+Business Media, New York
4. Siewert JR, Stein HJ (1998) Classification of adenocarcinoma of the oesophagogastric-junction. Br J Surg 85:1457-1459
5. Siewert JR, Feith M, Werner M et al (2000) Adenocarcinoma of the esophagogastric junction. Results of surgical therapy based on anatomical/topographic classification in 1,002 consecutive patients. Ann Surg 232:353-361
6. de Manzoni G, Pedrazzani C, Pasini F et al (2002) Results of surgical treatment of adenocarcinoma of the gastric cardia. Ann Thorac Surg 73:1035-1040
7. Pedrazzani C, de Manzoni G, Marrelli D et al (2007) It is time for a proper staging system for adenocarcinoma of the gastro-esopageal junction. J Clin Oncol 25:907-908
8. Marsman WA, Tytgat GNJ, ten Kate FJW et al (2005) Differences and similarities of adenocarcinomas of the esophagus and esophagogastric junction. J Surg Oncol 92:160-168
9. McColl KEL, Going JJ (2010) Aetiology and classification of adenocarcinoma of the gastro-esophageal junction/cardia. Gut 59:282-284
10. American Joint Committee on Cancer (2010) AJCC Cancer Staging Manual, 7th edn. Springer Science+Business Media, New York
11. Lagarde SM, ten Kate FJW, Reitsma JB et al (2006) Prognostic Factors in Adenocarcinoma of the Esophagus or Gastroesophageal Junction. J Clin Oncol 24:4347-4355
12. Rice TW, Zuccaro G, Adelstein DJ (1998) Esophageal carcinoma: depth of tumor invasion is predictive of regional lymph node status. Ann Thorac Surg 65:787-792
13. Ito H, Clancy TE, Osteen RT et al (2004) Adenocarcinoma of the gastric cardia: what is the optimal surgical approach? J Am Coll Surg 199:880-886
14. Pedrazzani C, de Manzoni G, Marrelli D et al (2007) Nodal staging in adenocarcinoma of the gastro-esophageal junction. Proposal of a specific staging system. Ann Surg Oncol 14:299-305
15. Sasako M, Sano T, Yamamoto S et al for the Japan Clinical Oncology Group (2006) Left thoracoabdominal approach versus abdominal transhiatal approach for gastric cancer of the cardia or subcardia: a randomised controlled trial. Lancet Oncol 7:644-651
16. Barbour AP, Rizk NP, Gonen M et al (2007) Adenocarcinoma of the gastroesophageal junction: influence of esophageal resection margin and operative approach on outcome. Ann Surg 246:1-6
17. Kurokawa Y, Sasako M, Sano T et al for the Japan Clinical Oncology Group (2011) Randomized controlled trials comparing postoperative changes in body weight, symptoms and respiratory function after estende surgery in gastric cancer patients. Br J Surg in press
18. Dresner SM, Lamb PJ, Bennett MK et al (2001) The pattern of metastatic lymph node dissemination from adenocarcinoma of the esophagogastric junction. Surgery 129:103-109
19. Pedrazzani C, de Manzoni G, Marrelli D et al (2007) Lymph node involvement in advanced gastro-esophageal junction adenocarcinoma. J Thorac Cardiovasc Surg 134:378-385
20. Peters CJ, Hardwick RH, Vowler SL et al for the Oesophageal Cancer Clinical and Molecular Stratification Study Group (2009) Generation and validation of a revised classification for oesophageal and junctional adenocarcinoma. Br J Surg 96:724-733
21. Nigro JJ, DeMeester SR, Hagen JA et al (1999) Node status in transmural esophageal adenocarcinoma and outcome after en bloc esophagectomy. J Thorac Cardiovasc Surg 117:960-968
22. Yuasa N, Miyake H, Yamada T et al (2006) Clinicopathologic comparison of Siewert type II and III adenocarcinomas of the gastroesophageal junction. World J Surg 30:364-371
23. Wijnhoven BPL, Siersema PD, Hop WCJ et al (1999) Adenocarcinomas of the distal oesophagus and gastric cardia are one clinical entity. Br J Surg 86:529-535
24. Roviello F, Pedrazzani C, Marrelli D et al (2010) Super-extended (D3) lymphadenectomy in advanced gastric cancer. Eur J Surg Oncol 36:439-446
25. Hsu CP, Wu CC, Chen CY et al (1997) Clinical experience in radical lymphadenectomy for adenocarcinoma of the gastric cardia. J Thorac Cardiovasc Surg 114:544-551
26. Kitamura K, Nishida S, Yamamoto K et al (1998) Lymph node metastasis in gastric cancer in the upper third of the stomach. Surgical treatment an the basis of the anatomical distribution of positive node. Hepatogastroenterology 45:281-285
27. Maeta M, Yamashiro H, Saito H et al (1999) A prospective pilot study of extended (D3) and superextended para-aortic lymphadenectomy (D4) in patients with T3 or T4 gastric cancer managed by total gastrectomy. Surgery 125:325-331
28. Wu CW, Hsiung CA, Lo SS et al (2006) Nodal dissection for patients with gastric cancer: a randomised controlled trial. Lancet Oncol 7:309-315
29. Songun I, Putter H, Kranenbarg EM et al (2010). Surgical treatment of gastric cancer: 15-year follow-up results of the randomised nationwide Dutch D1D2 trial. Lancet Oncol 11:404-405
30. Sasako M, Sano T, Yamamoto S et al (2008) Japan Clinical

Oncology Group. D2 lymphadenectomy alone or with para-aortic nodal dissection for gastric cancer. New Engl J Med 359:453-462
31. Di Leo A, Marrelli D, Roviello F et al (2007). Lymph node involvement in gastric cancer for different tumor's site and T stage. Italian Research Group for Gastric Cancer (IRGGC) experience. J Gastrointest Surg 11:1146-1153
32. Mariette C, Castel B, Baton JM et al (2003) Extent of oesophageal resection for adenocarcinoma of the oesophagogastric junction. Eur J Surg Oncol 29:588-593
33. Siewert JR, Bottcher K, Stein HJ (1995) Problem of proximal third gastric carcinoma. World J Surg 19:523-531
34. Collard JM (2001) Exclusive radical surgery for esophageal adenocarcinoma. Cancer 91:1098-1104
35. Mariette C, Castel B, Toursel H et al (2002) Surgical management of and long-term survival after adenocarcinoma of the cardia. Br J Surg 89:1156-1163
36. de Manzoni, Pedrazzani C, Pasini F et al (2003) Pattern of recurrence after surgery in adenocarcinoma of the gastro-oesophageal junction. Eur J Surg Oncol 29:506-510
37. Lerut T, Coosemans W, Decker G et al (2004) Extended surgery for cancer of the esophagus and gastroesophageal junction. J Surg Res 117:58-63
38. Wayman J, Bennett MK, Raimes SA et al (2002) The pattern of recurrence of adenocarcinoma of the oesophago-gastric junction. Br J Cancer 86:1223-1229
39. Barbour AP, Rizk NP, Gonen M et al (2007) Lymphadenectomy for adenocarcinoma of the gastroesophageal junction (GEJ): impact of adequate staging on outcome. Ann Surg Oncol 14:306-316

Surgical Treatment of Gastric Cancer in Elderly Patients

19

Pasquina M.C. Tomaiuolo, Andrea Mazzari, Ugo Grossi, and Antonio Crucitti

Abstract

Gastric adenocarcinoma is considered a disease of the elderly, with a peak incidence in the seventh and eighth decades of life. In the elderly, biochemical changes in tissues and in organ physiology, in association with *Helicobacter pylori* infection, lead to atrophic gastritis, with an increased risk of developing cancer. Gastric cancer in the elderly is often diagnosed at an advanced stage and is associated with a poor prognosis in terms of disease-free and overall survival. Surgical treatment of gastric cancer in these patients remains controversial due to the increased perioperative risk; instead, subtotal gastrectomy is preferred when feasible. Total gastrectomy with or without combined resections of adjacent organs is associated with higher rates of postoperative morbidity and mortality. For advanced cancer, palliative resection is preferable, whenever possible, to gastroenterostomy. Morbidity and mortality are higher in the elderly, probably related to the comorbidities in these patients. T stage, lymph node metastases, and depth of invasion of the primary tumor are recognized as independent prognostic factors in terms of overall survival. The impact of multimodality treatment in the elderly cannot be clearly evaluated; currently, adjuvant chemotherapy is recommended in otherwise healthy patients. In general, age alone has not been definitively confirmed as a negative prognostic factor in patients with gastric cancer and should not preclude gastric resection. After radical resection, elderly patients have the same chance of survival as middle-age patients.

Keywords

Elderly • Age • Gastric cancer • Gastrectomy • Lymphadenectomy • Comorbidity • Atrophic gastritis • Survival rate • Chemotherapy

19.1 Introduction

Although the incidence of gastric cancer has declined in the general population since the early 20th century, it remains the most common gastrointestinal malignancy in endemic areas (such as

A. Crucitti (✉)
Dept. of Surgery, General Surgery Unit,
Catholic University of Rome,
"A. Gemelli" Hospital,
Rome, Italy

G. de Manzoni, F. Roviello, W. Siquini (eds.), *Surgery in the Multimodal Management of Gastric Cancer*,

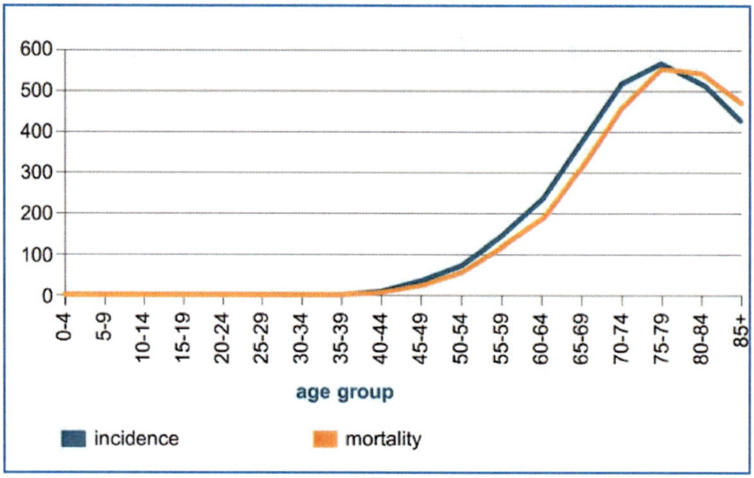

Fig. 19.1 Incidence and mortality for gastric cancer patients in Italy (1998–2002)

Japan and Latin American countries) and represents the second most frequent cause of cancer-related deaths in the world, thus constituting a major health problem [1].

In the area covered by the Italian Network of Cancer Registries, during 1998–2002, stomach cancer was the third most relevant cause of cancer death among males (8.0% of all cancer deaths), and the fifth (7.9%) among females [2]. It has been estimated that in Italy 9850 new cases of gastric cancer are annually diagnosed in men and 6604 in women (Fig. 19.1). With respect to time trends, stomach cancer has shown a relevant and stable decrease in incidence and mortality in both sexes.

In the USA, from 2003 to 2007, the median age at diagnosis for gastric cancer was 70 years. Approximately 24% of gastric cancer patients were diagnosed between age 65 and 74, 27% between 75 and 84, and 12% at 85 or older. The median age at death for gastric cancer was 73 years [3]; approximately 22% of these patients died between the ages of 65 and 74, 29% between 75 and 84, and 17% at 85 or older (Fig. 19.2).

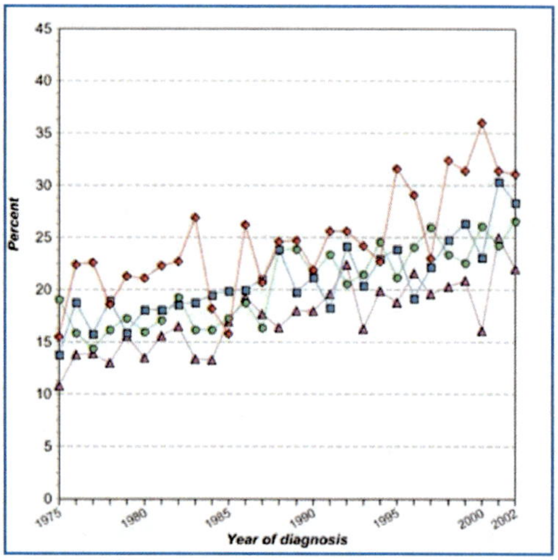

Fig. 19.2 Five-year survival for patients with gastric cancer by age at diagnosis in the USA

Gastric adenocarcinoma is considered a disease of the elderly, with a peak incidence in the seventh and eighth decades of life. Improvements in socioeconomic conditions, medical progress in the treatment of comorbidities, and better preventive medicine have led to an extended life span, as evidenced by the percentage of patients age 80 or older: 3–17% in Japan and 5–25% in Western countries [4]. Importantly, approximately 60% of patients diagnosed with cancer are > 65 years of age. Thus, despite a decrease in the global incidence of gastric cancer, the number of elderly patients with this disease is increasing. Indeed, data from a nationwide mass screening for gastric carcinoma in Japan show an increase of 2.3% compared to the previous decade in the incidence of gastric cancer in the elderly [5]. Consequently, more elderly patients will be candidates for major surgical operations for gastric carcinoma than in the past.

These epidemiologic findings raise several new clinical issues and highlight the importance of the correct approach to these patients. Many physicians are reluctant to perform surgery in older patients, even in those with operable gastric cancer. Radical gastric resection with extended lymph node dissection and chemo/radiotherapy are still a matter of controversy, because of their higher risk of complications in elderly patients, who frequently suffer from multiple comorbidities.

It is not clear whether there is a difference in the postoperative morbidity and mortality of elderly vs. younger patients. It is likewise unclear whether age represents a limiting factor due to comorbidity and differences in the response to major surgical procedures or whether it reflects differences in the cancer's characteristics in the older population [6]. Therefore, it is important to evaluate the clinicopathological characteristics of gastric cancer and the surgical outcomes in the elderly in order to identify prognostic factors that affect the survival rate of these patients.

19.2 Defining a Geriatric Patient

The "geriatric planet" has no clearly defined borders. American authors predict that 40% of the world population will be old in 2016; however defining an "old" patient is difficult, because the cut-off age is absolutely arbitrary and necessarily subjective, especially if we consider social, biological, or other criteria in the different populations. The age of 70, cited in most of scientific papers, may be acceptable in terms of biological or social patterns but the improved duration and quality of life make people in their 70s more similar to younger people of the previous decade. Instead, considering the 80-year-old patient as old might be of greater statistical relevance. With this cut-off age, estimated survival is lower such that the surgical option must be seriously considered, even if this is clinically feasible, in the interest of cancer healing.

Evaluation of the elderly patient may be difficult: a multitude of disease may have similar symptoms and the presentation of a true pathological process is often obscured by functional disorders. Moreover, multiple comorbidities and polypharmacy also confound clinical evaluation.

Older patients constitute a highly heterogeneous population. Many of them are malnourished and their general health is often compromised by one or more additional chronic conditions, such as cardiovascular and pulmonary diseases, hypertension, or diabetes mellitus. Furthermore, their functional reserve in various organs is often reduced. In addition, the elderly typically show a reduced adaptability to environmental changes. Furthermore, organ physiology clearly changes with increasing age. On a biochemical level, age-related tissue alterations are slowly becoming better understood, and several potential molecular markers of tissue aging have been identified.

Similarly, histological and functional changes have been observed in the stomach with increasing age, even though there is evidence in the literature that some of these changes represent pathological rather than physiological processes [7]. Gastric acid secretion declines as a consequence of normal aging. In addition, the cumulative effects of stress and exposure to the intraluminal contents, especially substances such as ethanol, nonsteroidal anti-inflammatory drugs (NSAIDs), and toxins, may damage the gastric mucosa. Many studies have also documented that gastric emptying of both solids and liquids slows with aging; consequently, gastric acid or agents injurious to the mucosa have prolonged contact with the mucosa [8]. Functionally, the loss of parietal cells, as part of the aging process, is thought to contribute to the higher rate of hypochlorhydria. All of these changes may led to atrophic gastritis, which is related to an increased risk of developing gastric cancer.

Another contributing factor is *Helicobacter pylori*, which is found in the stomach of > 75% of individuals over age 60. Acute infection with this bacterium is known to cause transient hypochlorhydria. In turn, the loss of gastric acidity favors the growth of *H. pylori*, thus adding another independent risk factor for gastric cancer. In fact, *H. pylori* is known to cause chronic gastritis and intestinal metaplasia, both precursors of neoplastic changes.

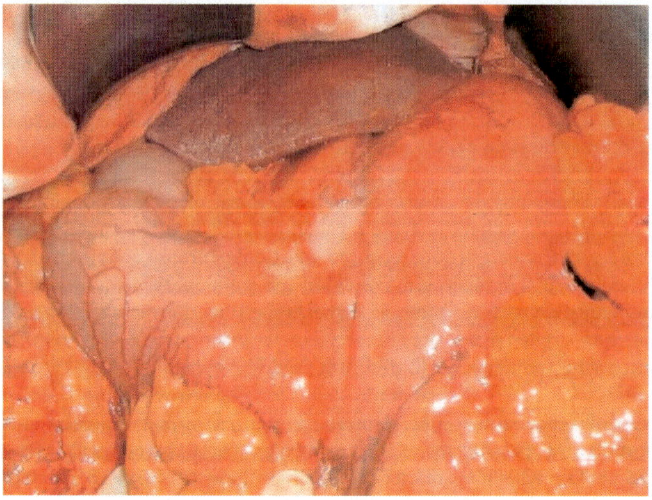

Fig 19.3 Locally advanced gastric tumor localized on the lesser curvature

19.3 Clinicopathological Characteristics

A number of distinguishing characteristics have been reported in elderly patients with gastric cancer, both in early and advanced stages of the disease.

19.3.1 Gender

In elderly patients, there is a male predominance whereas in younger patients (<40 years) a female prevalence has been consistently reported [1]. The cause of this gender difference is unclear, but the more frequent and prolonged exposure of elderly males to environmental carcinogens may be a predisposing factor. The positive correlation between female gender and the early development of gastric cancer must be viewed in terms of the presence of estrogen receptors and the poor survival of younger patients, suggesting a negative effect of female sex hormones in gastric cancer [9].

19.3.2 Tumor Location

Many studies have documented that gastric cancer in the elderly arises more frequently in the lower or distal third of the stomach (Fig. 19.3): 42 and 63% vs. 31–44% of the cases in younger patients [10], independent of pathological stage.

19.3.3 Macroscopic Appearance

The gross appearance of the tumor also seems to be influenced by age, in early and in advanced disease. As reported in the Japanese literature, almost 90% of the tumors comprising early gastric cancer in the general population are of the superficial depressed type, whereas in older patients this type accounts for 46% of the cases, a significant difference. Nonetheless, superficial depressed is the predominant macroscopic appearance of gastric cancers in older patients, followed by the superficial elevated type and polypoid type I.

Regarding advanced stage disease, according to Borrmann's classification, ulcerative tumors are the most prevalent type in elderly patients, while diffuse infiltrative tumors account for > 50% of the cases in the young population.

19.3.4 Histological Type

Regardless of tumor stage, gastric cancers in older patients seem to be mainly well-differentiated [11].

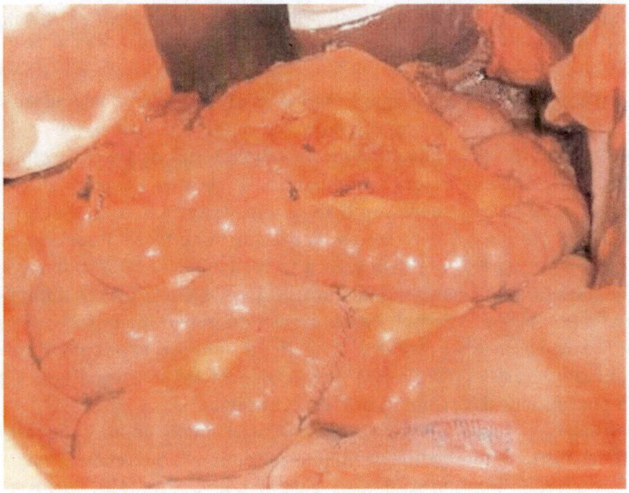

Fig 19.4 Roux-en-Y reconstruction after total gastrectomy

In the early stage of the disease, poorly differentiated and signet-ring cell types account for only 10% of the cases, whereas in the advanced stage the incidences of well-differentiated and poorly differentiated carcinomas are similar, even if these findings are generally limited to the superficial layers of the tumor. In other words, in older patients, gastric carcinoma seems to begin as a well-differentiated lesion that over time progresses to poorly differentiated carcinoma, while gastric cancer in younger patients often shows signs of histological non-differentiation beginning at a very early phase. These differences explain why gastric cancer in the elderly is less aggressive than in younger patients.

19.3.5 Synchronous Carcinomas

As reported in many studies [1], the incidence of synchronous gastric carcinomas is higher in older patients, accounting for 8–15% of cases. Endoscopically, these tumors appear as multiple elevated lesions, generally located in the lower third of the stomach and often converging to form a single giant lesion. Many authors have suggested that the higher rate of intestinal-type gastric cancer observed in this age group is associated with the underlying atrophic gastritis, thus explaining the high rate of multifocal cancerogenesis.

19.3.6 Patterns of Metastases

Well-differentiated carcinoma is usually associated with a high prevalence of vascular invasion, with a preferentially hematogenous diffusion. Thus, older patients usually have hematogenous metastases, predominantly involving the liver via tumor spread through the portal veins, whereas peritoneal invasion occurs less frequently.

Regarding lymph node metastases, there seems to be a lower incidence of lymph node involvement in patients older than 75, but this has yet to be confirmed.

19.4 Surgical Treatment

Radical resection, consisting of subtotal or total gastrectomy associated with D2 lymph node dissection, is the recommended treatment and the only modality potentially curative for gastric cancer. Indeed, R0 resection represents the most important indicator of long-term survival for this disease (Fig. 19.4). Nevertheless surgical treatment of gastric cancer in elderly patients remains controversial for several reasons. First of all, most older patients suffer from concomitant systemic disorders: hypertension is the most frequent comorbidity, followed by cardiovascular disease, diabetes mellitus, cerebrovascular disease, respiratory dysfunctions, and mild cirrhosis, either alone or in various combinations [12]. Many studies in the literature have confirmed a higher rate of elderly than younger ASA III–IV patients. Moreover, the elderly often have various grades of malnutrition, confirmed by the higher rate of patients with a low body mass index and hypoalbuminemia [13]. All these conditions seem to be more frequently associated with an increased pre-operative risk [14]. Second, gastric cancer in the elderly is often diagnosed at an advanced stage; this may be attributed to the lack of symptoms in the elderly population or to the absence of mass screening for this tumor. Finally, gastric cancer is generally associated with a poor prognosis in term of disease-free and overall survival.

For all these reasons, it is sometimes difficult to treat elderly patients with gastric cancer according to guidelines. The benefits of surgical treatment have to be balanced against postoperative morbidity and mortality such that physicians prefer a non-curative approach and less extensive lymph node dissection rather than radical resection.

Historically, resection rates for gastric cancer in patients over age 70 were very low. In the 1990s, overall resection rates were 25–35% in patients age 70–79 and < 10% in patients over 80, whereas curative resection rates were 16% and 4%, respectively [15]. In the last two decades, there has been a significant increase in overall resection rates, primarily due to an improvement in surgical and anesthetic techniques and perioperative care. Earlier endoscopic diagnosis, an overall higher standard of living, and wider health education of the elderly also may have played a role in changing these trends.

Recent Japanese and Asian studies report a resection rate of 72–88% and curative resection rates of 52–77% in patients over 80 years of age [16]. Similarly, in European reports, the rates of resection are 56–93% and those for curative resection 70–91% in patients over 75 years.

Regarding the type of gastric resection, surgeons are more likely to perform subtotal gastrectomy in the elderly, whenever feasible, mainly due to the fact that their tumors are predominantly located in the gastric distal third. Moreover, total gastrectomy is associated with higher rates of postoperative morbidity and mortality, especially in patients with preoperative comorbidities. Similarly, splenectomy or combined resections of adjacent organs are less frequently performed in this group.

Some authors [6, 17, 18] have suggested that minimally invasive surgery has a larger positive impact on the elderly in terms of fewer cardiorespiratory complications, shorter hospital stay, and more rapid return to daily activities, but to date there are no data confirming these observations.

With regard to the extent of lymphadenectomy, the vast majority of physicians prefer limited D1 lymph node dissection rather than D2 resection, especially in patients with serious comorbidities, while D3 lymphadenectomy is usually not performed in elderly patients.

For advanced cancer, many authors suggest that palliative limited resection is preferable, whenever possible, to gastroenterostomy [19], since relief from obstruction and ulcer symptoms and the prevention of bleeding may help to improve patients' nutritional status and their general well-being. Conversely, an extensive surgical approach such as total gastrectomy is generally not as well accepted as palliative treatment for patients with gastric cancer.

During the last several years, improvements in surgical techniques and perioperative intensive care, coupled with a more appropriate selection of patients, have resulted in a significant decline in postoperative morbidity and mortality in elderly patients with gastric cancer. The current morbidity rate after gastric resection in patients of advanced age ranges from 18 to 37% [18]. Nevertheless, a review of the literature suggests that morbidity remains slightly more frequent than in the younger age group, even though the majority of complications arising in the surgical management of elderly patients are not truly surgical but are often of a general nature. Whereas the most common surgically related cause of morbidity in both age groups is anastomotic leakage and abdominal abscess [6, 20], the most frequent complication in older patients seems to be respiratory failure, mainly due to aspiration pneumonia, and renal dysfunction [12].

Many studies have shown that the higher morbidity depends greatly on the number and severity of pre-existing concomitant disorders; therefore, preoperative comprehensive assessment is crucial to the optimal perioperative management of elderly patients. Some authors report a linear relationship between postoperative complications and the number of preoperative abnormal parameters [21]; for example, the elderly frequently show various degrees of hypoalbuminemia. Accordingly, preoperative nutritional support with intravenous hyperalimentation is essential in these patients. Interestingly, postoperative morbidity develops more frequently in the subset of patients who undergo palliative resection. In fact, elderly patients receiving palliative resection are frequently in poor health because of the advanced stage of the gastric cancer as well as physiological degeneration; therefore, they are more likely to develop complications.

The mortality rate after gastric resection is also higher in the elderly (3–10% in older vs. 1–3% in younger patients), probably as a result of lower patient tolerance to postoperative complications. This finding is more impressive in emergency than in elective surgery. Nonetheless, mortality following surgical resection has declined over the last few decades. Overall 5-year survival after curative resection in elderly patients varies between 44 and 65%, and disease-specific 5-year survival from 53 to 62%. Otherwise, in palliative resection no difference between overall and disease-specific survival has been determined in older vs. younger age groups. As in the general population, tumor stage, lymph node metastases, and depth of invasion of the primary tumor are independent prognostic factor negatively affecting the survival of elderly patients [22, 23].

19.5 Multimodality Treatment for Locally Advanced and Recurrent or Metastatic Gastric Cancer

As reported by the ESMO Guidelines Working Group, adjuvant chemotherapy and radiotherapy are recommended for patients with high-risk gastric cancer in an attempt to reduce local or distant recurrence and to improve survival after curative resection.

In the past, elderly patients with cancer were often excluded from clinical trials of adjuvant treatments as a result of an arbitrary upper age limit in the inclusion criteria. Chronological age is generally considered a risk factor for increased toxicity and reduced tolerance to chemotherapy, partly due to increased exposure to these drugs (e.g., because of the prolonged half-life for decreased elimination or impaired renal function) and to changes in pharmacodynamic features, such as distribution, excretion, and resorption.

Myelosuppression, mucositis, cardiac dysfunction, and central neurotoxicity are more common in elderly patients; however, the results of only a few trials have been adjusted for age-associated changes, such as impaired functional status and increased comorbidity, which also show an independent association with increased toxicity. This has led to several biases in the published data. Decision-making in cases involving elderly cancer patients should be based on the results of geriatric and oncologic assessments. In patients for whom definite cure is realistic, all efforts should be made to intensify supportive care in order to reduce the operative risk and to improve the curative potential. In patients treated by a non-curative approach and who have an increased risk of toxicity, dose reduction may be justified in order to minimize side effects.

To date, many trials of adjuvant postoperative chemotherapy have evaluated patients with locally advanced gastric cancer [24]. Protocols with postoperative fluorouracil plus leucovorin combined with radiotherapy, pre- and postoperative epirubicin, cisplatin and 5-fluorouracil (MAGIC trial), and S-1 adjuvant chemotherapy with an oral fluoropyrimidine all showed significantly better median overall survival and longer relapse-free survival. Nevertheless the impact of any multimodality treatment scheme in the elderly cannot be clearly assessed since the trials conducted so far have not reached any definitive conclusions regarding this age group. Currently, adjuvant chemotherapy alone is usually not recommended in Europe as it offers few survival benefits but considerable toxicity. Conversely, two viable options seem appropriate for elderly patients with operable gastric cancer: pre- and post-operative chemotherapy or postoperative chemo-radiotherapy.

With respect to the treatment of patient with recurrent or metastatic disease, palliative systemic chemotherapy, generally recommended for its survival advantages and better quality of life than supportive care alone, is still a matter of controversy in the elderly. Nevertheless, patients age >70 years with gastric cancer reportedly obtain similar benefits as younger patients, without increased toxicities from palliative chemotherapy in terms of symptomatic response, tumor regression, and survival [25].

Age alone is not a contraindication in the selection of patients for chemotherapy of gastric cancer; however, a geriatric assessment may help to classify elderly patients into different groups: those without significant co-morbidities who therefore can be treated similarly to younger patients, those who are vulnerable and need modified therapy, and those who are frail and cannot tolerate cytotoxic therapy. Cut-off levels to define these three groups will most likely depend on the underlying tumor entity and the kind and intensity of therapy that will be used.

19.6 Conclusions

Even though data in the literature regarding elderly patients are often limited and sometimes conflicting, the general opinion is that gastric cancer in older patients is not a more aggressive and advanced disease. After curative resection, elderly patients have the same chance of survival as middle-age patients; therefore, there may be no difference in the biological behavior of gastric cancer in patients of advanced age. Accordingly, surgical resection is warranted because the benefit to these patients is the same as for younger patients regarding early and long-term outcomes, with a similar return to normal work and daily activities in both age groups.

In general, age alone has not been definitively shown to be of prognostic significance for death for gastric cancer, and should not preclude gastric resection in the elderly. However, favorable outcome depends on appropriate clinical decision-making, careful judgment of the appropriate extent of lymph node dissection, and intensive treatment of comorbid conditions during hospital stays. In the elderly, the reasons for the poor prognosis of gastric carcinoma are linked to comorbidities, even in patients with early-stage tumors.

References

1. Saif MW, Makrilia N, Zalonis A et al (2010) Gastric cancer in elderly: an overview. EJSO 36:709-717
2. I tumori in Italia - Rapporto 2006. http://www.registri-tumori.it/incidenza1998/2002/rapporto/I%20dati%20dei%20registri%20tumori.html. Accessed 16 November 2010
3. Altekruse SF, Kosary CL, Krapcho M et al: SEER Cancer Statistics Review, 1975-2007, National Cancer Institute. Bethesda, MD. http://seer.cancer.gov/csr/1975_2007/index.html. Accessed 16 November 2010
4. Coniglio A, Tiberio GAM, Busti M et al (2004) Surgical treatment for gastric carcinoma in the elderly. J Surg Oncol 88:201-205
5. Dong-Yi K, Jae-Kyoon J, Seong-Yeob R et al (2005) Clinicopathologic characteristics of gastric carcinoma in elderly patients: a comparison with young patients. World J Gastroenterol 11:22-26
6. Orsenigo E, Tomajer V, Di Palo S et al (2007) Impact of age on postoperative outcomes in 1118 gastric cancer patients undergoing surgical tratment. Gastric Cancer 10:39-44
7. Levine JL, Zenilman ME (2001) Age-related physiologic changes in the gastrointestinal tract. In: Rosenthal RA (ed) Principles and practice of geriatric Surgery. Springer, New Jork, pp 511-527
8. Cima RR, Soybel DI (2001) Pathophysiology and treatment of benign disease of the stomach and duodenum. In: Rosenthal RA (ed) Principles and practice of geriatric Surgery. Springer, New Jork, pp 555-568
9. Furukawa H, Iwanaga T, Hiratsuka M et al (1994) Gastric cancer in young adults: growth accelerating effect of pregnancy and delivery. J Surg Oncol 55:3-6
10. Arai T, Esaki Y, Inoshita N et al (2004) Pathologic characteristics of gastric cancer in the elderly: a retrospective study of 994 surgical patients. Gastric Cancer 7:154-159
11. Kitamura K, Yamaguchi T, Taniguchi H et al (1996) Clinicopathological characteristics of gastric cancer in the elderly. Br J Cancer 73:798-802
12. Kunisaki C, Akiyama H, Nomura M et al (2005) Comparison of surgical outcomes of gastric cancer in elderly and middle-aged patients. The Am J Surg 191:216-224
13. Katai H, Sasako M, Sano T et al (2004) Gastric cancer surgery in the elderly without operative mortality. Surg Oncol 13:235-238
14. Oh J, Young-Kyu P, Seong-Yeob R et al (2010) Effect of age on surgical outcomes of extended gastrectomy with D2 lymph node dissection in gastric carcinoma: prospective cohort study. Ann Surg Oncol 17:1589-1596
15. Winslet MC, Mohsen YMA, Powell J (1996) The influence of age on the surgical management of carcinoma of the stomach. Eur J Surg Oncol 22:220-224
16. Eguchi T, Fujii M, Takayama T (2003) Mortality for gastric cancer in elderly patients. J Surg Oncol 84:132-136
17. Ozer I, Bostanci EB, Kou U et al (2010) Surgical treatment for gastric cancer in Turkish patients over age 70: early postoperative results and risk factors for mortality. Langenbecks Arch Surg 395:1101-1106

18. Saidi RF, Bell JL, Dudrick PS (2003) Surgical resection for gastric cancer in elderly patients: is there a difference in outcome? J Surg Res 118:15-20
19. Martella B, Militello C, Spirch A et al (2005) Palliative surgery for gastric cancer in elderly patients. Acta BioMed 76:49-51
20. Chew-Wun W, Su-Shun L, King-Han S et al (2000) Surgical mortality, survival and quality of life after resection for gastric cancer in the elderly. World J Surg 24:465-472
21. Hara H, Isozaki H, Nomura E et al (1999) Evaluation of treatment strategies for gastric cancer in the elderly according to the number of abnormal parameters on preoperative examination. Jpn J Surg 29:837-841
22. Hiroaki S, Tomohiro O, Daiki M et al (2006) Effect of age on prognosis in patients with gastric cancer. ANZ J Surg 76:458-461
23. Kubota H, Kotoh T, Dhar DK et al (2000) Gastric resection in the aged (> or =80 years) with gastric carcinoma: a multivariate analysis of prognostic factors. Aust N Z J Surg 70:254-257
24. Wedding U, Honecker F, Bokemeyer C et al (2007) Tolerance to chemotherapy in elderly patients with cancer. Cancer Control 14:44-56
25. Trumper M, Ross PJ, Cunningham D et al (2006) Efficacy and tolerability of chemotherapy in elderly patients with advanced oesophago-gastric cancer: a pooled analysis of three clinical trials. EJC 42:827-834

20 Cholecystectomy: Pros and Cons?

Marco Farsi, Marco Bernini, and Lapo Bencini

Abstract

The incidence of gallstones and gallbladder sludge is higher in patients after gastrectomy than in the general population, probably related to surgical dissection of vagus nerve branches and to the gastrointestinal anatomical reconstruction. Therefore, some surgeons routinely perform concomitant cholecystectomy during standard surgery for gastric malignancies. However, not all patients diagnosed with cholelithiasis after gastric cancer surgery will develop symptoms or require additional surgical treatment, and a standard laparoscopic cholecystectomy is often feasible even in those patients who have previously undergone gastric surgery. At present, there are no relevant randomized studies and decisions regarding gallbladder management are left to surgeons' individual preferences. However, routine cholecystectomy during gastric cancer surgery cannot be recommended in patients with a normal acalculous gallbladder.

Keywords

Incidental cholecystectomy • Routine cholecystectomy • Simultaneous cholecystectomy • Gastric cancer surgery • Gastrectomy • Gallbladder management

20.1 Introduction

The incidence of gallstones and gallbladder sludge in patients undergoing gastric surgery for malignancy or obesity is higher than in the general population (15–25% vs. 5–8%) [1-5]. This is probably related to surgical dissection of branches of the vagus nerve and to the gastrointestinal anatomical reconstruction [6, 7] (Fig. 20.1). The gallbladder's innervation is provided mainly by three sources: the anterior hepatic plexus, the posterior hepatic plexus, and the phrenic fibers. The lymph node stations located nearest these ramifications are those that include the right paracardial, lesser curvature, left gastric artery, celiac axis, and hepatic artery nodes. Thus, the regional anatomy accounts for the mechanism of injury to the vagal nerve (gastrectomy itself) or to the nerve fibers (through lymphadenectomy) (Fig. 20.2).

After gastric surgery, the mechanism of associated gallbladder dysfunction may be related to impaired filling/emptying of the gallbladder and impaired secretion of the hormone cholecys-

M. Farsi (✉)
Oncological Surgery,
Careggi University Hospital,
Florence, Italy

G. de Manzoni, F. Roviello, W. Siquini (eds.), *Surgery in the Multimodal Management of Gastric Cancer*,

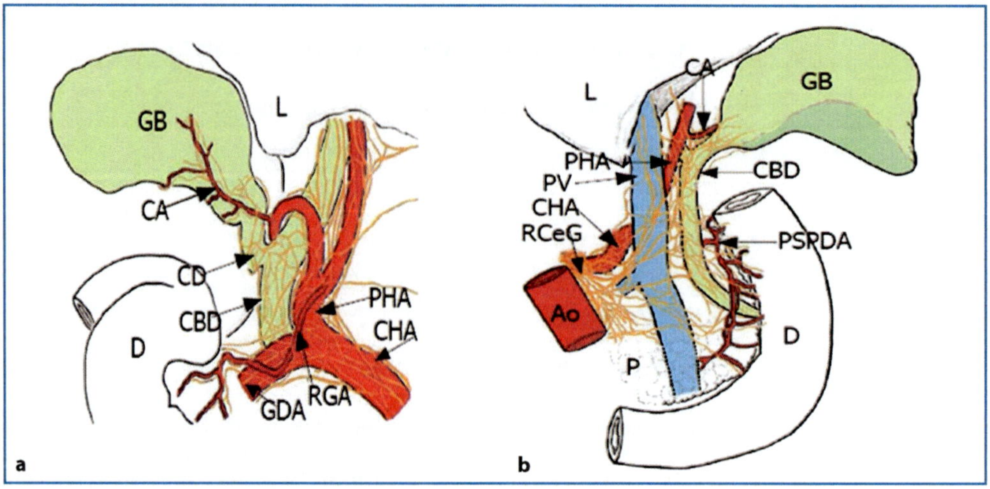

Fig. 20.1 Innervation of the gallbladder (*GB*) from the **a** ventral and **b** dorsal aspects. Branches innervating the GB originate from the anterior and posterior hepatic plexus and run along the cystic duct (*CD*) and cystic artery (*CA*). The hepatic divisions (*) of the vagus nerve join at the anterior hepatic plexus in the proper hepatic artery (*PHA*). *Arrows* indicate nerve branches. *CBD*, Common bile duct; *CHA*, common hepatic artery; *D*, duodenum; *GDA*, gastroduodenal artery; *L*, liver; *RGA*, right gastric artery; *Ao*, aorta; *IVC*, inferior vena cava; *PSPDA*, posterior superior pancreatoduodenal artery; *PV*, portal vein; *RCeG*, right celiac ganglion. (Modified from [7], with permission)

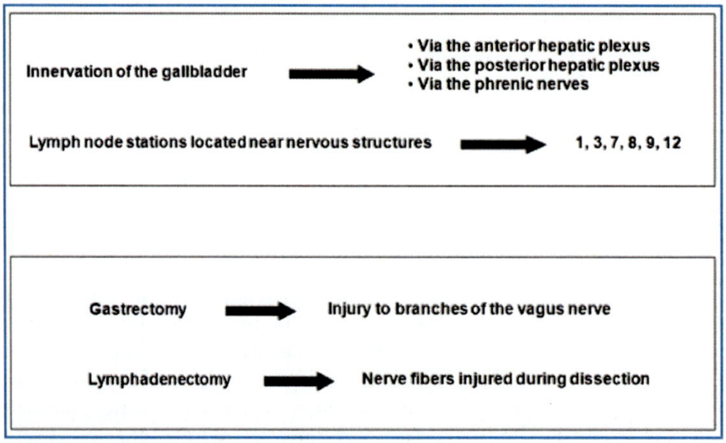

Fig. 20.2 The pathophysiology of the gallbladder and mechanism of injury to its innervation during gastric surgery for cancer

tokinin. Regardless of the pathogenesis, many surgeons routinely remove the gallbladder concomitantly during gastric surgery. In patients undergoing esophageal surgery, both pre- and/or postsurgical malnutrition, with a reduction in the total body mass index, and alcoholism have been demonstrated to play a role in the development of postoperative biliary complications [8, 9]. Given the lack of specific data and the contradictory results from various studies, some authors [4] recommend prophylactic cholecystectomy at the time of gastric surgery in order to spare patients postoperative complications and a worsening of the quality of life; however, this approach remains controversial [1, 10]. With the advent of more accurate statistical studies and the growing number of malpractice claims following unexpected bile duct injuries, prophylactic cholecystectomy has become increasingly questioned. Moreover, for surgically treated gastric malignancy patients, the poor survival rates that can be expected must be seriously taken into account. Although there is a strong consensus on the need for gallbladder removal when calculi are diagnosed at the time of surgery, there is little agreement in the case that the gallbladder is normal.

20.2 Why Remove a "Normal" Gallbladder?

Gallstones and gallbladder sludge are detected in 17% (mean value) of patients after gastric surgery, according to several studies [1–5, 10] (Fig. 20.3). Although in patients treated surgically for gastric cancer the 5-year survival rate is 24–42% in Europe [11], > 90% of those who will develop calculi do so within 2 years postoperatively [4]. Moreover the risk of subsequently developing gallstones may depend on the extent of the gastrectomy (subtotal or total) [1] and the lymphadenectomy (D1 or D2) during surgery for gastric cancer [4, 12, 13], with D2 representing the standard of care in Italian [14], Asian, and most European centers. For example, following partial gastrectomy the risk of developing calculi is < 8% while after total gastrectomy this risk may be three-fold higher [1]. In addition, the type of reconstruction seems to play a role in gallstone formation [1], occurring in 7% of patients who receive a Billroth I but in > 17% of those receiving a Roux-en-Y. The difference may be due to the exclusion of the duodenum, which leads to changes in the pattern of cholecystokinin secretion, resulting in decreased gallbladder contraction [6, 13].

In Akatsu's series of 805 surgically treated patients [13], the incidence of gallstone formation was 9.4% after D1 lymph node dissection, increasing to 17.8% with a standard D2 dissection, and ≥ 28% following extended dissection including station 12 lymph nodes, as reported by Kobayashi [1]. In those patients who developed gallstones, the need for further surgery (cholecystectomy) was higher following a D2 dissection (19 vs. 4% of D1-treated patients) [13]. Moreover, the interval between gastric surgery and gallstone formation was shorter in the presence of a more extended lymphadenectomy (19 months for D2 vs. 29 for D1) [13]. Interestingly, another study found that gallstone formation was independent of the length of follow-up [10].

The early postoperative gallbladder complications, such as acute cholecystitis [15, 16], described in many series after gastric and

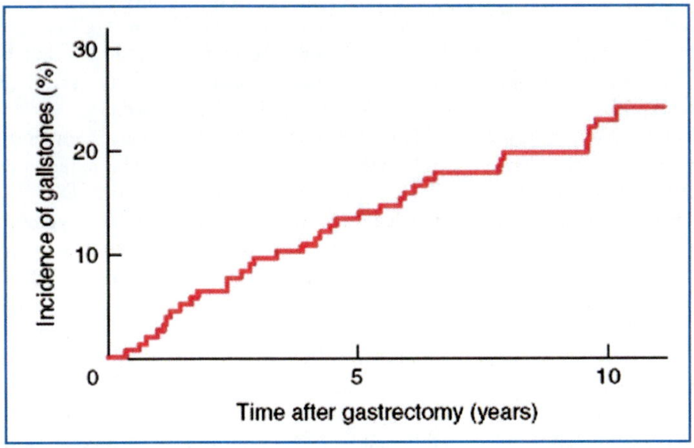

Fig. 20.3 Incidence of gallstones after gastrectomy. (Reproduced from [1], with permission)

esophageal [9] surgery are a cause for concern, as they imply the need for an additional hospital stay or reintervention, with increasing morbidity and mortality. Medium/long-term complications include symptomatic cholelithiasis, which may impair the quality of life and require further surgery. Moreover, cholecystectomy (in most cases attempted laparoscopically) is known to be more challenging after gastric surgery, with an increased risk of conversion and bile duct injuries, and a longer operating time [17, 18].

Concomitant cholecystectomy is not time-consuming and is substantially without additional risks to the patient because complications arising from an additional abdominal procedure performed as part of the main operation are known to be minimal. Assuming that the results of open concomitant cholecystectomy are at least equal to those achieved during a routine elective cholecystectomy, mortality is near 0% and morbidity is < 5% [19]. However, concomitant cholecystectomy has an even better outcome and involves a shorter procedure as it is performed in a larger exposed field and involves a normal gallbladder, without adherences or inflammation. The theoretical advantage of concomitant cholecystectomy is the avoidance of reintervention for perioperative gallbladder complications or long-term symptomatic cholelithiasis.

20.3 Why Not Remove a "Normal" Gallbladder?

Firstly, in a recent large European survey on the incidence and potential risk factors for developing gallstones disease in the general population, it was found that, after 5-years of follow-up, gastrointestinal symptoms and quality of life were substantially similar in the group that developed calculi and the group that did not [20]. Furthermore, not all patients who are diagnosed with cholelithiasis after gastric cancer surgery will develop symptoms or require additional surgical treatment [2–4] and a standard laparoscopic cholecystectomy is feasible even in those patients who previously underwent gastric surgery [17, 21]. A recent, highly thorough review article on incidental cholecystectomy during gastroesophageal resection was published by a German group [10]. The authors identified 16 studies on gallstone formation after upper gastrointestinal surgery, evaluating 3,735 patients. The reported incidence was between 5 and 60%, with an average of 17.5%, while in the general population it is 4% in men and 12% in women. However, the crucial finding was that < 5% of those patients who were operated on subsequently required a cholecystectomy, usually performed laparoscopically, for symptom treatment and they had minimal additional morbidity and mortality. Similarly, the issue of early postoperative gallbladder complications, e.g., acute cholecystitis, although well described [10, 15, 16] was found to be of minimal importance [10].

20.4 Discussion and Conclusions

To date, no randomized study on the need for cholecystectomy in gastric cancer patients has been published and gallbladder management is currently left to the surgeon. Most of the literature recommending prophylactic cholecystectomy during gastric surgery was published during the peptic ulcer era, more than 10 years ago, and thus has not been cited herein, while many more recent trials were conducted in the field of bariatric surgery [22]. In both cases, we are strongly convinced that the evidence for or against cholecystectomy can be applied to gastric cancer surgery, albeit with caution. Some studies demonstrated a lower incidence of gallstones in vagus-saving procedures due to a better contractile function of the gallbladder or unimpaired hormone secretion [12, 23], but none of these techniques have become the standard of care in Western gastric cancer surgery.

It is obvious that life expectancy is much lower in gastric cancer patients, while the pathophysiology of the remnant anatomy following lymphadenectomy may play a role in the development of postsurgical impairments. Moreover, some authors [24] have questioned whether cholecystectomy itself is truly the cause of symptom relief after surgery. Studies conducted on patients who underwent esophageal surgery [8, 9], although similar to procedures carried out for gastric cancer with respect to truncal vagotomy, are flawed due to the worse survival and greater perioperative morbidity of these patients, such as weight loss, malnutrition, and alcohol consumption, which are hardly comparable as risk factors for biliary complications.

The ideal patient who could benefit from a prophylactic cholecystectomy at the time of gastric cancer surgery should have a good life expectancy (younger age, few comorbidities) and be a candidate for total gastrectomy with radical D2 dissection, R0 surgery, and a Roux-en-Y.

The Oncological Surgery Division of Azienda Ospedaliero-Universitaria Careggi (Florence, Italy) is currently recruiting patients, together with many other centers, members of the GIRCG (Italian Research Group for Gastric Cancer), for the first controlled randomized trial (Registration: ClinicalTrials.gov ID. NCT00757640) addressing this issue [25]. The primary aim of this study is to determine whether patients who do not receive a prophylactic cholecystectomy and develop cholelithiasis eventually suffer from symptoms related to their gallstones, thus requiring another surgical intervention 5 years after gastrectomy. We will also evaluate the incidence of cholelithiasis in patients who have undergone gastric surgery and whether prophylactic cholecystectomy increases the complication rate, operative time, and postoperative stay.

Gallbladder disease is common after gastrectomy for cancer and any therapeutic improvements will benefit many patients, enhancing their quality of life and reducing morbidity, mortality, and hospital stay. Complications from cholecystectomy during a concomitant abdominal procedure are known to be minimal. At present, based on the literature data, we cannot recommend routine concomitant cholecystectomy during gastric cancer surgery, except in patients in whom calculi are demonstrated.

References

1. Kobayashi T, Hisanaga M, Kanehiro H, Yamada Y et al (2005) Analysis of risks factors for the development of gallstones after gastrectomy. Br J Surg 92:1399-1403
2. Sanders G, Kingsnorth AN (2007) Gallstones. BMJ 335: 295-299
3. Sakorafas GH, Milingos D, Peros G (2007) Asymptomatic cholelithiasis: is cholecystectomy really needed? Dig Dis Sci 52:1313-1325
4. Fukagawa T, Katai H, Saka M, Morita S et al (2009) Gallstone Formation after Gastric Cancer Surgery. J Gastrointest Surg 13:886-889
5. Vicky Ka Ming Li, Pulido N, Martinez-Suartez P, Fajnwaks P et al (2009) Symptomatic gallstones after sleeve gastrectomy. Surg Endosc 23:2488-2492
6. Qvist N (2000) Review article: gall-bladder motility after intestinal surgery. Aliment Pharmacol Ther 14 (s2): 35-38
7. Yi SQ, Ohta T, Tsuchida A, Terayama H et al (2007) Surgical anatomy of innervation of the gallbladder in humans and Suncus murinus with special reference to morphological understanding of gallstone formation after gastrectomy.World J Gastroenterol 14:2066-2071
8. Tachibana M, Kinugasa S, Yoshimura H, Dhar DK et al (2003) Acute cholecystitis and cholelithiasis developed after esophagectomy. Can J Gastroenterol 17:175-178
9. Tsunoda K, Shirai Y, Wakai T, Yokoyama N et al (2004) Increased risk of cholelithiasis after esophagectomy. J Hepatobiliary Pancreat Surg 11:319-323
10. Gillen S, Michalski CW, Schuster T, Feith M et al (2010) Simultaneous/Incidental cholecystectomy during gastric/esophageal resection: systematic analysis of risks and benefits. World J Surg 34:1008-1014
11. Lepage C, Sant M, Verdecchia A, Forman D et al (2010) Operative mortality after gastric cancer resection and long-term survival differences across Europe. Br J Surg 97:235-239
12. Tomita R, Tanjoh K, Fujisaki S (2004) Total gastrectomy reconstructed by interposition of a jejunal J pouch with preservation of hepatic vagus branch and lower esophageal sphincter for T2 gastric cancer without lymph node metastasis. Hepatogastroenterology 51:1233-1240
13. Akatsu T, Yoshida M, Kubota T, Shimazu M et al (2005) Gallstone disease after extended (D2) lymph node dissection for gastric cancer. World J Surg 29:182-186
14. Verlato G, Roviello F, Marchet A, Giacopuzzi S et al (2009) Indexes of surgical quality in gastric cancer surgery: experience of an Italian network. Ann Surg Oncol 16: 594-602
15. Oh SJ, Choi WB, Song J, Hyung WJ et al (2009) Complications requiring reoperation after gastrectomy for gastric cancer: 17 years experience in a single institute. J Gastrointest Surg 13:239-245
16. Liu XS, Zhang Q, Zhong J, Zhu KK et al (2010) Acute cholecystitis immediately after radical gastrectomy: a report of three cases. World J Gastroenterol 16:2702-2074
17. Sasaki A, Nakajima J, Nitta H, Obuchi T et al (2008) Laparoscopic cholecistectomy in atients with a history of gastrectomy. Surg Today 38:790-794
18. Fraser SA, Sigman H (2009) Conversion in laparoscopic cholecystectomy after gastric resection: a 15-year review. Can J Surg 52:463-466
19. Wolf AS, Nijsse BA, Sokal SM, Chang Y et al (2009) Surgical outcomes of open cholecystectomy in the laparoscopic era. Am J Surg 197:781-784
20. Halldestam I, Kullman E, Borch K (2009) Incidence of and potential risk factors for gallstone disease in a general population sample. Br J Surg 96:1315-1322
21. Kwon AH, Inui H, Imamura A, Kaibori M et al (2001) Laparoscopic cholecystectomy and choledocholithotomy in patients with a previous gastrectomy. J Am Coll Surg 193:614-619

22. Li VK, Pulido N, Fajnwaks P, Szomstein S et al (2009) Predictors of gallstone formation after bariatric surgery: a multivariate analysis of risk factors comparing gastric bypass, gastric banding, and sleeve gastrectomy. Surg Endosc 23:1640-1644
23. Hagiwara A, Imanishi T, Sakakura C, Otsuji E et al (2002) Subtotal gastrectomy for cancer located in the greater curvature of the middle stomach with prevention of the left gastric artery. Am J Surg 183:692-696
24. Berger MY, Olde Hartman TC, Bohnen AM (2003) Abdominal symptoms: do they disappear after cholecystectomy? Surg Endosc 17:1723-1728
25. Farsi M, Bernini M, Bencini L, Miranda E et al (2009) The CHOLEGAS study: multicentric randomized, blinded, controlled trial of gastrectomy plus prophylactic cholecystectomy versus gastrectomy only, in adults submitted to gastric cancer surgery with curative intent. Trials 10:32

21 Neoadjuvant Treatment for Resectable Locally Advanced Gastric Cancer

Domenico D'Ugo, Alberto Biondi, and Ferdinando Cananzi

Abstract

This chapter briefly reviews recent developments in pre-operative therapies for gastric carcinoma, stressing their safety and efficacy. The data and studies discussed in the following were obtained from PubMed, using the search terms "pre-operative chemotherapy," "pre-operative radiotherapy," "pre-operative chemoradiotherapy," "neoadjuvant treatment," and "gastric cancer." Only papers published in English from January 1970 through January 2010 were taken into consideration. Studies conducted over the last 20 years have progressed from the first "pioneering" chemotherapies for patients with non-resectable disease ("induction" therapy) to the most recent phase III trials on "neoadjuvant" therapies for resectable gastric neoplasms. There have also been several clinical trials examining pre-operative chemotherapy in the management of gastric cancer. While further evidence on the definitive role of neoadjuvant therapy is still needed, the most recent results of treatment using a multimodal approach to gastric adenocarcinoma are encouraging. In fact, most pre-operative multimodal regimens increase the likelihood that postponed tumor resection can still fulfill all the requirements of a true R0 resection.

Keywords

Neoadjuvant chemotherapy • Pre-operative chemotherapy, Peri-operative chemotherapy • Chemotherapy • Radiotherapy • Chemoradiotherapy • R0 resection • Down-staging • Pathologic response • Metabolic response

21.1 Introduction

Despite an incidence that has steadily declined over the past few decades, gastric carcinoma remains one of the most frequent malignancies worldwide [1], albeit with marked global variations in etiology and frequency. The natural course of this disease involves the early dissemination of tumor cells through the lymphatic system, blood, and peritoneum. Consequently, the likelihood that optimal surgery alone can be effectively curative is low, except in patients with early stage gastric cancers. In Japan and Korea, the introduction of screening for gastric cancer has indeed improved early detection, such that in

D. D'Ugo (✉)
Dept. of Surgery, General Surgery Unit,
Catholic University of Rome, "A. Gemelli" Hospital,
Rome, Italy

G. de Manzoni, F. Roviello, W. Siquini (eds.), *Surgery in the Multimodal Management of Gastric Cancer*,

almost half of all newly diagnosed patients the disease is detected at an early stage [2], which in turn has greatly impacted tumor management strategies in those countries. Due to the lower disease incidence in Europe and North America, large-scale screening programs have not been deemed cost-effective. Thus, in the Western world, two-thirds of the patients with gastric cancers have advanced-stage disease at presentation, often with lymph node metastasis or transmural progression of the primary tumor [3].

Under these circumstances, the clinical outcome is unsatisfactory, resulting in numerous attempts to improve survival, such as tailoring the extent of surgery or integrating surgery with pre-operative and/or post-operative treatments. Over the last 20 years, three large-scale randomized trials have proven the efficacy of different adjuvant therapies as an adjunct to optimal surgery: post-operative chemoradiation therapy (United States/INT-0116 trial) [4], postoperative single-drug chemotherapy (Japan/ACTS-GC trial) [5], and peri-operative three-drug combination chemotherapy (UK-Europe/MAGIC trial) [6]. Since the publication of the results of these trials, surgery alone is no longer considered the only treatment option for patients with resectable locally advanced gastric cancer; rather, any plan that is addressed at disease eradication must take into account that R0 resection is no longer a merely surgical target.

In this chapter, the theoretical rationale and state of the art of pre-operative neoadjuvant therapy are outlined in the light of new evidence and modern perspectives.

21.2 Neoadjuvant Treatment: Theoretical Rationale

The concept of pre-treating a tumor before surgical treatment has definitively led to higher curative resection rates in several cancers (e.g., rectum and breast). Provided that complete surgical resection remains the ultimate mainstay of curative treatment, pre-operative therapy of gastric adenocarcinoma appears to be similarly justified, even if with some drawbacks [7, 8].

21.2.1 Biological Rationale

Several observations provide the biological rationale for the pre-surgical treatment of gastric cancer. First, pre-operative therapy can down-stage the primary gastric tumor and possibly improve the likelihood of a curative R0 resection. Second, the administration of systemic therapy or radiation prior to the surgical procedure offers the theoretical advantage of treating an untouched cancer, with intact vessels and without fibrotic remodeling of the tumor bed following surgical removal ("surgeon-induced" resistance). Third, the malignant behavior of gastric tumors implies the possibility of unresected micrometastatic disease beyond the borders of surgical ablation. Pre-operative systemic therapy also targets micrometastases, as it is administered when the cellular growth fraction is high and the total tumor volume relatively low.

21.2.2 Up-front Randomization

Due to poor post-operative recovery, patients enrolled in randomized studies of adjuvant systemic therapy in gastric cancer must be relatively fit and reliably compliant. As a result, these patients are not representative of the entire population of patients who undergo resection with curative intent. In addition, frequent dose reductions and treatment delays weaken the ability to obtain homogeneous data. Conversely, randomized studies of pre-operative systemic therapy allow proper randomization without any pre-selection bias and with greater feasibility.

21.2.3 Pre-operative Staging

Unlike adjuvant therapy, which is based on the pathologic stage at the time of resection, the decision to administer pre-operative treatment necessarily relies on clinical staging. In gastric cancer, this assessment has been and remains difficult. The problem is currently being addressed through a variety of imaging techniques, i.e., endoscopic ultrasound, diagnostic laparoscopy, and PET scan, which are used to evaluate different stages of the disease.

21.2.4 Monitoring

While adjuvant therapy is administered without any possibility to assess its efficacy on an individual basis, the activity and efficacy of neoadjuvant therapy can be monitored, thus allowing treatment to be adjusted, changed, or abandoned according to the patient's individual response.

21.2.5 Delayed Surgery

Among the therapeutic options for gastric carcinoma, the concept of "delayed surgery" is relatively new. It has been shown that postponing resection in favor of systemic treatment does not exclude patients from the benefits of a potentially curative exeresis, nor does it statistically worsen surgical outcomes. Nevertheless, in a small number of cases there is the possibility of tumor progression during therapy. Disease progression remains the only aspect of delayed surgery that justifies the reluctance to pursue a multimodal pre-operative approach to gastric cancer. Actually, neoadjuvant therapy can be used to select patients who may benefit vs. those who are as unlikely to benefit from surgery as from any other treatment because of the unavoidable progression of "multi-resistant" and previously occult metastatic disease. Still, skepticism about this treatment option partially explains why, over the last 30 years, the acceptance of neoadjuvant therapies as a valid treatment for gastric cancer has been slow [7].

21.2.6 Contraindications

Neoadjuvant treatments are contraindicated in patients with obstructive or hemorrhagic tumors. Some cancers, particularly those in the cardia and pre-pyloric area, can be completely obstructive at diagnosis. Under these circumstances, up-front surgery is the recommended approach even if neoadjuvant therapy could be administered along with parenteral or enteral feeding through a jejunostomy. Acute bleeding from a gastric tumor is relatively infrequent but can be dramatic; in such cases, direct salvage surgery is mandatory.

21.2.7 Conclusions

In summary, the feasibility, biological rationale, randomization, and monitoring advantages make pre-operative therapy an attractive subject for investigation and for patient management. With this background, a search of the literature published during the last 30 years yields a relevant number of papers reporting the experiences of the various centers with pre-operative therapy for locally advanced gastric cancer (neoadjuvant chemotherapy, neoadjuvant radiotherapy, or a combination of modalities).

21.3 Pre-/Peri-operative Neoadjuvant Chemotherapy

Investigations into the efficacy and potential of pre-operative chemotherapy in patients with advanced gastric cancer began in the late 1970s. Encouraging results, however, were not reported until the early 1990s, when two independent studies in patients with non-resectable disease found that chemotherapy led to subsequent resection in 40–50% of patients, with an increase in total median survival of 18 months compared with patients whose tumors were not resected [9, 10]. These preliminary observations encouraged the introduction of pre-operative chemotherapy protocols not only for unresectable (Table 21.1) [9–15] but also for potentially resectable, locally advanced gastric cancers (Table 21.2) [6, 16–29]. However, the results of those first trials are questionable, mainly because of methodological biases. In fact, the reliance of several series on inaccurate pre-operative staging resulted in the recruitment of patients using non-homogeneous criteria. For example, patients with locally advanced disease and those with disease at unclear stages were enrolled in the same study, resulting in the lack of a fixed distinction between resectable and non-resectable tumors. In addition to the non-homogeneous recruitment, other biases in early trials included the use of variable chemotherapeutic regimens, non-standardized surgery or surgery of questionable quality, and missing or poorly detailed response criteria.

Table 21.1 Pre-operative chemotherapy in non-resectable gastric cancer

Author [Reference]	Regimen	Pts	Stage	R0 resection (%)	Median survival (months)
Wilkie [9]	EAP	34	NR	44	24
Plukker [10]	5FU+MTX	20	NR	40	22
Rougier [11]	5FU, P	30	NR	60	16
Kelsen [12]	FAMTX, IP 5FU-P	56	NR	61	15
Melcher [13]	ECF	27	R-NR	58 (patients with R) 10 (patients with NR)	10
Gallardo-Rincon [14]	P-ELF	60	NR	8.7	10
Cascinu [15]	EAFPLG	82	NR	45	17

5FU, 5-Fluorouracil; *EAFPLG*, epi-doxorubicin, 5FU, cisplatin, leucovorin, glutathione; *EAP*, etoposide, doxorubicin, cisplatin; *ECF*, epirubicin, cisplatin, 5FU; *FAMTX*, 5FU, doxorubicin, methotrexate; *IP*, intraperitoneal; *MTX*, methotrexate, 5FU; *NR*, non-resectable tumors; *P*, cisplatin; *P-ELF*, cisplatin, etoposide, leucovorin, 5FU; *R*, resectable tumors.

In 1993, the Dutch Gastric Cancer Group started the first randomized controlled trial of exclusively pre-operative chemotherapy for gastric cancer (patients with cardia tumors were excluded) [23]. The regimen used was FAMTX (fluorouracil, doxorubicin, and methotrexate), which was, at that time, the gold standard of treatment for adenocarcinoma of the stomach. This trial had many accrual problems and was prematurely stopped after an interim analysis showing that FAMTX was unlikely to achieve the goal of a 15% increase in curative resectability after pre-operative chemotherapy. Several biases have been outlined for the Dutch study, particularly the inaccuracy of the staging procedure, which included the optional use of CT and laparoscopy, and inadequate extension of lymphadenectomy. The investigators reported a high rate of tumor progression during treatment (36%) along with a reduction in curative resections (56 vs. 62%) and a decreased median survival (18 vs. 30 months) compared with untreated patients. However, even if all of the statistical differences in this study were insignificant, both the short-term and long-term results were discouraging [30].

In the late 1990s, other ambitious European phase III trials were designed with end-points allowing the efficacy of pre-operative treatments to be demonstrated. However, the adoption of strict selection criteria made patient selection so difficult that some studies were prematurely terminated (EORTC 40954 and SWS-SAKK-43/99 trials) [27, 29]. Thus, to date, only the MAGIC trial (started in the UK in 1994) and the FFCD 9703 trial (started in France in 1996) have been completed [6, 26] and their results published. These two studies have produced substantial evidence supporting the efficacy of peri-operative chemotherapy in terms of an increased survival rate (36 vs. 23% and 38 vs. 24%, estimated at 5 years for MAGIC and for the FFCD 9703, respectively; Table 21.2) along with a significantly higher curative resection rate in the treated than in the surgery-alone group (79 vs. 70%; p = 0·03 for MAGIC; 84 vs. 73% in arm 2; p = 0.04 for FFCD 9703) and without an increase in peri-operative morbidity or mortality. Increasing the R0 resection rate is an important goal of pre-operative chemotherapy [25]. In a phase II study, conducted by the authors of this chapter, of a peri-operative chemotherapy protocol, the achievement of a "true" R0 resection following pre-operative chemotherapy was shown to be the most significant prognostic indicator by univariate as well as multivariate analysis. Furthermore, R0 resection was the only independent variable in determining the probability of long-term survival of patients with locally advanced gastric carcinoma. The overall survival for all patients receiving curative resection was higher than reported in historical series in which patients were treated with surgery alone for locally advanced gastric cancer [25].

Table 21.2 Pre-operative chemotherapy in resectable gastric cancer

Author (year)	Phase	Selection criteria	Pre-operative	Post-operative	(N.)	R0[a](%)	Pathologic CR (%)	Median survival (months)
Ajani (1991) [16]	II	M0 *Resectable* (+ GEJ)	EFP × 2	EFP × 3	25	72	0	15
Leichman (1992) [17]	II	M0 *Resectable*	FPL × 2	IP FUDR + IP cisplatin × 2	38	88	8	>17
Kang (1992) [18]	III RCT	M0 *Locally advanced*	1. EFP × 3 2. None	EFP × 3-6	53 54	79 61	8 -	43 30
Ajani (1993) [19]	II	M0 *Resectable*	EAP × 3	EAP × 2	48	90	0	16
Rougier (1994) [20]	II	M0 *Loc. advanced* (+ GEJ)	FP × 6	None	30	78	0	16
Kelsen (1996) [21]	II	M0 *Loc. advanced*	FAMTX × 3	IP FP + F	56	77	n.r.	15
Crookes (1997) [22]	II	M0 *Resectable* (+ GEJ)	FPL × 2 IP cisplatin × 2	IP FUDR +	59	71	9	52
Songun (1999) [23]	II RCT	T2-T4; M0	1. FAMTX × 4 2. None	None	27 29	75 75	n.r. -	18 30
Schuhmacher (2001) [24]	II	III-IV; M0 (+ GEJ)	EAP	None	42	86	0	19
D'Ugo (2006) [25]	II	T3–T4 anyN; T≤2 N+; M0	EEP × 3 or ECF × 3	EEP × 3 or EEP × 3	34	82	3	>28
Cunningham (2006) [6]	III RCT	II-IV; M0 (+ GEJ)	1. ECF × 3 2. None	1. ECF × 3 2. None	250 253	74 68	n.r. -	18 30
Boige (2007) [26]	III RCT	*Resectable* (+ GEJ)	1. FP × 3 1. FP × 3	2. None 2. None	113 111	84 73	n.r. -	n.r.
Schuhmacher (2009) [27]	III RCT	*Locally advanced* T3-T4N × M0	1. FP × 2 2. None	None	72 72	81.9 66.7	n.r.	>36

(*cont.*)

Table 21.2 (*continued*)

Kinoshita (2009) [28]	II	Schirrous *Resectable*	TS-1 × 2	None	55	80.8	0	n.r.
Biffi (2010) [29]	III RCT	T3-4 any N or any M0 (+ GEJ)	1. TCF × 4 2. None	1. None 2. TCF × 4	34 35	85	11.7	n.r.

EL, exploratory laparotomies; *R0*, curative (R0) resections; *CR*, complete response; *EFP*, etoposide, fluorouracil, and cisplatin; *GEJ*, gastro-esophageal junction; *FPL*, fluorouracil, cisplatin, and leucovorin; *IP*, intraperitoneal; *FUDR*, 5-fluoro-2'-deoxyuridine; *RCT*, randomized controlled trial; *EAP*, etoposide, doxorubicin, cisplatin; *FP*, fluorouracil and cisplatin; *FAMTX*, fluorouracil, doxorubicin, methotrexate; *F*, fluorouracil; *n.r.*, not reported; *EEP*, etoposide, epirubicin, cisplatin; *ECF*, epirubicin, cisplatin, fluorouracil; *TCF*, docetaxel, cisplatin, fluorouracil.

[a]The R0 resection rate was calculated only among resection procedures after pre-operative chemotherapy.

21.4 Pre-operative Neoadjuvant Radio(chemo)therapy

Based on the results of the SWOG 9008/INT-0116 trial [4], the integration of chemotherapy with radiation applied in the pre-operative phase has gained substantial interest. The benefits of pre-operative radiotherapy for gastric cancer were reported in several pivotal randomized single-center studies. Zhang and co-workers [31] recruited 317 patients with adenocarcinoma of the cardia who were randomly assigned to either radiation therapy followed by surgery or surgery alone. This study indicated a significant 5-year survival benefit for patients treated with neoadjuvant radiotherapy compared with surgery alone (30.1 vs. 19.8%, respectively), with an improved rate of complete curative resection after radiotherapy (80 vs. 62%). A second mono-institutional trial, performed in the Ukraine, enrolled 293 patients with gastric cancer from February 1984 to May 1986 [32]. This three-arm study randomized patients into: (1) radiation therapy followed by surgery, (2) radiation therapy with local hyperthermia followed by surgery, or (3) surgery alone. With 5-year survival rates of 30.1, 44.7, and 51.5% for surgery alone, radiation therapy with surgery, and radiation therapy with hyperthermia followed by surgery, respectively, the combined approach using radiation therapy with hyperthermia followed by surgery was demonstrated to be significantly more effective than surgery alone ($p < 0.05$). A benefit of radiation therapy with surgery (vs. surgery alone) was also observed but did not reach significance. Finally, Skoropad et al. [33] reported the 20-year follow-up results of a randomized trial on pre-operative radiotherapy (given at a dose of 20 Gy) compared to surgery alone. Overall survival between the two treatment groups was not significantly different. A recent meta-analysis of these randomized studies on pre-operative radiotherapy, comprising a total of 832 patients, was reported by Fiorica et al. in 2007. The results suggested that surgery combined with preoperative radiotherapy compared to surgery alone significantly reduced the 3- and 5-year mortality rates [34].

Recently, published phase II studies have verified the efficacy of chemoradiotherapy in terms of complete pathologic response (up to 30% in some series) and increased long-term survival without an increase in morbidity or mortality (Table 21.3) [30–40].

Safran and colleagues reported that patients who received concurrent paclitaxel and radiation had an overall response of 56%, including a complete response in three patients (11%) with locoregional unresectable gastric cancer [35]. Two-year progression-free and overall survival were 29% and 31%, respectively.

In 2001, Lowy et al. reported a pilot study of neoadjuvant chemoradiotherapy (combined with intraoperative radiotherapy) for patients with gastric cancer [36]. The disease was determined to be potentially resectable using a staging protocol that included computed tomography, endoscopic ultrasonography, and staging laparoscopy. The treatment combined 45 Gy of external-beam radiation at 1.8 Gy per day and 5 days per week with continuous-infusion 5-FU (300 mg/m^2/day). Among the 24 patients treated for potentially resectable but poor-prognosis tumors (determined by endoscopic ultrasound to be T2 or higher), all but one were able to complete therapy. The radiation field included the entire stomach and regional lymph nodes. The tumors were restaged on the basis of a computed tomography scan at 4–6 weeks following treatment and before a planned resection. A spleen-preserving D2-gastrectomy was performed after completion of chemoradiotherapy in 19 (83%) patients. Intraoperative radiotherapy (10 Gy) was given at resection. Complete pathologic response was observed in two (11%) patients.

Finally, in a recent study by Ajani et al. [37], patients were treated with two courses of 5-FU, folinic acid, and cisplatin followed by 5FU-potentiated radiotherapy (45 Gy). In surgical resections performed after pre-operative chemoradiotherapy there was a non-significantly higher incidence of post-operative complications. Among the 34 patients with localized gastric adenocarcinoma who were enrolled in the study, 85% underwent resection. The pathologic complete response rate was remarkable (30%) and a partial response was seen in another 24%. Overall median survival was 33.7 months; however, patients who achieved a complete response had a median survival of 64 months, compared to 12.6 months in those who

Table 21.3 Pre-operative radio(chemo)therapy in gastric cancer

Author (year)	Study design	Selection criteria	Pre-operative	Pts	R0[a](%)	Pathologic CR (%)	Median survival
Zhang (1998) [31]	RCT	GEJ	1.40 Gy EBRT 2. None	171 199	89.5	0	5-year OS: 30% vs. 20%
Shchepotin (1994) [32]	RCT	M0 *resectable* and unresectable	1. None 2. 20 Gy EBRT 3. 20 Gy EBRT + Hy	98 100 95	n.r.	n.r.	5-year OS: 21.3%
Skoropad (2000) [33]	RCT	M0 *Resectable* (+GEJ)	1. 20 Gy EBRT + 20 Gy IORT 2. None	59 53	66	0	16 months
Safran (2000) [35]	Phase I	Unresectable M0	45 Gy EBRT + Paclitaxel	27	n.r.	11	2-year OS: 35%
Lowy (2001) [36]	Phase I	T>2 Any N M0	45 Gy EBRT, 5-FU; 10 Gy IORT	24	75	11	n.r.
Ajani (2004) [37]	Phase II	T>2 Any N M0	5FU, LV, P then 45 Gy EBRT, 5FU	33	70	30	34 months
Ajani (2005) [38]	Phase II	M0 *Resectable* (+GEJ)	FP, paclitaxel; 45 Gy EBRT, 5FU	41	78	20	> 36 months
Allal (2005) [39]	Phase I	T3-T4 N+	FP, Leucovorin 31.2– 45.6 Gy EBRT	19	n.r.	5	5-year OS: 35%
Ajani (2006) [40]	Phase II	M0 *Resectable*	FP, LV, P; 45 Gy EBRT, 5FU, cis	49	63	26	23 months

R0, curative (R0) resections; *CR*, complete response; *GEJ*, gastro-esophageal junction; *RCT*, randomized controlled trial; *EBRT*, external beam radiotherapy; *IORT*, intraoperative radiotherapy; *Hy*, hyperthermia; *FP*, fluorouracil, cisplatin; *5FU*, 5-fluorouracil; *LV*, leucovorin; *n.r.*, not reported.
[a]The R0 resection rate was calculated only among resection procedures after pre-operative chemotherapy.

had less than a complete response ($p < 0.05$). This study emphasizes that a durable survival benefit can be achieved in patients whose tumors respond to treatment and that chemoradiotherapy, when the added risk associated with age and obesity are carefully considered, can be safely performed in patients with gastric or gastro-esophageal cancer, with an acceptable operative morbidity and a low operative mortality. Similar findings were reported in two subsequent reports with different chemotherapy regimens [38, 40].

21.5 Induction of R0 Resection

All of the above results suggest that R0 resection is not an exclusive surgical target in locally advanced gastric cancer but that it can be facilitated or achieved by pre-operative therapy ("induction" of R0 resection).

Many answers are expected from ongoing trials exploring improved pre-operative treatment strategies for resectable gastric cancer [7]. The MAGIC B trial (UK National Cancer Research Institute ST03 trial) examines peri-operative epirubicin, cisplatin, and capecitabine, with or without the endothelial growth factor antibody bevacizumab. The CRITICS trial (ChemoRadiotherapy after Induction chemoTherapy In Cancer of the Stomach) is a phase III study that randomizes between pre-operative chemotherapy (three courses of epirubicin/cisplatin/capecitabine) and gastric surgery with limited lymph node dissection followed by post-operative chemotherapy (another three courses of epirubicin/cisplatin/capecitabine) or chemoradiotherapy. Two trials in Japan, the JCOG trial 0501 (Japan Clinical Oncology Group Study 0501 trial) and the KYUH-UHA-GC04-03 Kyoto trial, are testing pre-operative oral fluoropyrimidine S-1 together with cisplatin vs. post-operative oral fluoropyrimidine S-1.

21.6 Evaluation of the Response to Neoadjuvant Treatment

At present, there is no reliable morphological or functional surrogate parameter for grading the response to combined therapy in gastric cancer and thus for subsequently evaluating the efficacy of this approach. Although a large percentage of patients respond to neoadjuvant therapy in some clinically measurable way, an evaluation of clinical response is both highly variable and subjective [24, 41, 42]. Indeed, the evaluation criteria frequently used for metastatic disease have not been validated for localized tumors and for the tumor bed after surgical excision [42].

At present, the grade of pathologic response to pre-operative treatment has not been able to show a statistically irrefutable prognostic significance. Only a few studies in the literature have addressed both the pathologic response after neoadjuvant therapy and patient survival [25, 42] and most of them could not demonstrate any significant relationship. Becker et al. [43] determined a significant relationship between the grade of pathologic response and survival only when the patients' results were divided into three unconventional levels of response, concluding that the survival difference between responders and non-responders is not particularly convincing in gastric cancer. However, in the absence of a clear-cut pre-therapeutic histological baseline, only "complete" response and "nearly complete" response are demonstrable.

Based on our experience, we consider the measurement of clinical and pathologic tumor response to chemotherapy as an extremely variable phenomenon [25]. A "quantitative" evaluation of the pathologic response, which detects the percentage of residual vital tumor cells in surgical specimens, is difficult in gastric cancer; traditionally, response classes are used [43]. However, it is certainly possible to study the impact on survival using a more "qualitative" analysis, i.e., based on tumor down-staging induced by any grade of pathologic response [25]. Given the lack of standardized concepts for response evaluation, some authors claim that pathologic response after pre-operative treatments is essentially a surrogate endpoint, reflecting more than influencing local control or survival [42]. Similarly, in our experience, pathologic grading of the response has yet to reach the statistical relevance of a reliable prognostic indicator. Nevertheless, following the demonstration of a significant association between tumor down-staging and the achievement of a true R0 resection, in 2001 we decided to change our chemotherapeutic schedule of choice from epidoxorubicin, etoposide, and cisplatin (EEP) to epirubicin, cisplatin, and fluorouracil (ECF), as the latter has yielded better pathologic response rates [25].

More recently, measurement of the "metabolic" response to chemotherapy by means of FDG-PET performed early during treatment was tested in patients with esophago-gastric tumors (type I-II according to the Siewert classification)[44]. Theoretically, patients who did not exhibit an early response to the initial regimen could be shifted to a different or more intensive course of chemotherapy. In these studies, metabolic response predicted histological response and survival with sufficient accuracy, justifying a similar approach in gastric cancer [44, 45]. However, the relevant percentage (≤ 40%) of FDG-non-avid gastric carcinoma cases makes the issue more complicated. In these patients, histopathologic response and survival were not significantly better than in patients with FDG-avid metabolically non-responding tumors. In such cases, alternative treatment, such as immediate resection, or modified or potentially more intensive peri-operative chemotherapy regimens, might be considered [44, 46]. A response-based strategy is a very promising approach but the results of preliminary studies still need to be reproduced by larger sample sizes.

21.7 Conclusions

In gastric cancer, complete surgical resection offers the best chance for cure. As described by the term "R0," complete resection consists of the surgical removal of all cancer cells from the tumor bed, with no macroscopic or microscopic residual. However, distant and locoregional failure rates in most patients undergoing radical tumor resection, and especially in those with positive lymph nodes or serosal involvement, contradict this theoretical statement.

In gastric cancer, oncological research has proceeded slowly and standardization is still far from being settled. Geographic differences in epidemiology and treatment approaches and the lack of a universally accepted surgical gold standard have diverted attention from the pursuit of a multimodal approach. Still, a paradigm shift has rapidly advanced in the last 10 years following three pivotal studies, carried out in three different areas of the world (USA, Europe, and Japan), demonstrating that multimodal treatment strategies improve the prognosis of patients with resectable gastric cancer. The common target of all of these protocols was to improve prognosis so as to achieve a "truly curative" resection, with minimal morbidity and mortality. All current therapeutic efforts in resectable gastric cancer are directed toward the individualization of these therapeutic protocols, tailoring the extent of resection and the administration of pre-operative and post-operative treatment. Despite the need for further data regarding the definitive role of neoadjuvant chemoradiotherapy, the results of pre-operative chemotherapy in the multimodal treatment of gastric adenocarcinoma are now more than encouraging and the benefits seem unquestionable.

Modern concerns are identification of the optimal therapy regimen, the strict selection of study patients by accurate preoperative staging (to ensure the enrollment of homogeneous patients subgroups), the identification of early biomolecular and metabolic predictors of response (so as to exclude patients who will not respond to a multimodal approach and who are instead candidates for surgery alone), the standardization of surgical procedures, and the adoption of reliable criteria for response evaluation.

Newly designed trials are needed in order to identify the best treatment plan to be applied in the pre-operative setting and to understand how to combine conventional chemotherapeutic agents with new-generation molecules to achieve a therapeutic schedule tailored to the individual patient.

References

1. Kamangar F, Dores GM, Anderson WF (2006) Patterns of cancer incidence, mortality, and prevalence across five continents: defining priorities to reduce cancer disparities in different geographic regions of the world. J Clin Oncol 24:2137-2150
2. Kubota H, Kotoh T, Masunaga R, et al (2000) Impact of screening survey of gastric cancer on clinicopathological features and survival: retrospective study at a single institution. Surgery 128:41-47

3. Hundahl SA, Phillips JL, Menck HR (2000) The National Cancer Data Base Report on poor survival of U.S. gastric carcinoma patients treated with gastrectomy: Fifth Edition American Joint Committee on Cancer staging, proximal disease, and the "different disease" hypothesis. Cancer 88:921-932
4. Macdonald JS, Smalley SR, Benedetti J et al (2001) Chemoradiotherapy after surgery compared with surgery alone for adenocarcinoma of the stomach or gastroesophageal junction. N Engl J Med 345:725-730
5. Sakuramoto S, Sasako M, Yamaguchi T et al (2007) ACTS-GC Group. Adjuvant chemotherapy for gastric cancer with S-1, an oral fluoropyrimidine. N Engl J Med 357:1810-1820
6. Cunningham D, Allum WH, Stenning SP et al (2006) Perioperative chemotherapy versus surgery alone for resectable gastroesophageal cancer. N Engl J Med 355:11-20
7. D'Ugo D, Rausei S, Biondi A et al (2009) Preoperative treatment and surgery in gastric cancer: friends or foes? Lancet Oncol 10:191-195
8. August DA, Gannon C (2010) Guest editorial: Neoadjuvant therapy, predictors of response, and patient outcomes. J Surg Oncol 102:107-108
9. Wilke H, Preusser P, Fink U et al (1989) Preoperative chemotherapy in locally advanced and nonresectable gastric cancer: a phase II study with etoposide, doxorubicin and cisplatin. J Clin Oncol 7:1318-1326
10. Plukker JT, Mulder NH, Sleijfer DTH et al (1991) Chemotherapy and surgery for locally advanced cancer of the cardia and fundus: phase II study with methotrexate and 5-fl uorouracil. Br J Surg 78:955-958
11. Rougier P, Mahjoubi M, Lasser P et al (1994) Neoadjuvant chemotherapy in locally advanced gastric carcinoma—a phase II trial with combined continuous intravenous 5-fluorouracil and bolus cisplatinum. Eur J Cancer 30:1269-1275
12. Kelsen D, Karpeh M, Schwartz G et al (1996) Neoadjuvant therapy of high-risk gastric cancer: a phase II trial of preoperative FAMTX and postoperative intraperitoneal fluorouracil-cisplatin plus intravenous fluorouracil. J Clin Oncol 14:1818-1828
13. Melcher AA, Mort D, Maughan TS (1996) Epirubicin, cisplatin and continuous infusion 5-fluorouracil (ECF) as neoadjuvant chemotherapy in gastro-oesophageal cancer. Br J Cancer 74:1651-1654
14. Gallardo-Rincon D, Onate-Ocana LF, Calderillo-Ruiz G (2000) Neoadjuvant chemotherapy with P-ELF (cisplatin, etoposide, leucovorin, 5-fluorouracil) followed by radical resection in patients with initially unresectable gastric adenocarcinoma: a phase II study. Ann Surg Oncol 7:45-50
15. Cascinu S, Scartozzi M, Labianca R, et al (2004) Italian Group for the Study of Digestive Tract Cancer (GISCAD). High curative resection rate with weekly cisplatin, 5-fluorouracil, epidoxorubicin, 6S-leucovorin, glutathione, and filgastrim in patients with locally advanced, unresectable gastric cancer: a report from the Italian Group for the Study of Digestive Tract Cancer (GISCAD). Br J Cancer 90:1521-1525
16. Ajani JA, Ota DM, Jessup JM et al (1991) Resectable gastric carcinoma: an evaluation of preoperative and postoperative chemotherapy. Cancer 68:1501-1506
17. Leichman L, Silberman H, Leichman CG et al (1992) Preoperative systemic chemotherapy followed by adjuvant postoperative intraperitoneal therapy for gastric cancer: a University of Southern California pilot program. J Clin Oncol 10:1933-1942
18. Kang YK, Choi DW, Kim CW et al (1992) The effect of neoadjuvant chemotherapy on the surgical outcome of locally advanced gastric adenocarcinoma: interim report of a randomized controlled trial. Proc Am Soc Clin Oncol 11:173
19. Ajani JA, Mayer RJ, Ota DM et al (1993) Preoperative and postoperative chemotherapy for patients with potentially resectable gastric carcinoma. J Natl Cancer Inst 85: 1839-1844
20. Rougier P, Lasser P, Ducreux M et al (1994) Preoperative chemotherapy of locally advanced gastric cancer. Ann Oncol 5:59-68
21. Kelsen D, Karpeh M, Schwartz G et al (1996) Neoadjuvant therapy of highrisk gastric cancer: a phase II trial of preoperative FAMTX and postoperative intraperitoneal fluorouracil-cisplatin plus intravenous fl uorouracil. J Clin Oncol 14:1818-1828
22. Crookes P, Leichman CG, Leichman L et al (1997) Systemic chemotherapy for gastric carcinoma followed by postoperative intraperitoneal therapy: a final report. Cancer 79:1767-1775
23. Songun I, Keizer HJ, Hermans J et al (1999) Chemotherapy for operable gastric cancer: results of the Dutch randomised FAMTX trial. Eur J Cancer 35:558-562
24. Schuhmacher CP, Fink U, Becker K et al (2001) Neoadjuvant therapy for patients with locally advanced gastric carcinoma with etoposide, doxorubicin, and cisplatinum: closing results after 5 years of follow-up. Cancer 91:918-927
25. D'Ugo D, Persiani R, Rausei S et al (2006) Response to neoadjuvant chemotherapy and effects of tumor regression in gastric cancer. Eur J Surg Oncol 32:1105-1109
26. Boige V, Pignon J, Saint-Aubert B et al (2007) Final results of a randomized trial comparing preoperative 5-fluorouracil (F)/cisplatin (P) to surgery alone in adenocarcinoma of stomach and lower esophagus (ASLE): FNLCC ACCORD07-FFCD 9703 trial. J Clin Oncol ASCO Annual Meeting Proceedings 2007:4510
27. Schuhmacher C, Schlag P, Lordick F et al (2009) Neoadjuvant chemotherapy versus surgery alone for locally advanced adenocarcinoma of the stomach and cardia: Randomized EORTC phase III trial #40954. J Clin Oncol ASCO Annual Meeting Proceedings 2009:4510
28. Kinoshita T, Sasako M, Sano T et al (2009) Phase II trial of S-1 for neoadjuvant chemotherapy against scirrhous gastric cancer (JCOG 0002). Gastric Cancer 12:37-42
29. Biffi R, Fazio N, Luca F et al (2010) Surgical outcome after docetaxel-based neoadjuvant chemotherapy in locally-advanced gastric cancer. World J Gastroenterol 16:868-874
30. Hartgrink HH, van de Velde CJ, Putter H et al (2004) Cooperating Investigators of The Dutch Gastric Cancer Group. Neoadjuvant chemotherapy for operable gastric cancer: long term results of the Dutch randomised FAMTX trial. Eur J Surg Oncol 30:643-649
31. Zhang ZX, Gu XZ, Yin WB et al (1998) Randomized clinical trial of the combination of preoperative irradiation and surgery in the treatment of adenocarcinoma of the gastric cardia (AGC)-report on 370 patients. Int J Radiat Oncol Biol Phys 42:929-934

32. Shchepotin IB, Evans SR, Chorny V et al (1994) Intensive preoperative radiotherapy with local hyperthermia for the treatment of gastric carcinoma. Surg Oncol 3:37-44
33. Skoropad V, Berdov B, Zagrebin V (2002) Concentrated preoperative radiotherapy for resectable gastric cancer: 20-years follow-up of a randomized trial. J Surg Oncol 80:72-78
34. Fiorica F, Cartei F, Enea M et al (2007) The impact of radiotherapy on survival in resectable gastric carcinoma: a meta-analysis of literature data. Cancer Treat Rev 33:729-740
35. Safran H, King TP, Choy H et al (1997) Paclitaxel and concurrent radiation for locally advanced pancreatic and gastric cancer: a phase I study. J Clin Oncol 15:901-907
36. Lowy AM, Feig BW, Janjan N et al (2001) A pilot study of preoperative chemoradiotherapy for resectable gastric cancer. Ann Surg Oncol 8:519-524
37. Ajani JA, Mansfield PF, Janjan N et al (2004) Multi-institutional trial of preoperative chemoradiotherapy in patients with potentially resectable gastric cancer. J Clin Oncol 22:2774-2780
38. Ajani JA, Mansfield PF, Crane CH et al (2005) Paclitaxel-based chemoradiotherapy in localized gastric carcinoma: Degree of pathologic response and not clinical parameters dictated patient outcome. J Clin Oncol 23:1237-1244
39. Allal AS, Zwahlen D, Brundler MA et al Neoadjuvant radiochemotherapy for locally advanced gastric cancer: Longterm results of a phase I trial. Int J Radiat Oncol Biol Phys 63:1286-1289
40. Ajani JA, Winter K, Okawara GS et al (2006) Phase II trial of preoperative chemoradiation in patients with localized gastric adenocarcinoma (RTOG 9904) Quality of combined modality therapy and pathologic response. J Clin Oncol 24: 3953- 3958
41. Lowy AM, Mansfield PF, Leach SD et al (1999) Response to neoadjuvant chemotherapy best predicts survival after curative resection of gastric cancer. Ann Surg 229:303-308
42. Persiani R, Rausei S, Biondi A et al (2009) Perioperative chemotherapy for gastric cancer: how should we measure the efficacy? Ann Surg Oncol 16:1077-1079
43. Becker K, Mueller JD, Schuhmacher C et al (2003) Histomorphology and grading of regression in gastric carcinoma treated with neoadjuvant chemotherapy. Cancer 98:1521-1530
44. Ott K, Lordick F, Herrmann K et al (2008) The new credo: induction chemotherapy in locally advanced gastric cancer: consequences for surgical strategies. Gastric Cancer 11:1-9
45. Vallböhmer D, Hölscher AH, Schneider PM et al (2010) 18F]-fluorodeoxyglucose-positron emission tomography for the assessment of histopathologic response and prognosis after completion of neoadjuvant chemotherapy in gastric cancer. J Surg Oncol 102:135-140
46. Mezhir JJ, Tang LH, Coit DG (2010) Neoadjuvant therapy of locally advanced gastric cancer. J Surg Oncol 101:305-314

22 Neoadjuvant Treatment for Resectable Locally Advanced Gastric Cancer: European Ongoing Trials

William H. Allum

Abstract

Combination therapy has become the established treatment of gastric cancer. The challenge now is to select the appropriate combination for each clinical presentation. Current trials are designed to address specific issues. A consistent feature of these studies is the standardization of treatment so that the trial intervention can be assessed appropriately by minimizing the number of confounding variables. Support for these trials is essential if they are to reach the required study-population size, thus favouring multicentre collaborations. The results of these and future trials should provide more selective therapies aimed at improving the outcome for all patients undergoing radical treatment for gastric cancer. The inclusion of translational research projects may also increase our understanding of the biology and natural history of this heterogeneous disease.

Keywords

Gastric cancer • Clinical trials • Neoadjuvant and adjuvant chemotherapy • Chemoradiotherapy

22.1 Introduction

The results of clinical trials of perioperative and postoperative combination therapy in gastric cancer have established a role for these treatments. The Intergroup 116 trial from North America [1] has shown survival benefits with chemoradiotherapy after surgery. From Europe, the MAGIC Trial [2] and from France the FFCD Trial [3] have demonstrated similar 5 year survival advantages in patients receiving chemotherapy before and after surgery. The Japanese ACTS trial [4] reported a 10% survival improvement with adjuvant single-agent chemotherapy.

These trials have set the standard of care against which future studies should be compared. The North American and European trials were designed using treatments that had been established in the advanced disease setting in the early to mid 1990s. They were pragmatic trials to ensure recruitment and professional and patient compliance. Although the trials answered a number of questions, as with any research outcome, subsequent critical analysis has highlighted both the limitations of those studies and the need to resolve the outstanding issues as well as to develop further solutions.

W.H. Allum (✉)
Royal Marsden NHS Foundation Trust,
London, UK

G. de Manzoni, F. Roviello, W. Siquini (eds.), *Surgery in the Multimodal Management of Gastric Cancer*,

Criticism of MAGIC and of Intergroup 116 has focused on whether the combination therapies had instead compensated for less than adequate surgery. In both trials, preoperative staging was limited to external imaging. Both trials were developed in the era before routine laparoscopic staging and endoscopic ultrasound. Surgery was not standardized in either trial. In Intergroup 116, entry only occurred after surgery and 54% of patients had a D0 procedure. In MAGIC, the extent of surgery was left to the discretion of the surgeon and approximately 50% of the procedures reportedly included D2 lymphadenectomy. MAGIC also enrolled patients with T2N0 tumours, which many consider as treatable by surgery alone. There is thus a significant issue with the quality assurance of the surgery,

Although the trials' designs do not allow direct comparisons they do raise a number of questions. Would there be a further advantage combining the trial therapies? Since in MAGIC only 41% of the patients completed the postoperative therapy protocol, do the demonstrated benefits derive only from the preoperative cycles? Is there a role for other therapies? The limited number of complete responses and the modest survival benefit in MAGIC and FFCD raises the option of external imaging or functional assessment of treatment response. An important consideration in designing further trials in the light of the results of MAGIC, FFCD and Intergroup 116 is that the sample size will need to be much larger than previous ones in order to prove any benefit. Additionally, the option of multicentre recruitment has to be considered in new trial design to allow completion of the studies on an appropriate time scale.

There are currently three trials underway in Europe that have been designed to address many of these questions. In the UK, the ST03 Trial, the successor to MAGIC, is evaluating the addition of bevacizumab to chemotherapy. In Holland, the CRITICS trial has been developed to compare perioperative chemotherapy with preoperative chemotherapy and postoperative chemoradiotherapy. In Germany, the IMAGE trial has been designed to evaluate functional imaging assessment of chemotherapy response, with the non-responders then randomized to surgery and neoadjuvant chemoradiotherapy.

22.2 ST03 Trial

The STO3 Trial is a randomized phase II/III trial of perioperative chemotherapy with or without bevacizumab in patients with operable adenocarcinoma of the stomach or gastro-oesophageal junction. The combination chemotherapy is epirubicin, cisplatin and capecitabine (ECX). Capectabine substitutes for 5-FU, as used in MAGIC, given that the REAL-2 trial [5] showed the non-inferiority of capecitabine. A practical advantage is that capecitabine is an oral preparation and infusion devices are not required.

Bevacizumab is a monoclonal antibody against vascular endothelial growth factor (VEGF), a physiological and pathological regulator of angiogenesis and therefore of tumour growth. Bevacizumab has both a direct anti-angiogenic effect and an effect on tumour vasculature, with a decrease in elevated intra-tumoural interstitial pressure to improve delivery of the chemotherapeutic agent to tumour cells. In gastric cancer, VEGF expression has been shown to be indicative of a poor prognosis, correlating with poor 5 year survival rates, lymph node metastasis and vascular invasion [6]. In patients with advanced colorectal, lung and breast cancers, bevacizumab has been shown to improve survival. A randomized trial of capecitabine and cisplatin with or without bevacizumab showed a modest 2 month increase in survival in the arm including bevacizumab [7] but this did not reach statistical significance. The study authors noted the heterogeneity in the responses and postulated that it reflected the different subtypes of gastric cancer.

The trial design of ST03 is shown in Fig. 22.1. The primary end point of the trial is overall survival, with secondary endpoints including treatment-related morbidity, response rates, resection rates, disease-free survival, quality of life, and cost-effectiveness. The key inclusion criteria are adenocarcinoma of the stomach and Siewert type II and III gastro-oeosophageal junction cancers staged as Ib–IV (M0) (TNM 6th edn.) by CT, laparoscopy and endoscopic ultrasound. Patients should have adequate bone marrow, coagulation, liver and renal function with a performance status of 0–1, a left ventricular ejection fraction > 50%

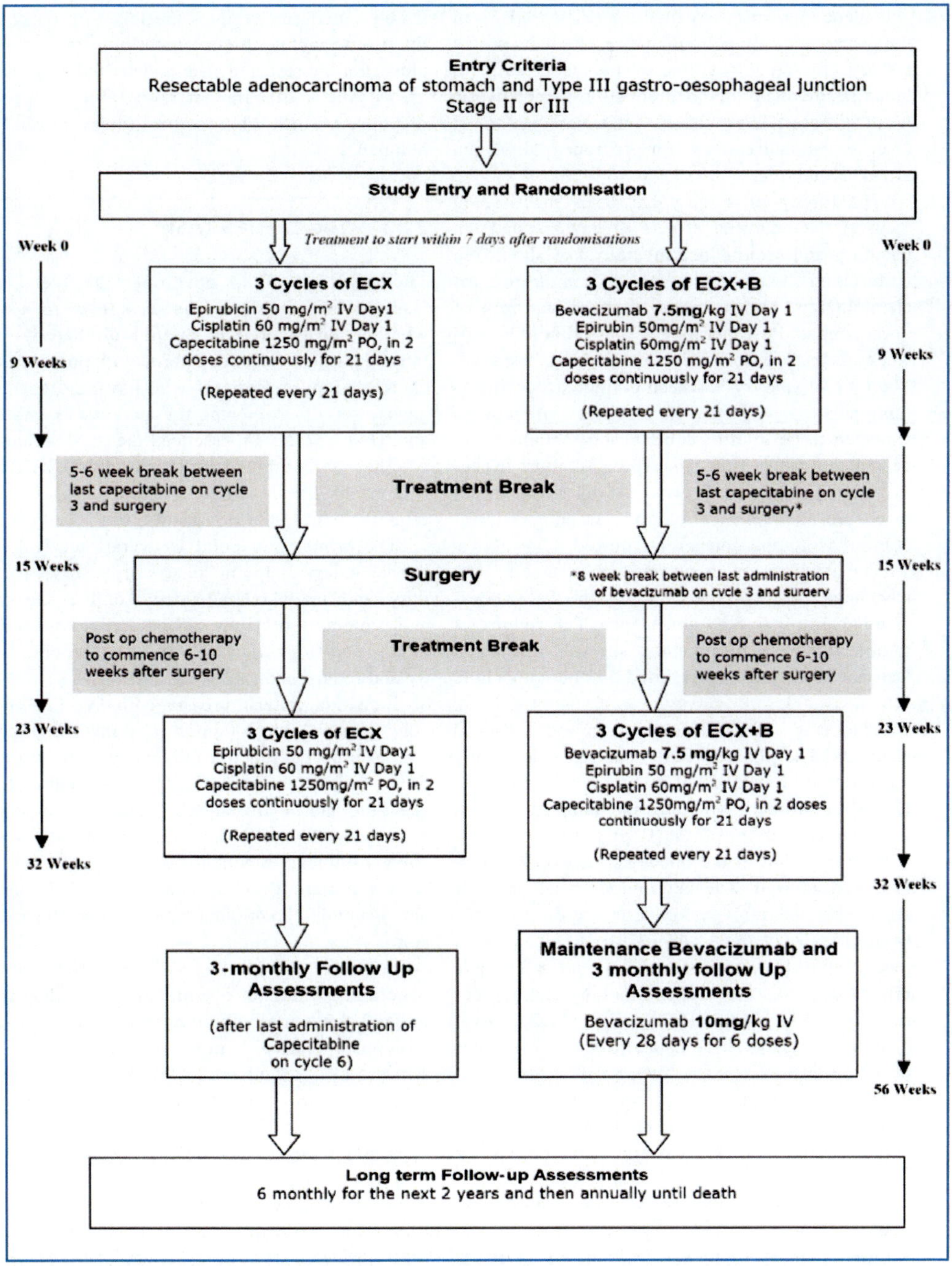

Fig. 22.1 Design of the UK National Cancer Research Institute STO3 Trial

and adequate respiratory function (FEV1 > 1.5l) in the presence of a junctional cancer. Patients with a history of a recent cardiac event, recent surgery, bleeding diathesis or coagulopathy, recent peptic ulcer disease, diverticulitis, inflammatory bowel disease, and/or treatment for previous malignancy are excluded.

The timing of surgery has been specified in view of the potential effects of bevacizumab on bleeding and wound healing. Surgery should be undertaken 5–6 weeks after completion of chemotherapy and 8 weeks after the last dose of bevacizumab. Postoperatively, there should be a 6-week interval before chemotherapy is restarted. The type of surgery has been defined according to tumour site, with the majority of procedures expected to be total or subtotal gastrectomy, with oesophago-gastrectomy for type II tumours if necessary to obtain a clear proximal margin. In order to ensure adequate pathological staging, a minimum of 15 lymph nodes are required.

The trial has been powered to detect a 10% advantage in 5-year survival for the ECX–bevacizumab arm with 80% confidence. This requires a sample size of 1100 patients. The trial opened in October 2007 and has recruited 402 patients (June 2011).

The design of ST03 combines phase II and III elements. The phase II part is aimed at assessing the safety and efficacy of adding bevacizumab to ECX. The protocol stipulates inclusion of the first 200 patients for the phase II part; these patients will be included in the phase III part once safety has been assured. The key endpoints of phase II are gastrointestinal perforations, cardiac events, wound healing, and gastrointestinal bleeding. A recent report [8] contained preliminary safety data related to preoperative chemotherapy and surgery in the first 104 patients (ECX ,$N = 51$; ECX–bevacizumab $N = 53$). These data showed similar rates of complications in the two arms in terms of haematological and symptomatic toxicities. In addition, there was a similar distribution of the key endpoints between the two arms (Table 22.1). A formal analysis of the safety data will be undertaken once the first 200 patients have completed treatment.

Also included in the design of the STO3 trial is a translational research study (Trans-STO3). Blood and tissue samples are taken on entry into the trial to include pretreatment biopsies and samples from the resected specimens. Studies aimed at identifying molecular markers able to predict response to the therapeutic interventions are planned as well.

22.3 The CRITICS Trial

The CRITICS Trial developed by the Dutch Gastric Cancer Group is designed to assess whether postoperative chemoradiotherapy prolongs overall survival compared with postoperative chemotherapy in patients who have had adequate gastric surgery following preoperative chemotherapy (Fig. 22.2). In essence, the trial examines whether the combined approaches of MAGIC and Intergroup 116 result in a therapy that is more effective than either treatment alone.

The primary endpoint is overall survival, and the secondary endpoints disease-free survival, toxicity, and health-related quality of life. Genomic and proteomic profiling of histological material is being used to predict the response to chemotherapy and recurrence risk.

Inclusion criteria are stage Ib–IVa (TNM 6th edn.) gastric cancer (which may involve the gastro-oesophageal junction) that is operable as determined by conventional staging assessment with CT scanning and laparoscopy. Patients should be performance status WHO 0 or 1, with satisfactory haematological, biochemical, cardiac, renal and liver function. Previous abdominal radiotherapy and systemic chemotherapy are reasons for exclusion.

It is expected that there will be a 10% survival benefit at 5 years for overall survival in the experimental arm combining preoperative chemotherapy with postoperative chemoradiotherapy. The sample size has been calculated at 788 patients to achieve 80% power to detect this difference at a significance level of 0.05.

The trial design has specifically considered two treatment quality issues. Firstly, surgeons are expected to carry out a standardized gastric resection with removal of at least 15 lymph nodes (described as a D1+), with avoidance of pancreatosplenectomy. It is recommended that surgery

Table 22.1 Adverse events in first 104 patients in the STO3 Trial

	ECX ($n = 51$)	ECX – B ($n = 53$)
Grade 3-4 venous thromboembolism events	5 (3 grade 4 PE, 1 grade 5 PE, 1 grade 3 renal vein thrombosis)	5 (4 grade 4 PE (1 during postoperative chemotherapy), 1 grade 3 DVT
Grade 3-4 arterial thromboembolic events	0	2 (1 grade 4 MI during postoperative chemotherapy, 1 grade 4 CVA postoperatively)
Wound healing complications:		
Anastomotic leak	2 (1 grade 3, 1 grade 4)	1 (grade 3)
Biliary leak	0	1 (grade 3)
Wound infection	3 (2 grade 2, 1 grade 3)	3 (1 grade 1, 1 grade 2, 1 grade 3)
Non-infectious wound complication	0	1 (1 grade 2)
GI perforation	1 (grade 4)	1 (grade 4)
Grade 3-4 haemorrhagic event	1 (upper GI bleed, grade 3)	1 (epistaxis grade 3)
Grade 3-4 hypertension	0	1 (grade 3)
Other clinically significant events	0	2 (1 grade 2 microvascular leukoencephalopathy; 1 grade 5 microngiopathic haemolytic anaemia due to marrow infiltration with carcinoma)

ECX, Epirubicin, cisplatin and capecitabine; *ECX–B*, ECX plus bevacizumab; *GI*, gastrointestinal; *PE*, pulmonary embolism; *DVT*, deep vein thrombosis; *MI*, myocardial infarction; *CVA*, cerebrovascular accident.

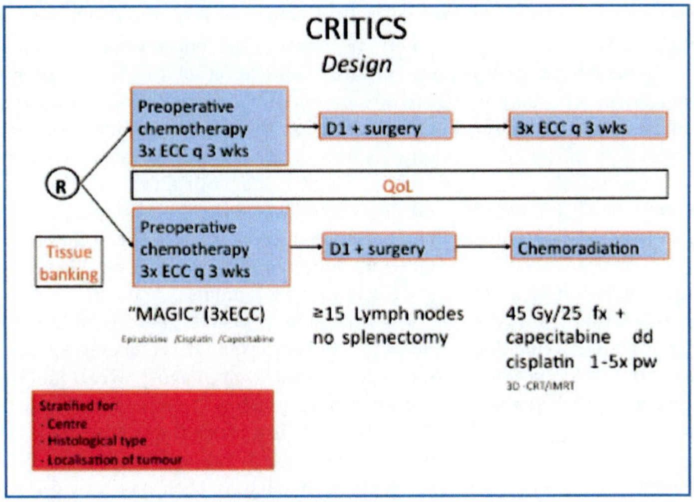

Fig. 22.2 Design of the CRITICS Trial. *ECC*, Epirubicin, cisplatin and capecitabine; *QoL*, quality of life; *fx* fraction; *dd*, daily; *pw*, weekly

should occur within 3–6 weeks after the last course of chemotherapy and that postoperative treatment should begin 4–12 weeks after surgery. The protocol justifies this recommendation based on the lack of benefit for extended lymphadenectomy in the Dutch [9] and MRC D1/D2 [10] trials, the trend for better survival in the subgroup with N2 disease after D2 dissection in the Dutch trial and the adverse effect of pancreatic resection and splenectomy.

Secondly, a standard radiotherapy planning technique is prescribed. Following gastric resec-

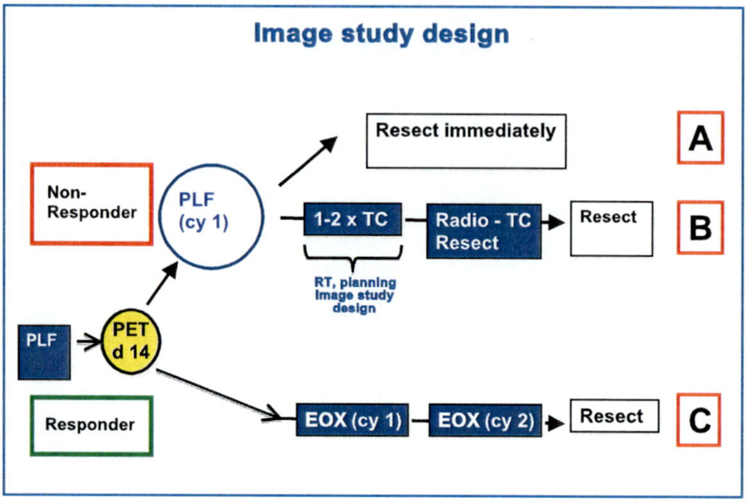

Fig. 22.3 Design of the IMAGE Trial

tion, the radiation-dose-limiting organs in the radiation field are the gastric remnant, the small intestine, the spinal cord, the kidneys and the liver. The selection of the radiation dose also needs to consider toxicity if the concurrent chemotherapy acts as a radiosensitizer. The trial management group has determined the dose from a phase I/II study in which maximal sparing of radiosensitive structures was achieved with adequate coverage of the clinical target volume. The method of administration of the radiation requires 3D conformal CT-based techniques or intensity modulated radiotherapy (IMRT).

The CRITICS trial opened for recruitment in 2007. Patients are being recruited from the Netherlands and Sweden with plans to include those from Denmark. So far, 318 patients (February 2011) have been recruited and planned interim analyses are awaited.

22.4 The IMAGE Study

The IMAGE study is designed to evaluate the use of functional imaging to determine response to chemotherapy and to assess the benefit of preoperative chemoradiotherapy in non-responders. The efficacy of functional imaging with positron emission tomography (PET) has been established in oesophago-gastric junctional cancers. Sequential imaging before and after 2 weeks of chemotherapy has been shown to predict histopathological response [11], which in turn allows identification of both responders and non-responders and thus appropriate modification of the treatment plans. The information provided by PET is limited in true gastric cancers as there is little or no uptake of the radiolabelled glucose by diffuse type or mucinous tumours. Kelsen and colleagues [12] confirmed that non-responders have a poorer prognosis and that continuation of ineffective chemotherapy may indeed be detrimental to survival by delaying surgery for resectable tumours .

The aim of the IMAGE study is to define the role of neodjuvant taxane based chemoradiation in locally advanced oesophago-gastric junctional cancers not responding to chemotherapy (Fig. 22.3). The study is a phase II design. Patients with Siewert type I and II tumours of the oesophagogastric junction that have been staged by CT, endoscopic ultrasound and PET as T3/T4 and/or N+ and are operable with R0 intent are eligible. All patients receive induction chemotherapy with cisplatin, 5-fluorouracil and leucovorin and undergo repeat PET scanning at 2 weeks. Responders continue with two further cycles of chemotherapy (epirubicin, oxaliplatin and capecitabine) and proceed to surgery (group C). Non-responders, according to PET criteria, are randomized to surgery (group A) or neo-adjuvant chemoradiotherapy with docetaxel and cisplatin and 45 Gy radiation in 25 fractions (group B).

The study has three objectives. Firstly, the effect of chemoradiotherapy in the non-responders will be determined by comparing the R0 resection rates between groups A and B. A sample size of 352 patients with 176 in each group is needed to demonstrate a 20% increase in R0 resections. Secondly, a comparison of the R0 resection rate of group A with that of group C will allow the prognostic value of the PET-determined response to be assessed. The third objective is to estimate the positive predictive value of the PET response by estimating the histopathological response in group C.

The trial is planned to recruit patients over a period of 30 months. A key component in the study is the quality assurance of the PET reporting.

22.5 Conclusions

Combination therapy has now become established in the treatment of gastric cancer. The challenge now is to select the appropriate combination for each clinical presentation. The current trials have been designed with specific issues to evaluate. A consistent feature of these studies is to standardize aspects of treatment so that the trial intervention can be assessed appropriately and minimize confounding variables. It is essential that the trials are supported and in order to reach the required study populations this would preferably be by multicentre collaboration. These and future trials should allow more selective therapies to improve the outcome for all patients undergoing radical treatment for gastric cancer. The inclusion of translational research projects may also increase our understanding of the biology and natural history of this hetereogeneous disease.

Acknowledgements
I thank my co-collaborators on the STO3 trial: Professor David Cunningham, Dr Alicia Okines and Dr Ruth Langley. I am also grateful to my colleagues Dr Henk Hartgrink and Dr Maurits Swellengrebel for information about the CRITICS trial, and to Professor Katja Ott for details of the IMAGE trial.

References

1. Macdonald JS, Smalley SR, Benedetti J et al (2001) Chemoradiotherapy after surgery compared with surgery alone for adenocarcinoma of the stomach or gastroesophageal junction. N Engl J Med 345:725-730
2. Cunningham D, Allum WH, Stenning SP et al (2006) Perioperative chemotherapy versus surgery alone for resectable gastroesophageal cancer. N Engl J Med 355:11-20
3. Ychou M, Boige V, Pignon et al (20011) Perioperative chemotherapy compared with surgery alone for resectable gastroesophageal adenocarcinoma: an FNCLCC and FFCD multicenter phase III trial. J Clin Oncol 29:1715-1721
4. Sakuramoto S, Sasako M, Yamaguchi T et al (2007) Adjuvant chemotherapy for gastric cancer with S-1, an oral fluoropyrimidine. N Engl J Med 357:1810-1820
5. Cunningham D, Starling N, Rao S et al (2008) Capecitabine and oxaliplatin for advanced esophagogastric cancer. N Engl J Med 358:36-46
6. Duff SE, Li C, Jeziorska M et al (2003) Vascular endothelial growth factors C and D and lymphangiogenesis in gastrointestinal tract malignancy. Br J Cancer 89:426-430
7. Kang Y, Ohtsu A, van Cutsem E et al (2010) AVAGAST: a randomized double blind placebo controlled phase III study of first line capecitabine and cisplatin plus bevacizuab or placebo in patients with advanced gastric cancer. J Clin Oncol 28 (18) supplement: 4007
8. Okines AF, Langley R, Cafferty FH et al (2010)Preliminary safety data from a randomized trial of perioperative epirubicin, cisplatin plus capecitabine (ECX) with or without bevacizumab (B) in patients with gastric or oesophagogastric adenocarcinoma. J Clin Oncol 28 (15) supplement: 4019
9. Bonenkamp JJ, Hermans J, Sasako M, van de Velde CJ (1999) Extended lymph node dissection for gastric cancer. Dutch gastric cancer group. NE J Med 340:908-914
10. Cuschieri A, Weeden S, Fielding J et al (1999) Patient survival after D1 and D2 resections for gastric cancer: long term results of the MRC randomised surgical trial. Surgical Cooperative group Br J Cancer 79:1522-1530
11. Lordick F, Ott K, Krause BJ et al (2007) PET to assess early metabolic response and to guide treatment of adenocarcinoma of the oesophago-gastric junction: the MUNICOM phase II trial. Lancet Oncol 8:797-805
12. Kelsen DP, Winter KA, Gunderson LL et al (2007) Longterm results of RTOG Trial 8911 (USA Intergroup 113): a random assignment trial comparison of chemotherapy followed by surgery compared with surgery alone for oesophageal cancer. J Clin Oncol 25: 3719-3725

The Role of Chemotherapy in Metastatic Disease

23

Felice Pasini, Anna Paola Fraccon, Giorgio Crepaldi, and Giovanni de Manzoni

Abstract

In the setting of metastatic or inoperable gastric cancer, chemotherapy has improved survival over that achieved with best supportive care. Randomized phase III trials showed better outcome for cisplatin-containing schedules, and in Western countries ECF is widely accepted as the reference regimen. Median survival in those studies was essentially < 1 year. However, recent phase III studies, also using new drugs, such as docetaxel, oxaliplatin, irinotecan, capecitabine, and S1, have likewise failed to demonstrate a major improvement. Promising data have been recently published for trastuzumab-containing therapy. In the 20–50% patients receiving 2nd-line chemotherapy, the results have been disappointing and survival is only 6–8 months. Thus, despite small signs of progress, metastatic gastric cancer remains an incurable disease and treatment should primarily consider the patient's quality of life. The best hope for the future is based on tailored interventions with new cytotoxic drugs, targeted therapies, and the integration of molecular determinants.

Keywords

Gastric cancer • Chemotherapy • Best supportive care • Cisplatin • Docetaxel • Oxaliplatin • Irinotecan • Capecitabine • S1 • Trastuzumab • Fluorouracil

23.1 Background

Despite improvements in the diagnosis of gastric cancer, in the Western world approximately two-thirds of the patients have inoperable disease at presentation or develop a recurrence within 5 years after surgery. These patients with inoperable, recurrent, or metastatic tumors are still incurable, with a prognosis of only a few months with best supportive care (BSC). The introduction of chemotherapy has been shown to prolong survival and improve symptom palliation in this group of patients, although, in the clinical setting, the benefits must be weighed against treatment-related toxicities.

First-generation chemotherapy protocols were based on 5-fluorouracil (5-FU), the most extensively single agent used, on cisplatin and anthracyclines but recent schedules evaluated in phase III trials include new drugs, such as capecitabine, oxaliplatin, docetaxel, paclitaxel, irinotecan, S-1, and monoclonal antibodies [1-6]. Other new drugs are currently under evaluation in phase II and III clinical studies.

F. Pasini (✉)
Dept. of Medical Oncology,
"Santa Maria della Misericordia" Hospital,
Rovigo, Italy

G. de Manzoni, F. Roviello, W. Siquini (eds.), *Surgery in the Multimodal Management of Gastric Cancer*,

In the setting of metastatic gastric cancer, current evidence shows that: (a) chemotherapy improves survival compared to BSC; (b) combination chemotherapy improves survival compared to single-agent 5-FU and produces a higher response rate, albeit at the cost of higher toxicity.

23.2 The Role of Chemotherapy: First Line Treatment

23.2.1 Chemotherapy vs. Best Supportive Care

In the 1980s and 1990s, many trials demonstrated the superiority of 5-FU-based regimens compared with BSC in terms of survival in patients with advanced gastric cancer [7-9]. Median survival of BSC (4.3 months) could be doubled by the administration of chemotherapy, resulting in a hazards ratio (HR) of 0.37 (95% CI 0.24–0.55) and a response rate of 33–50%. Since then, BSC is no longer considered an appropriate control arm in therapeutic trials [10].

23.2.2 Single-agent vs. Combination Therapy

A recent meta-analysis [10] demonstrated that combination chemotherapy had a statistically significant and consistent survival advantage compared with single-agent therapy (HR 0.80, 95% CI 0.72–0.89). Median survival was 8.3 vs. 6.7 months, median progression-free survival (PFS) 5.6 months vs. 3.6 months, and the pooled objective response rate (ORR) 35% vs. 18% in the combination and single-agent arms, respectively. Overall, toxicity was higher with combination chemotherapy but the difference was not statistically significant, probably because of the different reporting methods. The difference in toxic deaths was higher between treatment arms, with 1.9% for combination and 0.9% for single-agent 5-FU (OR 1.69; 95% CI 0.58–4.94).

23.2.3 Combination Regimens

Regimens Not Including Cisplatin

The FAM regimen (5-FU, doxorubicin, and mitomycin) was one of the first reference combinations used, with preliminary studies reporting a response rate of > 40% and a favorable toxicity profile [11, 12]. However, a randomized three-arm trial performed by the NCCTG, comprising 305 patients with advanced gastric and pancreatic cancer compared 5-FU as a single agent, 5-FU plus doxorubicin, and FAM. The response rate was higher in the combination arm than in the 5-FU alone arm, but survival was not statistically different [13].

The EORTC then compared the FAM and FAMTX (high-dose 5-FU, adriamicyn, and methotrexate) regimens. A significantly superior response rate and improved overall survival (OS) were obtained with FAMTX, which thus became the reference regimen [14].

Regimens Including Cisplatin

In turn, FAMTX was compared with other regimens (Table 23.1) [15–18]. In a small US study [15], FAMTX yielded similar results as EAP but was significantly less toxic. In a UK trial [16], ECF (epirubicin, cisplatin, 5-FU) was superior in terms of response rate (45% vs. 21%) and median survival (8.9 vs. 5.7 months). In the EORTC trial [17], there were no statistical differences in response rate and survival between FAMTX, FP (5-FU and cisplatin), and ELF (etoposide, leucovorin, 5-FU). The Italian trial [18] showed that PELF (cisplatin, epirubicin, leucovorin, 5-FU) was statistically superior in terms of response rate but not survival. A further UK study [19] compared ECF with the similar MCF regimen, in which the doses of 5-FU were increased and epirubicin was substituted for mitomycin. Survival and response rate were not statistically different, but quality of life (QoL) was better with ECF. The study concluded that ECF should remain the reference regimen.

As a whole, the meta-analysis [10] comparing the three-drug (FU/cisplatin/anthracycline) with the two-drug (5-FU/cisplatin or 5-FU/anthracy-

Table 23.1 Results of the randomized trials

	(N.)	Response (%)	Median survival[a]	1-year OS (%)	Author (year)
FAM	105	9	29 w	22	Wils (1991) [14]
FAMTX	108	41*	42 w*	41	
EAP	30	20	6.1	7	Kelsen (1992) [15]
FAMTX	30	33	7.3	17	
FAMTX	130	21	6.1	22	Waters (1999) [16]
ECF	126	46*	8.7*	37	
PF	134	20	7.2	27	Vanhoefer (2000) [17]
ELF	132	9	7.2	25	
FAMTX	133	12	6.7	28	
PELF	100	39*	7.7	30.8	Cocconi (2003) [18]
FAMTX	100	22	6.9	22.4	
MCF	285	44	8.7	32.7	Ross (2002) [19]
ECF	289	42	9.4	40.2	
PF	158	25	8.6	32	Van Cutsem (2006) [4]
TCF	159	37	9.2*	40	
FLO	112	35	10.7	45	Al-Batran (2008) [1]
FLP	108	24.5	8.8	40	
IF	172	32	9	37	Dank (2008) [3]
PF	165	26	8.7	31	
ECF	249	40.7	9.9	37.7	Cunningham (2008) REAL 2 [2]
ECX	241	46.6	9.9	40.8	
EOF	235	42	9.3	40.4	
EOX	239	47.9	11.2	46.8	
XP	160	46*	10.4	37	Kang (2009) [25]
PF	156	32	9.3	37	
S-1	160	31	11	46.7	Koizumi (2008) SPIRITS [27]
P-S1	156	54*	13*	54	
PF	508	32	7.9	30	Ajani (2010) FLAGS [28]
P-S1	521	29	8.6	30	
PF/PX	296	34.5	11.1	n.r.	Bang (2010) ToGA [5]
PF/PX-trastuzumab	298	47.3*	13.8*	n.r.	
PF/PX	387	29.5	10.1	n.r.	Kang (2010) AVAGAST [6]
PF/PX-bevacizumab	387	38*	12.1	n.r.	

OS, overall survival; *n.r.*, not reported.
For protocol abbreviations, see text.
*Statistically significant.
[a]Months, unless differently specified.

cline) regimens demonstrated a small but statistically significant benefit in OS in favor of the three-drug combinations (2 months and 1 month, respectively).

23.2.4 Regimens Including New Chemotherapy Agents

New agents, such as taxanes (docetaxel, paclitaxel), oxaliplatin, irinotecan, capecitabine, and S-1, have been recently tested in randomized trials. Many phase II studies have shown that taxanes (paclitaxel and docetaxel) produced a response rate of 22–65%. So far, no randomized phase III trials with paclitaxel have been published. By contrast, three phase II randomized studies evaluating docetaxel-based regimens demonstrated a response rate of around 40% and a median survival of 10 months [20-22].

Based on the findings of the phase II studies, docetaxel in combination with cisplatin and 5-FU (DCF) was tested in the V325 phase III trial against the standard PF [4]. The DCF arm demonstrated statistically superior time to progression (TTP) (6.6 vs. 3.7 months), response rate (37% vs. 25%), and OS (9.2 vs. 8.6 months). Compared with PF, DCF was also associated with a better preservation of QoL and maintenance of clinical benefit [23, 24]. Based on these results, the FDA approved DCF for the treatment of patients with advanced gastric cancer. However, it should be noted that in the DCF arm there was a higher rate of complicated neutropenia (29% vs. 12%), which prompted the authors to suggest prophylactic G-CSF support. Moreover, the median age of 55 years was well below the median age of the patients included in other trials and needs to be considered when applying these findings to the general population.

The same meta-analysis [10] pooled the results of three docetaxel-based protocols and reported that the HR for OS favored the docetaxel-containing regimens, but the difference did not reach statistical significance (HR 0.93, 95% CI 0.75–1.15). Also PFS was, on the whole, not statistically different but the results were flawed by differences in the schedules. The objective response rate was 36% in the docetaxel-containing arms vs. 31% in the control arms, corresponding to an OR of 1.30 (95% CI 0.98–1.72) with a non-significant advantage for the docetaxel-containing regimens.

Al-Batran et al. [1] compared the FLO (5FU, leucovorin, oxaliplatin) and FLP (5FU, leucovorin, cisplatin) regimens, finding only a trend in favor of FLO with respect to PFS (the primary end point) but no difference in OS. However, in the subset of patients older than 65 years, FLO resulted in significantly superior response rates (41.3% vs. 16.7%; $p = 0.012$), time to treatment failure (5.4 vs. 2.3 months; $p = 0.001$), PFS (6.0 vs. 3.1 months; $p = 0.029$), and an improved OS (13.9 vs. 7.2 months) compared with FLP. Overall, FLO was associated with reduced toxicity and in older adult patients perhaps with improved efficacy.

REAL-2 [2], a UK non-inferiority phase III trial, compared ECF, ECX (X: capecitabine), EOF (O: oxaliplatin), and EOX (O: oxaliplatin; X: capecitabine). Median survival in the ECF, ECX, EOF, and EOX groups was 9.9, 9.9, 9.3, and 11.2 months, respectively; survival rates at 1 year were 37.7, 40.8, 40.4, and 46.8%, respectively. Response rate (41–48%) and non-hematological toxicity were not statistically different. In the secondary analysis, OS was superior with EOX than with ECF (HR 0.80, 95% CI, 0.66–0.97; $p = 0.02$). There were significantly lower incidences of grade 3 or 4 neutropenia, thromboembolism, grade 2 alopecia, and elevation of serum creatinine levels in the oxaliplatin groups than in the ECF group. In the ML17032 trial, with participants largely drawn from the Asian population, XP (capecitabine, cisplatin) showed significant non-inferiority in terms of PFS when compared to PF. Overall survival favored the oral regimen (HR 0.85, 95% CI 0.65–1.11), resulting in median survival times of 10.4 and 9.3 months in favor of capecitabine but without reaching statistical significance [25]. These two trials [2, 25] consistently demonstrated the non-inferiority of capecitabine compared to 5-FU and suggested better outcome in patients receiving capecitabine.

A recent meta-analysis of individual patient data from the ML17032 and REAL-2 trials showed better OS in the 654 patients treated with capecitabine combinations than in the 664 patients treated with 5-FU combinations (HR 0.87 95% CI 0.77–0.98, $p = 0.02$) [26].

Recent data also emerged on the use of weekly

irinotecan in combination with 5-FU and leucovorin (IF protocol): IF did not yield a significant TTP or OS superiority over PF, and the results on the non-inferiority of IF were borderline. However, the toxicity profile favored the irinotecan arm over the PF arm in terms of discontinuation for toxicity (10.0% vs. 21.5%), febrile neutropenia (4.8% vs. 10.2%), and stomatitis (2% vs. 16.9%). The authors suggested that IF provides a viable, platinum-free front-line treatment alternative for patients with metastatic gastric cancer [3].

As for irinotecan, the meta-analysis reported that OS, response rate, TTP, and toxicity, while better with the irinotecan-containing regimens, were not statistically improved. The irinotecan-containing combinations resulted in an average median survival time of 9.8 vs. 8.3 months (HR 0.86, 95% CI 0.73–1.02), an ORR of 40 vs. 30% (OR 1.77, 95% CI 0.85–3.69), and a lower rate of treatment discontinuation and deaths due to toxicity. Therefore, irinotecan-containing regimens should be considered a suitable alternative to platinum combinations in consideration of the different toxicity profile (absence of neurotoxicity, no significant renal toxicity, less nausea and vomiting) and the lack of a need for hyperhydration.

The Japanese SPIRITS trial [27] tested S-1 plus cisplatin vs. S-1 alone. Median PFS (6.0 vs. 4.0 months; $p < 0.0001$) and OS (13.0 vs. 11.0 months; $p = 0.04$) were significantly longer in the combination group. Response was also significantly improved in patients with target tumors and assigned to S-1 plus cisplatin (54% vs. 31%). On the basis of these findings, S-1 plus cisplatin has become the standard of care in Japan. Although this was the first randomized trial to break the apparently insuperable wall of 12 months, it was criticized for not providing information about the advantage of S-1 over 5-FU when each drug was combined with cisplatin.

However, in a study of Western patients, the First-Line Advanced Gastric Cancer Study (FLAGS), comparing S-1 with 5-FU, both combined with cisplatin, failed to confirm the data reported in the Japanese study [28]. Median OS was 8.6 months in the cisplatin/S-1 arm and 7.9 months in the cisplatin/5-FU arm ($p = 0.2$). Statistically significant safety advantages for the S-1-based combination were obtained regarding the rates of G3–4 neutropenia (32% vs. 63.6%), stomatitis (1.3% vs. 13.6%), renal function (5.2% vs. 9.3%), and treatment-related deaths (2.5% vs. 4.9%). Thus, the future role of S-1 in gastric cancer is still unclear, but it is probably worth studying in the context of a three-drug regimen in order to improve the tolerability of DCF or ECF.

23.2.5 Regimens Including Targeted Agents

Phase III Studies

In recent years, different classes of targeted agents, such as monoclonal antibodies directed against epidermal growth factor receptors 1 (EGFR) and 2 (HER-2), tyrosine kinase inhibitors (TKIs), and angiogenesis inhibitors have been tested in clinical trials. So far, the TOGA trial [5] is the only published phase III study. It enrolled 594 patients with either immunohistochemically proven overexpression of HER2 or amplification of the HER2 gene as confirmed by fluorescence in-situ hybridization (FISH). HER2 was positive in 21% of gastric cancers and in 33.2% of gastro-esophageal junction cancers. The two treatment arms compared a chemotherapy regimen consisting of capecitabine or fluorouracil plus cisplatin given every 3 weeks for six cycles with or without trastuzumab, a monoclonal antibody directed against HER-2. The primary endpoint was OS. Median survival was 13.8 months (95% CI 12–16) in the trastuzumab arm compared with 11.1 months in the chemotherapy alone arm (HR: 0.74; 95% CI 0.60–0.91; p=0.0046). There was no difference in the rate of grade 3 or 4 adverse events and the percentage of cardiac events was identical in the two arms (<3%). Response rate was 47.3% and 34.5% (p=0.0017) in the trastuzumab and control arms, respectively. An explorative analysis showed that, in the subgroup of patients with high-HER2-expressing tumors, the HR was 0.65 (95% CI 0.51–0.83) and median survival 16.0 months (95% CI 15–19) in those receiving trastuzumab compared with 11.8 months (95% CI 10–13) in those assigned to chemotherapy alone. Thus, trastuzumab in combination with chemotherapy has been proposed as a new standard option for patients with HER2-positive advanced gastric or gastro-esophageal junction cancer.

The anti-VEGF (vascular endothelial growth

factor) monoclonal antibody bevacizumab was tested in the AVAGAST phase III trial [6], in which 774 patients were enrolled. The trial tested the combination of cisplatin and capecitabine (or fluorouracil) with or without bevacizumab, with OS as the primary end point. The difference was not statistically significant and therefore the trial failed to meet the primary endpoint. Median OS was 10.1 and 12.1 months in the control and bevacizumab arms, respectively (HR 0.87; $p = 0.1002$); however, there was a significant improvement in PFS (5.3 vs. 6.7 months) and ORR (29.5% vs. 38.%), with an acceptable safety profile for bevacizumab-treated patients; the only complications were hypertension (6.2% vs. 0.5%) and gastrointestinal tract perforation (2.3% vs. 0.3%).

Lapatinib (TKI of EGFR and HER-2), apatinib (TKI of the VEGF receptor), catumaxomab (anti-CD3 and anti- epithelial cell adhesion molecule monoclonal antibody), and ramucirumab (anti-VEGFR-2 monoclonal antibody) are at present under evaluation in phase III trials in metastatic gastric cancer [29].

Phase II Trials

Bevacizumab has been tested in combination with irinotecan-cisplatin [30] or with docetaxel-oxaliplatin [31], demonstrating a PFS and OS of 7–8 and of 11–12 months, respectively. Response rate was in the range of 65–79%; the most relevant toxicities consisted of neutropenia (34%) and gastrointestinal perforation (6–8%).

Cetuximab (anti-EGFR monoclonal antibody) was tested in different schedules (fluorouracil/capecitabine plus oxaliplatin or irinotecan, docetaxel plus oxaliplatin) [32-35]. The response rate was about 50% (range 41–65%) and the TTP 6 months (range 5–8 months). The principal toxicities were neutropenia (40%) and acne-like rash (20%). A phase III trial of capecitabine and cisplatin, with or without cetuximab, is now recruiting patients [29].

Panitumumab (anti-EGFR monoclonal antibody) is currently being tested in combination with EOX in the REAL-3 phase III trial; the end point is OS [29, 36].

The TKI Sunitinib was evaluated as single agent in ≥ 2nd-line setting but the studies were considered negative [37, 38]. However, another TKI, Sorafenib, in combination with docetaxel and cisplatin as a first-line treatment achieved a response rate of 41%, a PFS of 5.8 months, and an OS of 13.6 months. The toxicity was hematological, with a 64% incidence of severe neutropenia [39].

Everolimus (mTor inhibitor), in the 2nd- and 3rd-line setting [40], produced only disease stabilization in 56% of the patients and no objective responses; on the other hand, there were no unexpected toxicities. PFS and OS were 2.7 and 10.1 months, respectively. Two phase III trials in pretreated patients are ongoing [29].

23.2.6 Conclusions

Despite the positive impact of chemotherapy, the median OS of patients with advanced gastric cancer remains essentially below 12 months according to most of the larger clinical trials. Although small subsets of patients may benefit from survival prolongation, treatment options in advanced gastric cancer should primarily take into account QoL and quality-adjusted survival. It remains an open question whether the survival advantage conferred by three-drug vs. two-drug combinations compensates for the additional toxicity suffered by the patients. The hope for the future is that tailored interventions based on new cytotoxic drugs, targeted therapies, and the integration of molecular determinants will help to improve the current standard treatment.

23.3 The Role of Chemotherapy: Second Line Treatment

Phase II Trials

The role of second-line chemotherapy is even less defined than that of first-line chemotherapy, in terms of efficacy or toxicity profile. However, this information is meaningful because 20–50% of patients with advanced gastric cancer receive second-line chemotherapy [41-43]. A pooled analysis of 1080 patients from phase III studies testing first-line fluorouracil-based regimens suggested that about 20% of patients with disease progression received second-line treatment, with a response rate of 13.3% and median OS of 5.6 months after starting the second-line chemotherapy [44]. The critical points are that no relevant phase III trials have been conducted so far; rather, all of the studies were performed as phase II trials and no direct comparison with BSC is available.

Irinotecan has been tested mostly in combination with cisplatin and fluoropyrimidines (FOLFIRI/CAPIRI or similar schedules). The studies included a median of 33 patients each (range 8–131). Overall, the results were consistent, showing a median response rate of about 21% (0–52%) and a disease control rate ranging from 0 to 77% (median 47%). Median TTP and survival were reported to be approximately 3.3 (range 2.2–5.3) and 7.5 months (5–10.9), respectively. Neutropenia was the most common relevant toxicity (11–45%), followed by anemia (3–57%), diarrhea (3– 19%), and anorexia (12–17%) [45-61].

Docetaxel was mostly used in combination with other drugs (fluorouracil/capecitabine, cisplatin, epirubicin, oxaliplatin), achieving response rates ranging from 9 to 38% (median 17%), disease control rates of 50% (22–80%), a TTP of 3.9 months (2.4–5.2), and survival of 6.6 months (6–8.9). The most frequent G3–4 toxicities consisted of neutropenia in about 27% (12–71%) of the patients, febrile neutropenia in 11.5%, and fatigue-asthenia in 32% [62–76].

Paclitaxel was prevalently used as weekly single agent; only in a few studies was it combined with fluoropyrimidines. The studies included a median of 38 patients (range 4–85). The response rate was reported to be about 21% (0–35%), disease control rate between 25 and 77% (median 63.5%), median TTP 3.6 months (2.6–6.4), and survival 7.8 months (5–13.9). G3–4 toxicities were usually hematological, with neutropenia in about 23% (2–62%) and anemia in 12% (1–41%) of the patients. Peripheral neuropathy was generally reported to be < 10% [63, 77-87].

Oxaliplatin-fluorouracil combinations have also been tested as second- and third-line regimens for advanced gastric cancer, yielding response rates of 4–26%, disease control rates of about 50%, a TTP of 3–4 months, and survival of about 7 months. Severe neutropenia was reported in about 15% of the treated patients [88-90].

Some reports have been published evaluating the single agent S-1 [91-92], S-1 plus mitomycin [93], and fluorouracil plus mitomycin [94]. The disease control rate was about 50% and the TTP 3 months.

23.3.1 Conclusions

Due to a lack of sound randomized comparisons with placebo, it is unclear whether second-line chemotherapy confers a gain in survival over BSC alone. This is an important consideration in order to ensure that treated patients do not suffer from unnecessary toxicities without any benefit. The identification of predictive or prognostic markers is also essential to select patients likely to benefit from second-line treatment. In the clinical setting, the decision to treat patients with disease progression should rely on careful selection based on performance status, history of agents used, degree of response to the first-line therapy, and amount of metastatic disease. The use of other active agents not recognized for first-line therapy and the use of serial single agents rather than a combination of agents seems a reasonable approach in the absence of data showing a benefit of multi-agent therapy vs. monotherapy.

References

1. Al-Batran SE, Hartmann JT, Hofheinz R et al (2008) Phase III trial in metastatic gastroesophageal adenocarcinoma with fluorouracil, leucovorin plus either oxaliplatin or cisplatin: a study of the Arbeitsgemeinschaft Internistische Onkologie. J Clin Oncol 26:1435-1442
2. Cunningham D, Starling N, Rao S, Iveson et al; Upper Gastrointestinal Clinical Studies Group of the National Cancer Research Institute of the United Kingdom (2008) Capecitabine and oxaliplatin for advanced esophagogastric cancer. N Engl J Med 358:36-46
3. Dank M, Zaluski J, Barone C et al (2008) Randomized phase III study comparing irinotecan combined with 5-fluorouracil and folinic acid to cisplatin combined with 5-fluorouracil in chemotherapy naive patients with advanced adenocarcinoma of the stomach or esophagogastric junction. Ann Oncol 19:1450-1457
4. Van Cutsem E, Moiseyenko VM, Tjulandin S et al; V325 Study Group (2006) Phase III study of docetaxel and cisplatin plus fluorouracil compared with cisplatin and fluorouracil as first-line therapy for advanced gastric cancer: a report of the V325 Study Group. J Clin Oncol 24:4991-4997
5. Bang YJ, Van Cutsem E, Feyereislova A et al; ToGA Trial Investigators (2010) Trastuzumab in combination with chemotherapy versus chemotherapy alone for treatment of HER2-positive advanced gastric or gastro-oesophageal junc-

tion cancer (ToGA): a phase 3, open-label, randomised controlled trial. Lancet 376:687-697
6. Kang Y, Ohtsu A, Van Cutsem E et al (2010) AVAGAST: A randomized, double-blind, placebo-controlled, phase III study of first-line capecitabine and cisplatin plus bevacizumab or placebo in patients with advanced gastric cancer (AGC). J Clin Oncol 28, 18 suppl:LBA4007
7. Murad AM, Santiago FF, Petroianu A et al (1993) Modified therapy with 5-fluorouracil, doxorubicin, and methotrexate in advanced gastric cancer. Cancer 72:37-41
8. Glimelius B, Hoffman K, Haglund U et al (1994) Initial or delayed chemotherapy with best supportive care in advanced gastric cancer. Ann Oncol 5:189-190
9. Pyrhonen S, Kuitumen T, Nyandoto P et al (1995) Randomized comparison of fluorouracil, epidoxorubicin and methotrexate (FEMTX) plus best supportive care alone in patients with non-resectable gastric cancer. Br J Cancer 71:587-591
10. Wagner AD, Unverzagt S, Grothe W et al (2010) Chemotherapy for advanced gastric cancer. Cochrane Database Syst Rev 17 CD004064
11. MacDonald JS, Schein PS, Woolley PV et al (1980) 5-Fluorouracil, doxorubicin, and mitomycin (FAM) combination chemotherapy for advanced gastric cancer. Ann Intern Med 93:533-536
12. Douglass HO, Lavin PT, Goudsmit A et al (1984) An Eastern Cooperative Oncology Group evaluation of combinations of methyl-CCNU, mitomycin C, adriamycin, and 5-fluorouracil in advanced measurable gastric cancer (EST 2277). J Clin Oncol 2:1372-1381
13. Cullinan SA, Moertel CG, Fleming TR et al (1985) A comparison of three chemotherapeutic regimens in the treatment of advanced pancreatic and gastric carcinoma. Fluorouracil vs fluorouracil and doxorubicin vs fluorouracil, doxorubicin, and mitomycin. JAMA 253:2061-2067
14. Wils JA, Klein HO, Wagener DJ et al (1991) Sequential high-dose methotrexate and fluorouracil combined with doxorubicin—a step ahead in the treatment of advanced gastric cancer: a trial of the European Organization for Research and Treatment of Cancer Gastrointestinal Tract Cooperative Group. J Clin Oncol 9: 827-831
15. Kelsen D, Atiq OT, Saltz L et al (1992) FAMTX versus etoposide, doxorubicin, and cisplatin: a random assignment trial in gastric cancer. J Clin Oncol 10:541-548
16. Waters JS, Norman A, Cunningham D et al (1999) Long-term survival after epirubicin, cisplatin and fluorouracil for gastric cancer: results of a randomized trial. Br J Cancer 80:269-272
17. Vanhoefer U, Rougier P, Wilke H et al (2000) Final results of a randomized phase III trial of sequential high-dose methotrexate, fluorouracil, and doxorubicin versus etoposide, leucovorin, and fluorouracil versus infusional fluorouracil and cisplatin in advanced gastric cancer: A trial of the European Organization for Research and Treatment of Cancer Gastrointestinal Tract Cancer Cooperative Group. J Clin Oncol 18:2648-2657
18. Cocconi G, Carlini P, Gamboni A et al; Italian Oncology Group for Clinical Research (2003) On behalf of the Italian Oncology Group for Clinical Research Cisplatin, epirubicin, leucovorin and 5-fluorouracil (PELF) is more active than 5-fluorouracil, doxorubicin and methotrexate (FAMTX) in advanced gastric carcinoma. Ann Oncol 14:1258-1263
19. Ross P, Nicolson M, Cunningham D et al (2002) Prospective randomized trial comparing mitomycin, cisplatin, and protracted venous-infusion fluorouracil (PVI 5-FU) With epirubicin, cisplatin, and PVI 5-FU in advanced esophagogastric cancer. J Clin Oncol 20:1996-2004
20. Roth AD, Fazio N, Stupp R et al; Swiss Group for Clinical Cancer Research (2007) Docetaxel, cisplatin, and fluorouracil; docetaxel and cisplatin; and epirubicin, cisplatin, and fluorouracil as systemic treatment for advanced gastric carcinoma:a randomized phase II trial of the Swiss Group for Clinical Cancer Research. J Clin Oncol 25:3217-3223
21. Ajani JA, Fodor MB, Tjulandin SA et al (2005) Phase II multi-institutional randomized trial of docetaxel plus cisplatin with or without fluorouracil in patients with untreated, advanced gastric, or gastroesophageal adenocarcinoma. J Clin Oncol 23:5660-5667
22. Thuss-Patience PC, Kretzschmar A, Repp M et al (2005) Docetaxel and continuous-infusion fluorouracil versus epirubicin, cisplatin, and fluorouracil for advanced gastric adenocarcinoma: a randomized phase II study. J Clin Oncol 23:494-501
23. Ajani JA, Moiseyenko VM, Tjulandin S et al (2007) Quality of life with docetaxel plus cisplatin and fluorouracil compared with cisplatin and fluorouracil from a phase III trial for advanced gastric or gastroesophageal adenocarcinoma: the V-325 Study Group. J Clin Oncol 25:3210-3216
24. Ajani JA, Moiseyenko VM et al (2007) Clinical benefit with docetaxel plus fluorouracil and cisplatin compared with cisplatin and fluorouracil in a phase III trial of advanced gastric or gastroesophageal cancer adenocarcinoma: the V-325 Study Group. J Clin Oncol 25:3205-3209
25. Kang YK, Kang WK, Shin DB et al (2009) Capecitabine/cisplatin versus 5-fluorouracil/cisplatin as first-line therapy in patients with advanced gastric cancer: a randomised phase III non inferiority trial. Ann Oncol 20:666-673
26. Okines AF, Norman AR, McCloud P et al (2009) Meta-analysis of the REAL-2 and ML17032 trials: evaluating capecitabine-based combination chemotherapy and infused 5-fluorouracil-based combination chemotherapy for the treatment of advanced oesophago-gastric cancer. Ann Oncol 20:1529-1534
27. Koizumi W, Narahara H, Hara T et al (2008) S-1 plus cisplatin versus S-1 alone for first-line treatment of advanced gastric cancer (SPIRITS trial): a phase III trial. Lancet Oncol 9:215-221
28. Ajani JA, Rodriguez W, Bodoky G et al (2010) Multicenter phase III comparison of cisplatin/S-1 with cisplatin/infusional fluorouracil in advanced gastric or gastroesophageal adenocarcinoma study: the FLAGS trial. J Clin Oncol 8:1547-1553
29. http://www.cancer.gov/search/ResultsClinicalTrials.aspx?protocolsearchid=8608536. Accessed 27 November 2010
30. Shah MA, Ramanathan RK, Ilson DH et al (2006) Multicenter Phase II Study of Irinotecan, Cisplatin, and Bevacizumab in Patients With Metastatic Gastric or Gastroesophageal Junction Adenocarcinoma. J Clin Oncol 24:5001-5006
31. El-Rayes BF, Zalupski M, Bekai-Saab T et al (2010) A phase II study of bevacizumab, oxaliplatin, and docetaxel in locally advanced and metastatic gastric and gastroesophageal junction cancers. Ann Oncol 21:1999-2004
32. Kim C, Lee JL, Ryu MH et al (2009) A prospective phase

II study of cetuximab in combination with XELOX (capecitabine and oxaliplatin) in patients with metastatic and/or recurrent advanced gastric cancer. Invest New Drugs Dec 9 [Epub ahead of print]
33. Lordick F, Luber B, Lorenzen S et al (2010) Cetuximab plus oxaliplatin/leucovorin/5-fluorouracil in first-line metastatic gastric cancer: a phase II study of the Arbeitsgemeinschaft Internistische Onkologie (AIO). Br J Cancer 102:500-505
34. Pinto C, Di Fabio F, Siena S et al (2007) Phase II study of cetuximab in combination with FOLFIRI in patients with untreated advanced gastric or gastroesophageal junction adenocarcinoma (FOLCETUX study). Ann Oncol 18:510-517
35. Pinto C, Di Fabio F, Barone C et al (2009) Phase II study of cetuximab in combination with cisplatin and docetaxel in patients with untreated advanced gastric or gastro-oesophageal junction adenocarcinoma (DOCETUX study). Br J Cancer 101:1261-1268
36. Okines A, Ashley SE, Cunningham D et al (2010) Epirubicin, Oxaliplatin, and Capecitabine With or Without Panitumumab for Advanced Esophagogastric Cancer:Dose-Finding Study for the Prospective Multicenter, Randomized, Phase II/III REAL-3 Trial. J Clin Oncol 28:3945-3950
37. Bang YJ, Kang YK, Kang WK et al (2010) A Phase II study of sunitinib as second-line treatment for advanced gastric cancer. Invest New Drugs May 12 [Epub ahead of print]
38. Moehler MH, Hartmann JT, Lordick F et al (2010) An open-label, multicenter phase II trial of sunitinib for patients with chemorefractory metastatic gastric cancer. J Clin Oncol 28, 15 suppl:e14503
39. Sun W, Powell M, O'Dwyer PJ et al (2010) Phase II study of sorafenib in combination with docetaxel and cisplatin in the treatment of metastatic or advanced gastric and gastroesophageal junction adenocarcinoma: ECOG 5203. J Clin Oncol 28:2947-2951
40. Doi T, Muro K, Boku N et al (2010) A Multicenter phase II study of everolimus in patients with previously treated metastatic gastric cancer. J Clin Oncol 28:1904-1910
41. Wesolowski R, Lee C, Kim R (2009) Is there a role for second-line chemotherapy in advanced gastric cancer? Lancet Oncol 10:903-912
42. Catalano V, Graziano F, Santini D et al (2008) Second-line chemotherapy for patients with advanced gastric cancer: who may benefit? Br J Cancer 99:1402-1407
43. Ji SH, Lim do H, Yi SY et al (2009) A retrospective analysis of second-line chemotherapy in patients with advanced gastric cancer. BMC Cancer 9:110:1-6
44. Chau I, Norman AR, Ross PJ (2004) Multivariate prognostic factor analysis and second-line treatment in locally advanced and metastatic oesophago-gastric cancer, pooled analysis of 1080 patients from three multicentre randomised controlled trials using individual patient data. ASCO GI 2004; Abs 5
45. Assersohn L, Brown G, Cunningham D et al (2004) Phase II study of irinotecan and 5-fluorouracil/leucovorin in patients with primary refractory or relapsed advanced oesophageal and gastric carcinoma. Ann Oncol 15:64-69
46. Baek JH, Kim JG, Sohn SK et al (2005) Biweekly irinotecan and cisplatin as second-line chemotherapy in pretreated patients with advanced gastric cancer: a multicenter phase II study. J Korean Med Sci 20:966-970
47. Chun JH, Kim HK, Lee JS et al (2004) Weekly irinotecan in patients with metastatic gastric cancer failing cisplatin-based chemotherapy. Jpn J Clin Oncol 34:8-13
48. Giuliani F, Molica S, Maiello E et al (2005) Irinotecan (CPT-11) and mitomycin-C (MMC) as second-line therapy in advanced gastric cancer: a phase II study of the Gruppo Oncologico dell' Italia Meridionale (prot. 2106). Am J Clin Oncol 28:581-585
49. Kanat O, Evrensel T, Manavoglu O et al (2003) Single-agent irinotecan as second-line treatment for advanced gastric cancer. Tumori 89:405-407
50. Kim SG, Oh SY, Kwon HC et al (2007) A phase II study of irinotecan with bi-weekly, low-dose leucovorin and bolus and continuous infusion 5-fluorouracil (modified FOLFIRI) as salvage therapy for patients with advanced or metastatic gastric cancer. Jpn J Clin Oncol 37:744-749
51. Kim SH, Lee GW, Il Go S et al (2010) A Phase II Study of Irinotecan, Continuous 5-fluorouracil, and leucovorin (folfiri) combination chemotherapy for patients with recurrent or metastatic gastric cancer previously treated with a fluoropyrimidine-based regimen. Am J Clin Oncol Jan 29 [Epub ahead of print]
52. Kim ST, Kang WK, Kang JH et al (2005) Salvage chemotherapy with irinotecan, 5-fluorouracil and leucovorin for taxane- and cisplatin-refractory, metastatic gastric cancer. Br J Cancer 92:1850-1854
53. Leary A, Assersohn L, Cunningham D et al (2009) A phase II trial evaluating capecitabine and irinotecan as second line treatment in patients with oesophago-gastric cancer who have progressed on, or within 3 months of platinum-based chemotherapy. Cancer Chemother Pharmacol 64:455-462
54. Lorizzo K, Fazio N, Radice D et al (2009) Simplified FOLFIRI in pre-treated patients with metastatic gastric cancer. Cancer Chemother Pharmacol 64:301-306
55. Seo MD, Lee KW, Lim JH et al (2008) Irinotecan combined with 5-fluorouracil and leucovorin as second-line chemotherapy for metastatic or relapsed gastric cancer. Jpn J Clin Oncol 38:589-595
56. Shimada S, Yagi Y, Kuramoto M et al (2003) Second-line chemotherapy with combined irinotecan and low-dose cisplatin for patients with metastatic gastric carcinoma resistant to 5-fluorouracil. Oncol Rep 10:687-691
57. Sun Q, Hang M, Xu W et al (2009) Irinotecan plus capecitabine as a second-line treatment after failure of 5-fluorouracil and platinum in patients with advanced gastric cancer. Jpn J Clin Oncol 39:791-796
58. Suzuki S, Harada N, Takeo Y et al (2007) Bi-weekly irinotecan hydrochloride and cisplatin as a second-line chemotherapy for patients with advanced gastric cancer. Gan To Kagaku Ryoho 34:2245-2248
59. Takahari D, Shimada Y, Takeshita S et al (2010) Second-line chemotherapy with irinotecan plus cisplatin after the failure of S-1 monotherapy for advanced gastric cancer. Gastric Cancer 13:186-190
60. Ueda S, Hironaka S, Boku N et al (2006) Combination chemotherapy with irinotecan and cisplatin in pretreated patients with unresectable or recurrent gastric cancer. Gastric Cancer 9:203-207
61. Yoshida T, Yoshikawa T, Tsuburaya A et al (2006) Feasibility study of biweekly CPT-11 plus CDDP for S-1- and paclitaxel-refractory, metastatic gastric cancer. Anticancer Res 26:1595-1598

62. Barone C, Basso M, Schinzari Get al (2007) Docetaxel and oxaliplatin combination in second-line treatment of patients with advanced gastric cancer. Gastric Cancer 10:104-111
63. Chon HJ, Rha SY, Im CK et al (2009) Docetaxel versus paclitaxel combined with 5-FU and leucovorin in advanced gastric cancer: combined analysis of two phase II trials. Cancer Res Treat 41:196-204
64. Giuliani F, Gebbia V, De Vita F et al (2003) Docetaxel as salvage therapy in advanced gastric cancer: a phase II study of the Gruppo Oncologico Italia Meridionale (G.O.I.M.). Anticancer Res 23:4219-4222
65. Jo JC, Lee JL, Ryu MH et al (2007) Docetaxel monotherapy as a second-line treatment after failure of fluoropyrimidine and platinum in advanced gastric cancer: experience of 154 patients with prognostic factor analysis. Jpn J Clin Oncol 37:936-941
66. Kunisaki C, Imada T, Yamada R et al (2005) Phase II study of docetaxel plus cisplatin as a second-line combined therapy in patients with advanced gastric carcinoma. Anticancer Res 25:2973-2977
67. Lee JL, Ryu MH, Chang HM et al. A phase II study of docetaxel as salvage chemotherapy in advanced gastric cancer after failure of fluoropyrimidine and platinum combination chemotherapy. Cancer Chemother Pharmacol 2008; 61(4): 631-637
68. Nakajima Y, Suzuki T, Haruki S et al (2008) A pilot trial of docetaxel and nedaplatin in cisplatin-pretreated relapsed or refractory esophageal squamous cell cancer. Hepatogastroenterology 55:1631-1635
69. Nguyen S, Rebischung C, Van Ongeval J et al (2006) Epirubicin-docetaxel in advanced gastric cancer: two phase II studies as second and first line treatment. Bull Cancer 93:E1-E6
70. Park SH, Kang WK, Lee HR et al (2004) Docetaxel plus cisplatin as second-line therapy in metastatic or recurrent advanced gastric cancer progressing on 5-fluorouracil-based regimen. Am J Clin Oncol 27:477-480
71. Polyzos A, Tsavaris N, Kosmas C et al (2006) Subsets of patients with advanced gastric cancer responding to second-line chemotherapy with docetaxel-cisplatin. Anticancer Res 26:3749-3753
72. Rosati G, Bilancia D, Germano D et al (2007) Reduced dose intensity of docetaxel plus capecitabine as second-line palliative chemotherapy in patients with metastatic gastric cancer: a phase II study. Ann Oncol 18 Suppl 6:128-132
73. Shin SJ, Kim MK, Lee KH et al (2004) The Efficacy of Docetaxel and Cisplatin Combination Chemotherapy for the Treatment of A dvanced Gastric Cancer after Failing to 5-Fluorouracil Based Chemotherapy. Cancer Res Treat 36: 367-371
74. Sym SJ, Chang HM, Kang HJ et al (2008) A phase II study of irinotecan and docetaxel combination chemotherapy for patients with previously treated metastatic or recurrent advanced gastric cancer. Cancer Chemother Pharmacol 63:1-8
75. Yildiz R, Kalender ME, Dane F et al (2010) Docetaxel combined with oral etoposide as second-line treatment for advanced gastric carcinoma after failure of platinum- and fluoropyrimidine-based regimens. J Oncol Pharm Pract 16:173-178
76. Zhong H, Zhang Y, Ma S et al (2008) Docetaxel plus oxaliplatin (DOCOX) as a second-line treatment after failure of fluoropyrimidine and platinum in Chinese patients with advanced gastric cancer. Anticancer Drugs 19:1013-1018
77. Arai W, Hosoya Y, Hyodo M et al (2007) Doxifluridine combined with weekly paclitaxel for second-line treatment in patients with gastric cancer resistant to TS-1. Int J Clin Oncol 12:146-149
78. Baize N, Abakar-Mahamat A, Mounier N et al (2009) Phase II study of paclitaxel combined with capecitabine as second-line treatment for advanced gastric carcinoma after failure of cisplatin-based regimens. Cancer Chemother Pharmacol 64:549-555
79. Hironaka S, Zenda S, Boku N et al (2006) Weekly paclitaxel as second-line chemotherapy for advanced or recurrent gastric cancer. Gastric Cancer 9:14-18
80. Im CK, Rha SY, Jeung HC et al (2009) A phase II feasibility study of weekly paclitaxel in heavily pretreated advanced gastric cancer patients with poor performance status. Oncology 77:349-357
81. Kodera Y, Ito S, Mochizuki Y et al (2007) A phase II study of weekly paclitaxel as second-line chemotherapy for advanced gastric Cancer (CCOG0302 study). Anticancer Res 27:2667-2671
82. Koizumi W, Akiya T, Sato A et al (2009) Second-line chemotherapy with biweekly paclitaxel after failure of fluoropyrimidine-based treatment in patients with advanced or recurrent gastric cancer: a report from the gastrointestinal oncology group of the Tokyo cooperative oncology group, TCOG GC-0501 trial. Jpn J Clin Oncol 39:713-719
83 Matsuda G, Kunisaki C, Makino H et al (2009) Phase II study of weekly paclitaxel as a second-line treatment for S-1-refractory advanced gastric cancer. Anticancer Res 29:2863-2867
84. Rino Y, Yukawa N, Murakami H et al (2010) Phase II study of S-1 monotherapy as a first-line combination therapy of s-1 plus cisplatin as a second-line therapy, and weekly paclitaxel monotherapy as a third-line therapy in patients with advanced gastric carcinoma: a second report. Clin Med Insights Oncol 4:1-10
85. Shimoyama R, Yasui H, Boku N et al (2009) Weekly paclitaxel for heavily treated advanced or recurrent gastric cancer refractory to fluorouracil, irinotecan, and cisplatin. Gastric Cancer 12:206-211
86. Takiuchi H, Goto M, Imamura H et al (2008) Multi-center phase II study for combination therapy with paclitaxel/doxifluridine to treat advanced/recurrent gastric cancer showing resistance to S-1 (OGSG 0302) Jpn J Clin Oncol 38:176-181
87. Yamaguchi K, Nakagawa S, Yabusaki H et al (2007) Combination chemotherapy with 5-fluorouracil, cisplatin and paclitaxel for pretreated patients with advanced gastric cancer. Anticancer Res 27:3535-3539
88. Kim DY, Kim JH, Lee SH et al (2003) Phase II study of oxaliplatin, 5-fluorouracil and leucovorin in previously platinum-treated patients with advanced gastric cancer. Ann Oncol 14:383-387
89. Seo HY, Kim DS, Choi YS et al (2008) Treatment outcomes of oxaliplatin, 5-FU, and leucovorin as salvage therapy for patients with advanced or metastatic gastric cancer: a retrospective analysis. Cancer Chemother Pharmacol 63:433-439
90. Jeong J, Jeung HC, Rha SY et al (2008) Phase II study of combination chemotherapy of 5-fluorouracil, low-dose leucovorin, and oxaliplatin (FLOX regimen) in pretreated advanced gastric cancer. Ann Oncol 19:1135-1140

91. Jeung HC, Rha SY, Shin SJ et al (2007) A phase II study of S-1 monotherapy administered for 2 weeks of a 3-week cycle in advanced gastric cancer patients with poor performance status. Br J Cancer 97:458-463
92. Ono A, Boku N, Onozawa Y et al (2009) Activity of S-1 in advanced or recurrent gastric cancer patients after failure of prior chemotherapy, including irinotecan + cisplatin or fluorouracil (except S-1) Jpn J Clin Oncol 39:332-335
93. Park SH, Kim YS, Hong J et al (2008) Mitomycin C plus S-1 as second-line therapy in patients with advanced gastric cancer: a noncomparative phase II study. Anticancer Drugs 19:303-307
94. Hartmann JT, Pintoffl JP, Al-Batran SE et al (2007) Mitomycin C plus infusional 5-fluorouracil in platinum-refractory gastric adenocarcinoma: an extended multicenter phase II study. Onkologie 30:235-240

Adjuvant Treatment After Surgical Resection

24

Mario Scartozzi, Walter Siquini, Elena Maccaroni, Maristella Bianconi, Riccardo Giampieri, Rossana Berardi, and Stefano Cascinu

Abstract

In patients with gastric cancer, radical gastrectomy with D2 lymphoadenectomy, when feasible, remains the cornerstone of any curative procedure.

The prognosis of patients with locally advanced gastric cancer is poor, even after potentially curative resection, with locoregional and/or distant recurrence reported in almost 60% of patients who undergo R0 resection.

It is therefore clear that surgery alone is unable to eradicate all locoregional disease. Instead, there is a need for well-evaluated complementary strategies to prevent disease relapse and thus improve the survival of gastric cancer patients, either pre-, peri- or post-operatively.

Keywords

Resectable gastric cancer • Peri-operative chemotherapy • Adjuvant chemotherapy • Chemo-radiotherapy • Neoadjuvant therapy

24.1 Introduction

Despite its declining incidence in Western countries, gastric cancer is a common and highly fatal disease, with current 5-year survival rates of < 20%. In fact, in Europe in 2006, there were 159,900 new cases and 118,200 deaths, representing the fifth highest incidence and fourth highest cause of cancer-related death. Although the incidence of gastric cancer is decreasing, there has been a relative increase in the incidence of tumors of the esophagogastric junction (EGJ) and gastric cardia [1].

Surgical resection remains the cornerstone of any curative procedure and radical gastrectomy with D2 lymphadenectomy is now recognized as a reasonably safe procedure in experienced centers. However, the prognosis for patients with locally advanced gastric cancer remains poor, even after potentially curative resection, with a high risk of locoregional and/or distant recurrence, affecting almost 60% of the patients who undergo R0 resection [2]. This underlines the fact that surgery alone is unable to eradicate all locoregional disease and supports the need for the evaluations of complementary strategies to prevent relapse and to improve survival for gastric cancer patients, either pre-, peri-, or post-operatively.

M. Scartozzi (✉)
Dept. of Medical Oncology,
"Ospedali Riuniti" University Hospital,
Polytechnic University of Marche,
Ancona, Italy

G. de Manzoni, F. Roviello, W. Siquini (eds.), *Surgery in the Multimodal Management of Gastric Cancer*,

Data regarding the role of additional treatments has recently become available, offering new perspectives for improved outcome in patients with gastric cancer [3, 4]. These treatments, the indications for their use, and the results obtained thus far are the subject of this chapter.

24.2 Indications for Adjuvant Treatment

In gastric cancer patients who have undergone complete surgical resection of their tumors, adjuvant treatment is still a matter of debate. Chemotherapy alone or in combination with radiotherapy, post-operative or peri-operative treatment, and which chemotherapeutic regimen are some of the issues that still must be solved. A wider consensus has been reached in international and national guidelines regarding which patients should be treated after surgery. There is no indication to treat patients with resected Tis, T1, and T2, N0 tumors. These patients have a 5-year survival of 70–80% after surgery alone. In such cases, adjuvant treatment can be considered only in the presence of high-risk features, such as: poorly differentiated or higher-grade cancers, lymphovascular invasion, or neural invasion. By contrast, expert panels recommend that patients with T3–T4 tumors or any positive lymph node category receive adjuvant treatment. Nonetheless, there is little agreement as to the best therapeutic strategy. In the USA, guidelines recommend a combined treatment of concurrent radiochemotherapy for patients with no or microscopic residual disease at the surgical margins. European authors, however, have critically viewed studies favoring combined treatment and most have concluded that this approach is not feasible for all patients [5, 6].

24.3 Adjuvant Systemic Chemotherapy

The role of adjuvant therapy in gastric cancer has been extensively studied during the past three decades in attempts to improve the prognosis of patients with gastric cancer who have undergone curative surgery. However, the results have been for the most part disappointing. Indeed, to date, no definitive conclusions have been drawn from randomized clinical trials of adjuvant chemotherapy. Few studies have shown a significant positive impact on survival compared with surgery alone. However, these studies usually randomized a low number of patients and are clearly underpowered. More favorable results were reported in Asian studies, but differences in tumor location, prevalence of early stages, extent of pre-operative staging evaluation, and a more extensive lymphadenectomy may also account for those results. Differences in drug metabolism between Asian and Western patients should also be considered as a confounding factor.

24.3.1 Adjuvant Chemotherapy with Cisplatin-based Regimens

Several studies have evaluated the role of cisplatin-based combination therapy in the adjuvant treatment of gastric cancer. In 2002, the Italian Trials in Medical Oncology (ITMO) group reported the 5-year results of an adjuvant randomized study comparing surgery alone (gastric resection) plus the adjuvant EAP (etoposide, adryamicin, platinum) chemotherapy regimen followed by 5-FU and leucovorin (according to the Machover schedule). The study population consisted of 274 patients with poor prognostic factors, the majority (90%) of whom had N+ disease. All patients underwent a subtotal or total gastrectomy with D2 dissection. After a median follow-up of 66 (range 2–83) months, the results of the study were rather disappointing: adjuvant treatment produced only a not statistically significant benefit in 5-year overall survival (OS) (52% in the treatment group vs. 48% in the control group, $p = 0.869$) and in disease-free survival (DFS) (49% in the treatment group vs. 44% in the control group, $p = 0.421$). Although this study failed to reach statistical significance, in the presence of widespread nodal involvement (N+ >6) the OS of the patients receiving chemotherapy was significantly better than that of the control patients (42 vs. 20%). However, the ITMO trial was designed to detect a 15% difference in 5-year survival (from 30% in the control arm to 45% in the treatment arm) but 5-year OS in both groups was significantly better than expected on the basis of previously published data. In fact, the data from this trial seem to suggest that D2 surgery has a favorable impact on OS [7].

A few years later, the 7-year results of the FFCD (Federation Francophone de la Cancerologie Digestive) randomized trial were published. In this study, 260 gastric cancer patients, after curative resection, were randomly assigned to post-operative chemotherapy with 5-fluorouracil and cisplatin or surgery alone. The study closed prematurely due to poor accrual. Also, at 97.8 months of median follow-up, it failed to demonstrate a benefit in terms of survival in the adjuvant treatment arm: in fact, 5- and 7-year OS rates were 41.9 and 34.9% in the control group vs. 46.6 and 44.6% in the chemotherapy group ($p = 0.22$). However, a risk reduction in recurrence was observed (HR = 0.70; 95% CI 0.51–0.97; $p = 0.032$) [8].

In 2007, the GISCAD (Gruppo Italiano per lo Studio dei Carcinomi dell'Apparato Digerente) study investigated the efficacy of weekly PELF (cisplatin, epirubicin, leucovorin, and 5-FU) as adjuvant treatment for 400 high-risk gastric cancer patients who underwent radical resection. In this study, 201 patients were randomly assigned to receive the PELFw regimen, with the support of filgrastim, while 196 patients were assigned to a regimen consisting of six monthly administrations of a 5-day course of 5-FU (according to the Machover schedule). Final analysis, performed after the planned extent of follow-up (median follow-up 54 months), showed that DFS and OS were virtually identical in the two study arms and that the use of adjuvant PELFw did not reduce the risk of death (HR = 0.95, 95% CI = 0.70–1.29) or relapse (HR = 0.98, 95% CI = 0.75–1.29). It is important to note the unexpectedly high survival rate in both treatment arms, possibly due to the high quality of the gastric surgery performed; thus, the statistical power of the study to detect differences in outcomes was limited [9].

Similar results were obtained in the GOIRC (Gruppo Oncologico Italiano di Ricerca Clinica) study, in which 258 patients with gastric adenocarcinoma were randomized to receive surgery alone or surgery followed by four cycles of PELF. Also in this study, adjuvant chemotherapy based on a PELF regimen did not improve DFS (HR of recurrence= 0.92, 95% CI= 0.66–1.27) or OS (HR of death= 0.90, 95% CI= 0.64–1.26) [10].

24.3.2 Adjuvant Chemotherapy without Cisplatin-containing Regimens

In 2006, a planned combined analysis of two trials was performed consisting of 397 untreated patients, 206 from 23 European Organization for Research and Treatment of Cancer (EORTC) institutions and 191 from 16 International Collaborative Cancer Group (ICCG) institutions. The patients were randomly assigned to surgery alone or surgery followed by fluorouracil, doxorubicin, methotrexate (FAMTX) or fluorouracil, epirubicin, methotrexate (FEMTX). The results showed no significant differences between the treatment and control arms with respect to either DFS (HR 0.98, $p = 0.87$) or OS (HR 0.98, $p = 0.86$). Moreover, the 5-year OS was 43% in the treatment arm and 44% in the control arm and the 5-year DFS was 41 and 42%, respectively [11].

In 2007, the Gruppo Oncologico Italia Meridionale (GOIM) group conducted a randomized, multicenter, phase III trial study aimed at evaluating the efficacy and safety of epirubicin, leucovorin, 5-fluorouracil, and etoposide (ELFE regimen) as adjuvant therapy for gastric cancer patients treated by radical resection. The trial enrolled 228 stage IB–IIIB gastric cancer patients. All patients received a total or subtotal gastrectomy, with at least a D1 lymphadenectomy, and were randomized to receive surgery alone or surgery followed by chemotherapy. With a median follow-up of 60 months, the 5-year OS was 48% in the treatment arm and 43.5% in the control arm (HR 0.91; 95% CI 0.69–0.21; $p = 0.610$); the 5-year DFS was 44% in the treatment arm and 39% in the control arm (HR 0.88; 95% CI 0.66–0.17; $p = 0.305$). In node-positive patients, the 5-year OS was 41% in the treatment arm and 34% in the control arm (HR 0.84; 95% CI 0.69–0.01; $p = 0.068$), while the 5-year DFS was 39% in the treatment arm and 31% in the control arm (HR 0.88; 95% CI 0.78–0.91; $p = 0.051$). The authors concluded that these data do not support the use of adjuvant treatment with the ELFE regimen in patients with radically resected gastric cancers [12].

Recently, the ACTS-GC group phase III trial randomized 1059 patients with stage II or III gastric cancer, who had undergone gastrectomy with D2 lymph node dissection, to S-1 monotherapy vs.

surgery alone. At 3 years, the OS for all randomly assigned patients was 80.1% in the S-1 group and 70.1% in the surgery-only group ($p = 0.0024$) [13]. Due to these impressive results, this regimen was proposed as the standard treatment for stage II/III gastric cancer patients after curative D2 dissection in Japan. However, these data for the use of S-1 should be interpreted with caution, particularly with respect to the implications for clinical practice in a non-Japanese population, which can harbor different polymorphisms in genes crucial for the metabolism of several chemotherapeutic agents. These considerations have been confirmed also in the metastatic setting.

24.3.3 Meta-analysis

Since 1993, several meta-analyses regarding adjuvant chemotherapy in gastric cancer have been published, showing only a small benefit of adjuvant chemotherapy on OS and a 12–18% reduction in the risk of death (Table 24.1). However, those studies analyzed older chemotherapy regimens, such as FAM or FAM-like, designed before the introduction of cisplatin into the treatment of metastatic disease [14-17].

Recently, a new meta-analysis was conducted by the GASTRIC (Global Advanced/Adjuvant Stomach Tumour Research International) group, in order to quantify the potential benefit of chemotherapy after complete resection over surgery alone in terms of OS and DFS, and to further study the role of monochemotherapy, combined chemotherapy, and other regimens. Trials were eligible if they were randomized, ended patient recruitment before 2004, and compared any adjuvant therapy after curative resection with surgery alone. Trials testing radiotherapy; neoadjuvant, peri-operative, or intra-peritoneal chemotherapy; or immunotherapy were excluded. Although 31 eligible trials (6390 patients) were identified, at the time of analysis (2010) individual patient data were available from only 17 (3838 patients, representing 60%of the targeted data), with a median follow-up exceeding 7 years.

There were 1000 deaths among 1924 patients assigned to chemotherapy groups and 1067 deaths among 1857 patients assigned to surgery-only groups. Adjuvant chemotherapy was associated with a statistically significant benefit in terms of OS (HR 0.82; 95% CI, 0.76–0.90; $p = 0.001$) and DFS (HR 0.82; 95% CI, 0.75–0.90; $p = 0.001$). There was no significant heterogeneity for OS across randomized clinical trials ($p = 0.52$) or the four regimen groups (p=0.13). An increase in the 5-year OS from 49.6 to 55.3% with chemotherapy was determined. The authors concluded that, among the studies examined, post-operative adjuvant chemotherapy based on fluorouracil combinations was associated with a reduced risk of death from gastric cancer compared with surgery alone and is recommended for patients who have not received peri-operative treatments after complete resection of their gastric cancer [18].

24.3.4 Peri-operative Approach

Adjuvant chemotherapy in gastric cancer has so far been shown to confer only a slight advantage regarding survival or relapse control. Moreover, a post-operative approach seems less tolerable for gastric patients who have undergone resection. In

Table 24.1 Results of meta-analyses regarding adjuvant treatment in gastric cancer patients

Author (year)	Studies (N.)	Patients (N.)	Hazard ratio for overall survival (95% CI)	Mortality reduction (%)
Hermans (1993)	11	2096	0.82 (0.78–1.08)	18
Earle (1999)	13	1990	0.80 (0.66–0.97)	20
Mari (2000)	20	3568	0.82 (0.75–0.89)	18
Panzini (2002)	17	2913	0.72 (0.62–0.84)	28
Janunger (2002)	21	3962	0.84 (0.74–0.96)	16
GASTRIC (2010)	17	3838	0.82 (0.76–0.90)	18

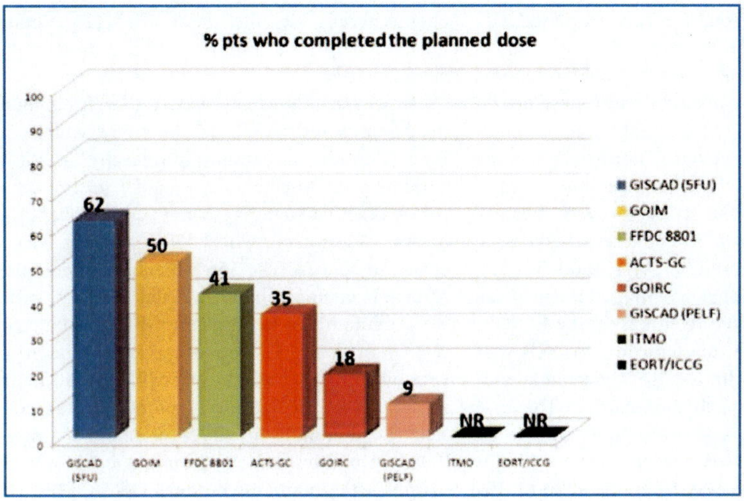

Fig. 24.1 Treatment compliance by patients enrolled in adjuvant treatment trials

fact, the proportion of patients completing adjuvant chemotherapy in Western trials is usually disappointing (Fig. 24.1). These considerations have led some authors to evaluate different approaches to treatment, such as peri-operative chemotherapy. Recently, two important trials have supported the use of this treatment to improve clinical outcome in gastric cancer patients (Table 24.2). The MAGIC (Medical Council Adjuvant Gastric Infusional Chemotherapy) trial randomized 504 patients with resectable stomach, lower esophagus, or EGJ adenocarcinoma to receive surgery alone or peri-operative chemotherapy consisting of three cycles of epirubicin-cisplatin-5-fluorouracil (ECF), given pre- and post-operatively [19]. Patients receiving peri-operative chemotherapy had a significantly better OS, with a 36% survival rate at 5 years compared to 23% in patients treated with surgery only. Peri-operative chemotherapy showed significant results also in tumor down-sizing, 3 cm in the chemotherapy group vs. 5 cm in the surgery alone group ($p < 0.001$), and an improved R0 resection rate (79 vs. 70%, $p = 0.03$).

These results were confirmed by a French trial (ACCORD07-FFCD 9703) that evaluated another chemotherapy regimen, with 5-fluorouracil and cisplatin [20]. The 224 patients were randomized to surgery alone or surgery and peri-operative chemotherapy (2–3 neoadjuvant cycles and 3–4 post-operative cycles). Peri-operative chemotherapy improved R0 resection (84 vs. 73%, $p = 0.04$), 5-year DFS (34 vs. 21%), and OS (38 vs. 24%) rates. The magnitude of these benefits is similar to that observed in the MAGIC trial (a 13% higher rate of survival after 5 years). In both studies, about 85% of patients in the chemotherapy arm completed neoadjuvant treatment while < 50% received the planned adjuvant part of systemic therapy. A possible explanation is the decreased tolerance to chemotherapy observed after gastrectomy.

Table 24.2 Peri-operative chemotherapy trials

Trial	Patients (N.)	Chemotherapy regimen	Hazard ratio for disease-free survival	Hazard ratio for overall survival	5-year overall survival (%)
MAGIC	504	ECF	0.66 (0.53–0.81)	0.75 (0.60–0.93)	36 vs. 23
FFCD 9703	224	5FU, CDDP	0.63 (0.46–0.86)	0.69 (0.50–0.95)	38 vs. 24
EORTC 40954	144	PLF	0.66(0.42–1.03)	0.84 (0.52–1.35)	NR

Moreover, the SAKK group recently presented data that docetaxel-based pre-operative chemotherapy is better tolerated than post-operative chemotherapy. This trial compared pre-operative with post-operative treatment using docetaxel, cisplatin, and fluorouracil (TCF) for four cycles; unfortunately, the study was prematurely closed but the dose intensity in the two arms of the study was significantly different: 93.2% in the pre-operative schedule vs. 81.8% in the post-operative one ($p < 0.0003$) [21]. At the 2009 ASCO annual meeting, the European Research Group presented results from the EORTC 40954 trial. This was a randomized phase III trial that enrolled patients with locally advanced adenocarcinoma of the stomach and cardia. The 144 patients, who had comparable baseline characteristics, were randomized between primary surgery or two 48-day cycles of weekly folinic acid and 5-FU plus biweekly cisplatin (PLF) followed by surgery. OS between the two arms did not differ (HR = 0.84; 95% CI: 0.52–1.35; $p = 0.466$). Median survival exceeded 36 months in both arms. Due to low accrual, this trial was stopped prematurely; however, the unexpectedly long median survival in the surgery arm would have made the primary objective difficult to reach anyway. Difference in time to progression was borderline significant (HR = 0.66; 95% CI: 0.42–1.03; $p = 0.065$). The response rate to chemotherapy was 35.2% (95% CI: 23.7–45.7%). The R0 resection rate was 81.9% after pre-operative chemotherapy compared to 66.7% with surgery alone ($p = 0.036$). There were no major differences in intra- or post-operative complications [22].

24.4 Radiation Therapy

Adjuvant radiotherapy alone has failed over the last decades to improve treatment results and patient outcome [23], as concluded by two randomized trials of adjuvant radiotherapy vs. surgery alone [24, 25]. In the three-arm randomized trial reported by the British Stomach Cancer Group [24], adjuvant chemotherapy (5FU, doxorubicin, mitomycin) and adjuvant radiotherapy were compared to surgery alone. No survival advantage was shown for the 436 patients randomized to surgery only, or surgery with 45–50 Gy radiotherapy, or surgery with FAM chemotherapy. In the other trial [25], patients received adjuvant intra-operative radiotherapy or surgery alone.

However, this debate was further stimulated by the findings of the SWOG 9008 group, which examined combined chemoradiotherapy (CRT) in patients with resected stage IB–IV gastric cancers [6]. A practice-changing benefit for adjuvant therapy was determined, with CRT enhancing local and systemic control. The 556 patients with completely resected adenocarcinoma of the stomach or EGJ were randomized to adjuvant 5-FU and leucovorin (5-FU/LV)-based CRT or observation. The primary endpoint of the trial was survival, with an increase in median survival from 27 months in the control arm to 36 months in the experimental arm ($p = 0.005$). However, toxicity from the regimen was not insignificant, with three toxic deaths (1%), 41% grade 3 toxicity, and 32% grade 4 toxicity. Following presentation of the data in 2001, adjuvant CRT became a widely accepted practice, mainly in the USA, although the trial was criticized for the quality of the surgery included. Only 10% of patients underwent the recommended D2 resection, with a further 36% undergoing D1 resection and 54% D0 resection only. This led some investigators to question whether radiotherapy had compensated for inadequate surgery, and hence whether it was unnecessary after D2 resection. No significant difference in the outcome of patients by level of dissection was reported, in terms of DFS or OS ($p = 0.80$). While in the multimodality arm, the local relapse rate was reduced from 90 to 29%, there was no difference in the risk of distant metastasis. In addition, Park and colleagues investigated a similar protocol in 290 patients, all of whom were curatively resected with extensive D2 lymph node dissection [26]. After a median follow up of 49 months, 43% of patients had experienced a relapse, with 67% local relapses and 36% distant metastases. The 5-year overall and relapse-free survival rates were 60 and 57%, respectively, better than in the SWOG trial [17]. Therefore, it is unclear whether Japanese or Western patients undergoing D2 resection benefit from post-operative chemoradiation.

There are phase II data to suggest that adjuvant CRT can be optimized by the addition of cisplatin and possibly paclitaxel [27], but confirmatory phase III data are awaited.

24.5 Conclusions

Based on the conclusions of recently published trials, peri-operative chemotherapy or post-operative CRT should be recommended for patients presenting with resectable, locally advanced tumors of the stomach or EGJ (stages II and III). In Europe, the recommendation favors peri-operative chemotherapy, consisting of 8–9 weeks of pre-operative platin-fluoropyrimidine-based chemotherapy. The same duration of post-operative chemotherapy using the same regimen should be considered if tolerated by the patient. Post-operative CRT should be considered in patients who have recovered from a gastrectomy, in whom a pT3 or pT4 or pTxN+ tumor was resected, and who did not receive pre-operative chemotherapy, and especially in those in whom a less than optimal lymph node resection was performed [28]. Adjuvant chemotherapy should be considered an option for high-risk patients who underwent resection but who were not treated pre-operatively.

References

1. Crew KD, Neugut AI (2006) Epidemiology of gastric cancer. World J Gastroenterol 12:354-362
2. Bouvier AM, Haas O, Piard F et al (2002(How many nodes must be examined to accurately stage gastric carcinomas. Cancer 94:2862-2866
3. Van de Velde CJ, Peeters KC (2003) The gastric cancer treatment controversy. J Clin Oncol 21:2234-2236
4. Roth AD (2003) Curative treatment of gastric cancer: towards a multidisciplinary approach? Crit Rev Oncol Hematol 46:59-100
5. Van Cutsem E, Van de Velde C, Roth A et al (2008) Expert opinion on management of gastric and gastro-oesophageal junction adenocarcinoma on behalf of the European Organisation for Research and Treatment of Cancer (EORTC) - gastrointestinal cancer group. Eur J Cancer 44:182-194
6. Macdonald JS, Smalley SR, Benedetti J et al (2001) Chemoradiotherapy after surgery compared with surgery alone for adenocarcinoma of the stomach or gastroesophageal junction. N Engl J Med 345:725-730 (SWOG/INT-0116)
7. Bajetta E, Buzzoni R, Mariani L et al (2002) Adjuvant chemotherapy in gastric cancer: 5-year results of a randomized study by the Italian Trials in Medical Oncology (ITMO) Group. Ann Oncol 13:299-307
8. Bouche`O, Ychou M, Burtin P et al (2005) Adjuvant chemotherapy with 5-fluorouracil and cisplatin compared with surgery alone for gastric cancer: 7-year results of the FFCD randomized phase III trial (8801). Ann Oncol 16:1488-1497
9. Cascinu S, La bianca R, Barone C et al (2007) adjuvant treatment of high-risk, radically resected gastric cancer patients with 5-fluorouracil, leucovorin, cisplatin, and epidoxorubicin in a randomized controlled trial. J Natl Cancer Inst 99:601-607
10. Di Costanzo F, Gasperoni S, Manzione L et al (2008) Adjuvant chemotherapy in completely resected gastric cancer: a randomized phase III trial conducted by GOIRC. J Natl Cancer Inst 100:388-398
11. Nitti D, Wils J, Dos Santos Guimares J et al (2006) Randomized phase III trial of FAMTX or FEMTX compared with surgery alone in resected gastric cancer. A combined analysis of the EORTC GI Group and ICCG. Ann Oncol 17:262-269
12. De Vita F, Giuliani F, Orditura M et al (2007) Adjuvant chemotherapy with epirubicin, leucovorin, 5-fluorouracil and etoposide regimen in resected gastric cancer patients: a randomized phase III trial by the Gruppo Oncologico Italia Meridionale (GOIM 9602 Study). Ann Oncol 18:1354-1358
13. Sakuramoto S, Sasako M, Yamaguchi T et al (2008) for the ACTS-GC Group. Adjuvant Chemotherapy for Gastric Cancer with S-1, an Oral Fluoropyrimidine. N Eng J Med 357:1810-1820
14. Hermans J, Bonekamp JJ, Bon MC et al (1993) Adjuvant therapy after resection for gastric cancer: meta-analysis of randomized trials. J Clin Oncol 11:1441-1447
15. Earle CC, Maroun JA (1999) Adjuvant chemotherapy after resection for gastric cancer in non-Asian patients. Revisiting a meta-analysis of randomized trials. Eur J Cancer 35:1059-1064
16. Mari M, Floriani I, Tinazzi A et al (2000) Efficacy of adjuvant chemotherapy after curative resection for gastric cancer: a meta-analysis for published randomised trials. A study of the GISCAD (Gruppo Italiano per lo Studio dei Carcinomi dell'Apparato Digerente). Ann Oncol 11:837-843
17. Panzini I, Gianni L, Fattori PP et al (2002) Adjuvant chemotherapy in gastric cancer: a meta-analysis of randomized trials and a comparison with previous meta-analyses. Tumori 88:21-27
18. GASTRIC (Global Advanced/Adjuvant Stomach Tumor Research International Collaboration) Group, Paoletti X, Oba K, Burzykowski T et al (2010) Benefit of adjuvant chemotherapy for resectable gastric cancer: a meta-analysis. JAMA 303:1729-1737
19. Cunningham D, Allum WH, Stenning SP et al (2006) MAGIC Trial Participants. Perioperative chemotherapy versus surgery alone for resectable gastroesophageal cancer. N Engl J Med 355:11-20
20. Boige V, Pignon J, Saint-Aubert B et al (2007) Final results of randomized trial comparing preoperative 5-fluorouracil (F)/cisplatin (P) to surgery alone in adenocarcinoma of the stomach and lower esophagus (ASLE): FNLCC ACCORD07-FFCD 9703 trial. 2007 ASCO Annual Meeting, abstr 4510
21. Roth A, Biffi R, Stup R et al (2007) Comparative evaluation in tolerance of neoadjuvant versus adjuvant docetaxel based chemotherapy in resectable gastric cancer in a randomised trial of the Swiss Group for Clinical Cancer Research (SAKK) and the European Institute of Oncology (EIO). Ann Oncol 18:S7

22. Schuhmacher C, Schlag P, Lordick F et al (2009) Neoadjuvant chemotherapy versus surgery alone for locally advanced adenocarcinoma of the stomach and cardia: Randomized EORTC phase III trial 40954. 2009 ASCO Annual Meeting, Abs: 4510
23. Moehler M, Lyros O, Gockel I et al (2008) Multidisciplinary management of gastric and gastroesophageal cancers. World J Gastroenterol 14(24):3773-3780
24. Hallissey MT, Dunn JA, Ward LC, Allum WH (1994) The second British Stomach Cancer Group trial of adjuvant radiotherapy or chemotherapy in resectable gastric cancer: five-year follow-up. Lancet 343:1309–1312
25. Kramling HJ, Wilkowski R, Duhmke E et al (1996) Adjuvant intraoperative radiotherapy of stomach carcinoma. Langenbecks Arch Chir Suppl Kongressbd 113:211–213
26. Park SH, Kim DY, Heo JS et al (2003) Postoperative chemoradiotherapy for gastric cancer. Ann Oncol 14: 1373-1377
27. Kooby DA, Suriawinata A, Klimstra DS et al (2003) Biologic predictors of survival in node-negative gastric cancer. Ann Surg 237:828-835 discussion 835-837
28. Van Cutsem E, Dicato M, Arber N et al (2006) The neoadjuvant, surgical and adjuvant treatment of gastric adenocarcinoma. Current expert opinion derived from the Seventh World Congress on Gastrointestinal Cancer, Barcelona 2005. Ann Oncol 17:vi13–vi18

25 Follow-up and Treatment of Recurrence

Daniele Marrelli, Stefano Caruso, and Franco Roviello

Abstract

About two-thirds of patients with advanced gastric cancer treated by R0 resection develop tumor relapse during the follow-up, and most of them will die from the disease. The main patterns of dissemination are peritoneal, hematogenous, and locoregional, and their incidence differs according to multiple clinical, surgical, and pathological factors. The main purpose of follow-up is to diagnose tumor relapse as early as possible. An ideal follow-up program is one that is individualized according to the predicted risk, timing, and site of recurrence. However, the real clinical utility of these programs is affected by the low chance of cure for recurrent gastric cancer. Surgical treatment has a limited role and is indicated only in a few cases of resectable locoregional recurrences, isolated liver metastases, or limited peritoneal carcinomatosis. Currently, the prevention of recurrence is probably more important than its early detection. A correct surgical procedure and the selection of pre-, peri- or post-operative systemic and/or locoregional treatments could improve the prognosis of gastric cancer patients. The Italian Research Group for Gastric cancer has developed an individualized follow-up program based on the risk of recurrence and patients' compliance with follow-up. Three different schedules (mild, moderate, or intensive) are proposed.

Keywords

Gastric cancer • Follow-up • Survival • Loco-regional recurrence • Liver metastases • Peritoneal carcinomatosis • Gastric stump carcinoma • Score systems • Gastrectomy • Lymphadenectomy • HIPEC • Lauren histotype

25.1 Introduction

About two-thirds of patients with advanced gastric cancer (GC) treated by R0 resection develop tumor relapse during the follow-up, and most of them will die from the disease. Recurrences are seen in most cases within the first 2 years after surgery, with only a minority diagnosed after 5 years [1–4].

D. Marrelli (✉)
Dept. of Human Pathology and Oncology,
Section of General Surgery and Surgical Oncology,
Translational Research Laboratory,
University of Siena,
Siena, Italy

G. de Manzoni, F. Roviello, W. Siquini (eds.), *Surgery in the Multimodal Management of Gastric Cancer*,

The main patterns of dissemination are peritoneal, hematogenous (mainly the liver), and loco-regional (lymph node, gastric stump, gastric bed, anastomosis). However, marked differences in the incidence and distribution of recurrences have been reported in the literature. This may be explained by several factors: different study populations and disease stages, lack of standardized definitions of recurrence or of the methods used for diagnosis, and different treatment approaches (extent of lymphadenectomy, additional therapies, etc.).

25.2 Pathogenesis

Locoregional recurrence results from lymphatic spread or direct tumor propagation within the abdominal cavity. Four types of local recurrence can be differentiated according to location and origin: lymph node metastasis, extraluminal recurrence, recurrence within the gastric remnant, and anastomotic recurrence following total gastrectomy [5].

Peritoneal carcinomatosis originates mainly from local propagation within the abdominal cavity, with free tumor cells exfoliating as a consequence of direct invasion by the primary tumor. Subsequently, the cells become implanted on the peritoneal surface in a process mediated by adhesion molecules. Another mechanism is the transport of malignant cells through lymphatic fluid or venous blood within the peritoneal cavity. A third possibility is surgical manipulation/trauma [6].

Hematogenous metastases develop through a complex process in which cancer cells detach from the primary site, invade the vasculature by degradation of the surrounding tissue, and migrate to the secondary organ, where the cells transmigrate through the endothelial cell layer and develop into metastatic lesions. Biological factors and surface molecules may strongly affect the site of GC recurrence [7, 8].

25.3 Pattern of Recurrence

There are few definitive studies regarding recurrence patterns, as their methods of diagnosis differ and patient cohorts are heterogeneous. Studies based on autopsy findings typically describe end-stage disease. By contrast, clinical studies are generally able to demonstrate the early modes of recurrence based on clinical, surgical, and radiological examinations [1, 4, 9].

The incidence and site of recurrence may also depend on multiple demographic, clinical, and pathological factors. In Western countries, there is a greater frequency of local recurrence than in Asia [9-11]. In contrast, studies from Asian countries report the liver and peritoneum as the main sites of recurrence (Fig. 25.1) [1, 3, 4, 12, 13]. This may be related to the fact that extended lymphadenectomy is routinely performed, which would improve local control of the disease. Indeed, in those Western centers where D2 lymphadenectomy is the procedure of choice [3, 4], the rates of local recurrence are more similar to those of Asian series and notably lower than in series of Western patients treated by limited lymph node dissection [10, 11]. In the re-evaluation of the Dutch trial, local recurrences were significantly higher in the D1 than in the D2 group [11]. A recent retrospective evaluation of two prospective studies concluded that the addition of postoperative chemoradiotherapy (CRT) had a major impact on local recurrence after D1 surgery but probably not after D2 [14]. The potential impact of CRT on local relapse after limited lymphadenectomy was also suggested by the results of the INT-0116 trial [10].

25.4 Timing of Recurrence

Most recurrences of GC occur in the first few years after R0 resection. In the study conducted by the Italian Research Group for Gastric Cancer (GIRCG), the median time to recurrence was 13 months, and about two-thirds of the recurrences were detected in the first 2 years (Fig. 25.2) [4]. Similar findings were reported by other studies [1, 3]. Among the clinical and pathological factors predictive of early relapse are depth of invasion, lymph node involvement, macroscopic type, tumor size, extent of lymphadenectomy and gastrectomy [1].

In general, locoregional recurrences tend to occur later than hematogenous or peritoneal recurrences [1, 4]. Five years postoperatively, recurrences are primarily locoregional; a second primary

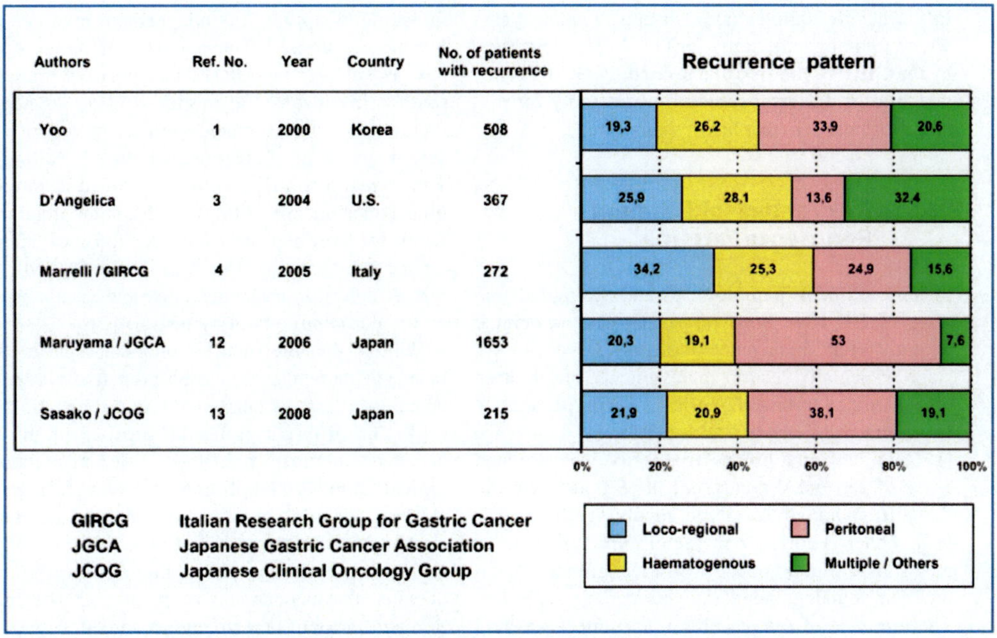

Fig. 25.1 Pattern of recurrence after R0 resection for GC according to the main series in the literature

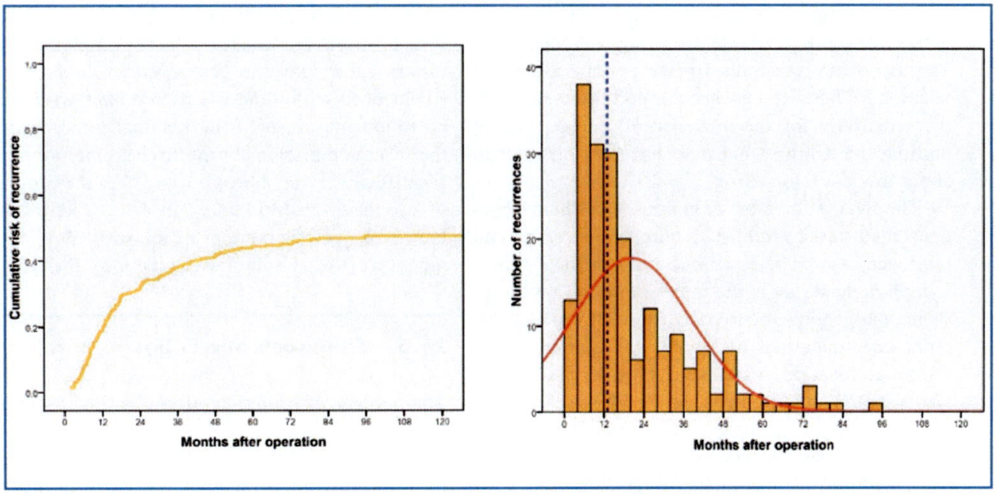

Fig. 25.2 Cumulative risk and timing of recurrence after R0 resection for GC (GIRCG study). *Dotted line* indicates median time to recurrence

in the gastric stump may also appear many years after subtotal gastrectomy for GC. In a recent study by the GIRCG, the risk of a secondary GC was estimated to be 4% after subtotal gastrectomy for distal gastric cancer (manuscript submitted).

25.5 Risk Factors for Different Recurrence Patterns

Specific clinical, pathological, and biological features of GC have been reported to be associated with different recurrence patterns. Advanced pT stage (especially serosal involvement), and Lauren diffuse-mixed or undifferentiated histotypes are the main factors associated with peritoneal recurrence [1, 3, 15, 16]. In a prospective study, we estimated a risk of peritoneal recurrence of 69% at 5 years in the diffuse-mixed histotype involving the serosa [16]. Other reported risk factors are lymph node metastasis, tumor size, infiltrative growth, distal location, female gender, and younger age [1, 3, 16]. The presence of tumor cells in peritoneal washing (cy+) is another recognized strong predictor of peritoneal recurrence [17]; in fact, positive peritoneal cytology is now included in stage IV in the new TNM classification. However, the incidence of cy+ cases in the absence of macroscopic peritoneal metastases is rather low, due to frequent false-negatives; consequently, cy+ does not emerge as an independent prognostic factor in some studies [18]. The use of reverse transcriptase polymerase chain reaction (RT-PCR) has been reported to increase the sensitivity for the presence of cancer cells in peritoneal washings, but it is currently difficult to apply in a clinical setting.

The liver is the most common site of hematogenous metastases from GC; lung, bone, skin, and brain can also be affected but at much lower rates. Lymph node status is the most important predictor of hematogenous recurrence from GC; pT stage, older age, intestinal histotype, vascular invasion, proximal location, expansive growth, and tumor size are other reported risk factors [1, 3, 7, 15]. In a single-center experience, we estimated a cumulative risk of liver metastases of 16% at 5 years after R0 resection [7]. Logistic regression identified lymph node involvement, preoperative positivity of tumor markers (CEA, CA 19-9, or CA 72-4), and intestinal histotype as independent predictors of hepatic recurrence. The majority of patients who developed liver metastases had positive preoperative marker levels, and in almost all cases hepatic recurrence was associated with an increase in the serum levels of these markers during follow-up. Tumor markers are molecules involved in intercellular adhesion; for example, CEA is an attachment factor for liver metastases. Some biological characteristics, such as the overexpression of growth factors or adhesion molecules, also have been reported to be related to liver metastasis [8].

Unlike the intestinal histological type, the diffuse type demonstrates a high propensity to metastasize to distant organs, avoiding the hepatic filter [15]. The different molecular profiles of the two histotypes could explain their different epidemiological, clinical, and prognostic features. In general, the association between peritoneal carcinomatosis and liver metastases as initial failure is infrequent. This probably reflects biological differences between the mechanisms of peritoneal dissemination and those of hematogenous spread.

As previously stated, the surgical approach may affect the locoregional recurrence of GC. Nodal status, depth of invasion, proximal location, tumor size, histotype, and advanced age are other potential risk factors [1, 3]. Lymph nodes, anastomosis, and the gastric bed account for most of these recurrences, mainly due to the progression of residual lymph node metastases or the implantation of tumor cells into the resection area [1, 5, 19]. Recurrence within the gastric remnant after partial resection may result from residual tumor cells on the resection margins or multifocal carcinomas [5]. Multifocality was shown not to affect the prognosis of esophago-gastric cancer in a large series [20]. However, gastric stump neoplasms may appear many years after subtotal gastrectomy for GC.

25.6 Diagnosis and Follow-up Protocols

The purpose of follow-up after curative resection is mainly to assess long-term complications, to collect data on survival and the clinical evolution of the disease, and to diagnose as early as possible any potential recurrence [9]. However, the real clinical utility of follow-up programs is notably reduced by the limited chance of cure for recurrent GC. An ideal follow-up program should be individualized according to the predicted risk, timing, and site of recurrence. Ideally, recurrence should be diagnosed in an asymptomatic and still treatable stage of disease.

To diagnose GC recurrence, several types of investigations can be used, based mainly on endoscopy, radiology, and blood tests. The diagnostic accuracy of endoscopy is limited to cases of intraluminal recurrences in the gastric stump or anastomosis. Imaging, specifically, ultrasound (US), computed tomography (CT), magnetic resonance (MRI), and positron emission tomography (PET), undoubtedly has the most important role in the follow-up of GC patients. Abdominal US may show liver metastases or ascites but its accuracy is notably reduced for locoregional recurrence or small peritoneal nodules. However, it has the advantage of limited costs and good patient compliance. Hematogenous metastases are better detected by CT, MRI, or PET. Modern multi-slice CT has notably increased the diagnostic accuracy for hematogenous, lymph nodal, locoregional, and peritoneal recurrences of GC; however, the detection rates remain low in the early stage of recurrent disease [9, 21]. Locoregional and peritoneal recurrences are generally difficult to diagnose in the early phase despite intensive follow-up programs [9]. Recent studies suggested PET-CT as the most reliable diagnostic procedure for this purpose; however, the high costs and potential false-positives limit the indications for this combined modality to selected cases only. Furthermore, frequent false-negatives have been reported, mainly in signet-ring cell and non-solid type poorly differentiated carcinoma [22]. Diagnostic laparoscopy could be indicated for the detection of early-stage peritoneal recurrence in patients with equivocal radiologic or clinical findings.

Recently, the use of serum tumor markers in the follow-up of GC patients has increased. In an observational study, we investigated the diagnostic accuracy of CEA, CA 19-9, and CA 72-4 after R0 resection [23]. Marker sensitivity for recurrence was 44% for CEA, 56% for CA 19-9, and 51% for CA 72-4; the combined sensitivity was 87%. Sensitivity was 90% for locoregional recurrences, 96% for hematogenous recurrences, and 67% for peritoneal recurrences. The increase in marker levels preceded clinical diagnosis in most cases. Interestingly, marker sensitivity in patients with positive preoperative levels was 100%. However, false CEA, CA 19-9, and CA 72-4 elevations in disease-free patients were observed in 21, 26, and 3% of cases, respectively. We concluded that the combined assay of tumor markers may be useful for the early diagnosis of recurrence of GC, but only CA 72-4 positivity should be considered a specific indicator of tumor recurrence during follow-up. These results have been confirmed in other studies [7]. Moreover, despite the intensive follow-up program, a potentially curative treatment was possible in only a minority of patients with recurrent GC [6].

Concerning the potential survival benefit of follow-up, only retrospective or observational studies are available [2, 9, 24, 25]. Several papers suggest that although an intensive follow-up program is able to detect a higher proportion of asymptomatic recurrences, the early detection of recurrence in an asymptomatic phase does not result in improved survival [2, 24], mainly due to the lack of effective treatments for recurrent GC.

Hence, there are no universally shared guidelines on what type of follow-up is to be implemented in GC patients. Furthermore, follow-up intervals and the choice of tests also differ considerably among clinicians. In the absence of national and international guide-lines, follow-up protocols vary widely among different centers. The National Comprehensive Cancer Network (NCCN) suggests a minimal follow-up: in the absence of specific symptoms, a check-up consisting solely of blood chemistry parameters and tumor markers every 4–6 months for 3 years, and annually thereafter [26]. Conversely, more intensive follow-up protocols have been promoted in other centers [4, 25]. An interesting option was offered by the National Cancer Center in Tokyo, where follow-up programs differ depending on disease stage [9].

25.7 Treatment of Recurrence

In spite of the many reports available in the literature on the incidence and sites of recurrence, there are very few studies concerning the treatment options for recurrent GC. This is, in most cases, a condition with an unfavorable prognosis [1, 3, 19]. Systemic chemotherapy may prolong survival compared with best supportive care but does not offer any chance of cure [9, 27]. There are no reports in the literature demonstrating potential benefit for the earlier delivery of chemotherapy in patients with asymptomatic vs. symptomatic disease recurrence [2, 9]. New chemotherapeutic agents are strongly awaited in the near future to improve survival results.

Surgical treatment has a limited role in recurrent GC. Yoo et al. reported that of 508 patients who developed a recurrence, 48 (9%) underwent further resection, but in only 19 (3.7%) was curative treatment possible [1]. In a recent report from the USA, 7459 medical records of patients with gastric or gastro-esophageal cancer were reviewed. In only 60 patients was an operation for recurrent tumor attempted, and less than half of these cases involved resectable tumors [19].

Hematogenous metastases from GC are generally not suitable for curative treatment, and median survival does not exceed 9 months [1]. Nonetheless, surgical resection could be indicated in selected cases. Retrospective studies suggested a chance of cure in patients with hepatic recurrence who underwent liver resection, with overall survival rates ranging between 11 and 42% [8, 9]. Still, relatively few cases involve isolated hepatic recurrences and only a minority of these are resectable with curative intent. In a recent GIRCG study, 73 patients who developed liver metastases after R0 resection for GC were analyzed [28]. Surgical resection was possible in 11 patients, with a subsequent 5-year survival of 20%. This suggests that hepatic resection is indicated when R0 resection is still possible, but this applies to only a minority of cases.

Similarly, peritoneal carcinomatosis of GC is a fatal disease, with a reported median survival after diagnosis of only 6 months [1, 6]. In recent years, normothermic (EPIC) or hyperthermic intraperitoneal chemotherapy (HIPEC), associated with cytoreductive surgery, has been proposed as a potentially effective treatments to improve survival or prevent peritoneal recurrence from GC. A recent French multi-institutional study reviewed 159 patients treated with surgical cytoreduction and HIPEC or EPIC [29]. The overall median survival was 9.2 months with a 5-year survival of 13%. The only independent prognostic indicator was the completeness of cytoreductive surgery: CCR-0 resulted in a median survival of 15 months and a 5-year survival of 23%. However, we underline that only a minority of patients with peritoneal carcinomatosis from GC are candidates for complete cytoreduction [6]. As such, in our opinion, HIPEC and EPIC should be focused on the prevention of peritoneal recurrence after an R0 resection for primary GC. In this setting, both techniques were reported to be potentially effective [30]. High-risk groups, such as patients with diffuse-mixed type tumors involving the serosa or patients with positive peritoneal cytology, may particularly benefit from this approach.

Local recurrence, if detected at an early stage, is amenable to surgical resection more often than hematogenous or peritoneal failures but often requires the resection of adjacent organs and is thus associated with high morbidity and mortality [1, 5, 19, 27]. Recurrence in the gastric stump is generally the only condition associated with a chance of cure. Lymph node or extraluminal recurrences can rarely be operated on with curative intent and reports of successful treatment are anecdotal [5]. Anastomotic recurrences after total gastrectomy are detectable by endoscopy and could be amenable to surgical resection in a few selected cases. In summary, the number of patients with locally recurrent GC in whom surgery may be attempted with curative intent is low, and even in these selected cases, median survival rarely surpasses 24 months [5, 19, 27].

At present, therefore, prevention of recurrence is probably more important than its early detection. A correct surgical procedure and the selection of systemic and/or locoregional pre-, peri-, or postoperative treatments, based on the predicted risk of recurrence pattern, is the more reasonable approach to improve the prognosis of patients with GC.

25.8 The GIRCG Follow-up Program

On the basis of data on the recurrence of GC, an individualized follow-up program has been proposed by the GIRCG. The intensity of follow-up is

MILD

Months	3	6	9	12	15	18	21	24	27	30	33	36	42	48	54	60
Tumor markers*		X		X		X		X		X		X	X	X	X	X
Abdominal Ultrasound		X		X		X		X		X		X	X	X	X	X
Chest X-ray				X				X				X				
Thoraco-abdominal CT scan																
Endoscopy				X				X				X				X

* CEA, CA 19-9, CA 72-4
CT scan: increase of tumor marker levels, clinical or radiological suspicion of recurrence

MODERATE

Months	3	6	9	12	15	18	21	24	27	30	33	36	42	48	54	60
Tumor markers*	X	X	X	X	X	X	X	X		X		X	X	X	X	X
Abdominal Ultrasound		X				X				X			X		X	X
Chest X-ray																
Thoraco-abdominal CT scan				X				X				X		X		
Endoscopy				X				X				X				X

* CEA, CA 19-9, CA 72-4

INTENSIVE

Months	3	6	9	12	15	18	21	24	27	30	33	36	42	48	54	60
Tumor markers*	X	X	X	X	X	X	X	X	X	X	X	X	X	X	X	X
Abdominal Ultrasound													X		X	
Chest X-ray																
Thoraco-abdominal CT scan		X		X		X		X		X		X		X		X
Endoscopy				X				X				X				X

* CEA, CA 19-9, CA 72-4

Fig. 25.3 Follow-up protocols proposed by the GIRCG, on the basis of recurrence risk and patients' compliance with follow-up. The model to calculate the GIRCG prognostic score can be downloaded from the website: www.gircg.it

based on the risk of recurrence after R0 resection and patients' compliance with follow-up. The risk of recurrence is calculated according to the prognostic score described in Chap. 6. Three different schedules (mild, moderate, or intensive) are proposed (Fig. 25.3):

- Mild: risk of recurrence < 10% or low compliance with follow-up
- Moderate: risk between 10 and 50%
- Intensive: risk > 50%

After 5 years, clinical monitoring and annual examinations are carried out on request. Screening for other primaries is advisable in long-term survivors.

References

1. Yoo CH, Noh SH, Shin DW et al (2000) Recurrence following curative resection for gastric carcinoma. Br J Surg 87:236-242
2. Kodera Y, Ito S, Yamamura Y et al (2003) Follow-up surveillance for recurrence after curative gastric cancer surgery lacks survival benefit. Ann Surg Oncol 10:898-902
3. D'Angelica M, Gonen M, Brennan MF et al (2004) Patterns of initial recurrence in completely resected gastric adenocarcinoma. Ann Surg 240:808-816
4. Marrelli D, De Stefano A, de Manzoni G et al (2005) Prediction of recurrence after radical surgery for gastric cancer: a scoring system obtained from a prospective multicenter study. Ann Surg 241:247-255
5. Lehnert T, Rudek B, Buhl K et al (2002) Surgical therapy for loco-regional recurrence and distant metastasis of gastric cancer. Eur J Surg Oncol 28:455-461
6. Roviello F, Caruso S, Marrelli D et al (2011) Treatment of peritoneal carcinomatosis with cytoreductive surgery and hyperthermic intraperitoneal chemotherapy: state of the art and future developments. Surg Oncol 20:e38-54
7. Marrelli D, Roviello F, De Stefano A et al (2004) Risk factors for liver metastases after curative surgical procedures for gastric cancer: a prospective study of 208 patients treated with surgical resection. J Am Coll Surg 198:51-58
8. Kakeji Y, Morita M, Maehara Y (2010) Strategies for treating liver metastasis from gastric cancer. Surg Today 40:287-294
9. Whiting J, Sano T, Saka M et al (2006) Follow-up of gastric cancer: a review. Gastric Cancer 9:74-81
10. Macdonald JS, Smalley SR, Benedetti J et al (2001) Chemoradiotherapy after surgery compared with surgery

alone for adenocarcinoma of the stomach or gastroesophageal junction. N Engl J Med 345:725-730
11. Songun I, Putter H, Kranenbarg EM et al (2010) Surgical treatment of gastric cancer: 15-year follow-up results of the randomised nationwide Dutch D1D2 trial. Lancet Oncol 11:439-449
12. Japanese Gastric Cancer Association Registration Committee (2006) Gastric cancer treated in 1991 in Japan: data analysis of nationwide registry. Gastric Cancer 9:51–66
13. Sasako M, Sano T, Yamamoto S et al (2008) D2 lymphadenectomy alone or with para-aortic nodal dissection for gastric cancer. N Engl J Med 359:453-462
14. Dikken JL, Jansen EP, Cats A et al (2010) Impact of the extent of surgery and postoperative chemoradiotherapy on recurrence patterns in gastric cancer. J Clin Oncol 28:2430-2436
15. Marrelli D, Roviello F, de Manzoni G et al (2002) Different patterns of recurrence in gastric cancer depending on Lauren's histological type: longitudinal study. World J Surg 26:1160-1165
16. Roviello F, Marrelli D, de Manzoni G et al (2003) Prospective study of peritoneal recurrence after curative surgery for gastric cancer. Br J Surg 90:1113-1119
17. Mezhir JJ, Shah MA, Jacks LM et al (2010) Positive peritoneal cytology in patients with gastric cancer: natural history and outcome of 291 patients. Ann Surg Oncol 17:3173-3180
18. de Manzoni G, Verlato G, Di Leo A et al (2006) Peritoneal cytology does not increase the prognostic information provided by TNM in gastric cancer. World J Surg 30:579-584
19. Badgwell B, Cormier JN, Xing Y et al (2009) Attempted salvage resection for recurrent gastric or gastroesophageal cancer. Ann Surg Oncol 16:42-50
20. Morgagni P, Marfisi C, Gardini A et al (2009) Subtotal gastrectomy as treatment for distal multifocal early gastric cancer. J Gastrointest Surg 13:2239-2244
21. Marrelli D, Mazzei MA, Pedrazzani C et al (2011) High Accuracy of Multislices Computed Tomography (MSCT) for Para-Aortic Lymph Node Metastases from Gastric Cancer: A Prospective Single-Center Study. Ann Surg Oncol (In press)
22. Shimada H, Okazumi S, Koyama M et al (2011) Clinical utility of (18)F-fluoro-2-deoxyglucose positron emission tomography in gastric cancer. A systematic review of the literature. Gastric Cancer (In press)
23. Marrelli D, Pinto E, De Stefano A et al (2001) Clinical utility of CEA, CA 19-9, and CA 72-4 in the follow-up of patients with resectable gastric cancer. Am J Surg 181:16-19
24. Bennett JJ, Gonen M, D'Angelica M et al (2005) Is detection of asymptomatic recurrence after curative resection associated with improved survival in patients with gastric cancer? J Am Coll Surg 201:503-510
25. Hur H, Song KY, Park CH (2010) Follow-up strategy after curative resection of gastric cancer: a nationwide survey in Korea. Ann Surg Oncol 17:54-64
26. Jensen EH, Tuttle TM (2007) Preoperative staging and postoperative surveillance for gastric cancer. Surg Oncol Clin N Am 16:329-342
27. Nunobe S, Hiki N, Ohyama S et al (2011) Outcome of surgical treatment for patients with locoregional recurrence of gastric cancer. Langenbecks Arch Surg 396:161-166
28. Tiberio GA, Coniglio A, Marchet A et al (2009) Metachronous hepatic metastases from gastric carcinoma: a multicentric survey. Eur J Surg Oncol 35:486-491
29. Glehen O, Gilly FN, Arvieux C et al (2010) Peritoneal carcinomatosis from gastric cancer: a multi-institutional study of 159 patients treated by cytoreductive surgery combined with perioperative intraperitoneal chemotherapy. Ann Surg Oncol 17:2370-2377
30. Yan TD, Black D, Sugarbaker PH et al (2007) A systematic review and meta-analysis of the randomized controlled trials on adjuvant intraperitoneal chemotherapy for resectable gastric cancer. Ann Surg Oncol 14:2702-2713

Endoscopic and Surgical Palliation of Unresectable Gastric Cancer

26

Giovanni de Manzoni, Alberto Di Leo, Luca Rodella, Francesco Lombardo, and Filippo Catalano

Abstract

Chemotherapy is the standard treatment in patients with unresectable gastric cancer, but is not an option for those with malignant gastric outlet obstruction. Instead, in these cases gastrojejunostomy is the most commonly used palliative treatment. Recently, endoscopic stent placement has been introduced as an alternative, safe, and effective procedure for palliative treatment of malignant strictures involving the gastroduodenal region. The results of different studies suggest that gastrojejunostomy is associated with better long-term results and is therefore the optimal treatment in patients with good performance status and relatively long life expectancy. However, in patients with a relatively short life expectancy and poor performance status, endoscopic stent placement is the treatment of choice.

Keywords

Gastric outlet obstruction (GOO) • Open gastrojejunostomy (OGJ) • Laparoscopic gastrojejunostomy (LGJ) • Stomach-partitioning gastrojejunostomy (SPGJ) • Endoscopic stenting (ES) • Delayed gastric emptying (DGE) • Esophago-gastric junction

26.1 Surgical Palliation

Most patients with incurable advanced gastric cancer (AGC) or recurrent gastric cancer die within 1 year after diagnosis. These patients often receive systemic chemotherapy, which has become the standard palliative treatment [1]. However, treatment is complicated since these patients often present with symptoms such as anorexia, abdominal pain, nausea/vomiting, and gastric or bowel obstruction, due to primary tumor progression and/or peritoneal dissemination [2]. Effective and appropriate palliative surgery in patients with unresectable gastric tumor remains controversial and specific indications from the literature are often based on the results of retrospective studies. Nevertheless, in patients with an acceptable life expectancy [3-5], palliative bypass surgery could be useful, especially in cases of gastric outlet obstruction and good performance status according to the guidelines of the Eastern Cooperative Oncology Group (ECOG) (Table 26.1) [3, 6].

G. de Manzoni (✉)
Dept. of Surgery,
Upper G.I. Surgery Division,
University of Verona,
Verona, Italy

G. de Manzoni, F. Roviello, W. Siquini (eds.), *Surgery in the Multimodal Management of Gastric Cancer*,

Table 26.1 ECOG performance status

Grade	ECOG
0	Fully active, able to carry on all pre-disease performance without restriction
1	Restricted in physically strenuous activity but ambulatory and able to carry out work of light or sedentary nature, e.g., light house work, office work
2	Ambulatory and capable of all self-care but unable to carry out any work activities. Up and about more than 50% of waking hours
3	Capable of only limited self-care, confined to bed or chair more than 50% of waking hours
4	Completely disabled. Cannot carry on any self-care. Totally confined to bed or chair
5	Dead

26.1.1 Gastric Outlet Obstruction Due to the Primary Tumor

Gastric outlet obstruction (GOO) is a problem especially in patients with AGC located in the distal part of the stomach, but it can also occur when the tumor extends widely within the stomach. If curative resection is not possible, the GOO should be treated to avoid the poor clinical condition (vomiting, dehydration, and malnutrition) that rapidly develops in these patients. Furthermore, adequate oral intake and weight loss prevention are essential for subsequent systemic chemotherapy [7]. Indeed, patients in whom oral intake is adequately restored can be treated with chemotherapy by oral administration [8].

The most common palliative bypass operation is conventional open gastrojejunostomy (OGJ), with retrocolic or antecolic anastomosis. When cancer invades the great part of the stomach, except the fundus and the esophago-gastric junction, gastric fundus jejunostomy is another option. In a multicenter, randomized trial of palliative treatment for malignant GOO, both OGJ and laparoscopic gastrojejunostomy (LGJ) provided better long-term results than endoscopic stent placement. Although stent placement resulted in a more rapid improvement of food intake, shorter hospital stay, and lower costs, gastrojejunostomy was recommended as the treatment of choice in patients with a life expectancy ≥2 months. In fact, after a longer follow-up, surgical bypass had better results with respect to food intake and fewer major complications, recurrent obstructive symptoms, and reinterventions [9].

OGJ undertaken through laparotomy provides good results but it carries the risk and discomfort associated with this procedure. Moreover, in patients with GOO, OGJ has been associated with delayed gastric emptying (DGE) in up to 16% of cases and with an 8% reintervention rate. Morbidity is approximately 25% and mortality ranges between 8 and 17% [10, 11]. In the past few years, improvements in laparoscopic techniques have led surgeons to explore the feasibility of performing LGJ for the palliation of GOO. The procedure can be carried out safely, with efficient relief from symptoms and earlier recovery of bowel movements than obtained with OGJ. Minimally invasive surgery also provides less suppression of immune function and can prevent postoperative adhesions [12].

In 1997, Kaminishi et al. described a different procedure for OGJ, stomach-partitioning gastrojejunostomy (SPGJ), which achieved an improved quality of life and a better prognosis than OGJ in patients with GOO. SPGJ has been indicated as an effective treatment for DGE and for the prevention of hemorrhage from the tumor caused by contact with retained food. In this bypass operation, the upper third of the stomach is partitioned from the greater curvature to a point located 2 cm from the lesser curvature, leaving the latter with a lumen of about one finger's width. Finally, the partitioned proximal part of the stomach is anastomosed to the jejunum [13]. In a series of patients suffering from malignant GOO due to different unresectable primary tumors, Kubota et al. reported that SPGJ achieved improved quality of life (intake of solid food and fewer complications) and a better prognosis than stenting procedures, even though patients comprising the stent group probably had worse performance status or more advanced tumors [14]. In another group of patients with unresectable pancreatobiliary cancer, 65% of whom had GOO, morbidity rates were 38% after SPGJ and 50% after OGJ, with 23 and 40% of patients suffering DGE, respectively. Recently, the laparoscopic approach to SPGJ was reported to be a useful technique for treating GOO in patients with unresectable antral AGC [15] and could be successfully adopted in patients with malignant pyloroduodenal obstruction due to different tumors [16].

26.1.2 Gastric Outlet Obstruction Due to Recurrent Tumor

In patients who have previously undergone subtotal gastrectomy for gastric cancer, locoregional recurrence may involve the gastric bed, causing anastomotic obstruction and GOO. In the presence of resectable disease, surgical resection can result in improved overall survival in selected patients [17-19], whereas the finding of unresectable disease is associated with a high risk of morbidity and mortality after palliative surgery [19]. These patients are usually poor surgical candidates because of advanced malignancy, poor performance status, and malnutrition; moreover, they generally have a relatively short life expectancy. In such cases, a less invasive procedure is preferred and endoscopic stent insertion has become widely accepted. Recent studies have reported that endoscopic insertion of a self-expandable metal stent provides safe and effective palliation of a recurrent anastomotic stricture caused by gastric cancer, with a technical success rate that is comparable to that achieved with a primary malignant GOO [20-22].

26.2 Endoscopic Palliation

The traditional approach to palliating malignant GOO has been OGJ. More recently, significant advantages have been reported for endoscopic stenting (ES). A systematic review of different methods to palliate GOO [23-25] showed that among the 12 studies comparing ES and OGJ (244 and 218 patients, respectively), more favorable results were obtained with ES, specifically, earlier oral intake after the procedure (mean difference 7 days) and earlier discharge from the hospital (mean difference 12 days). After OGJ, patients had more severe complications, especially medical ones (myocardial infarction, respiratory infections, and renal failure). Complications after ES were related to the procedure (stent migration, obstruction by tumor in- or overgrowth or by food impaction, bleeding, perforation, or fracture). No differences were found in length of survival or mortality at 30 days.

Only a few studies have compared ES with LGJ. Faster relief of symptoms, reduced time of oral intake, fewer complications, and shorter length of hospital stay were observed after ES, while fewer recurrences of obstructive symptoms and less need for reintervention were seen with LGJ [26, 27]. Both procedures showed significant advantages compared to OGJ, as mortality was higher with the latter than with ES and LGJ (2.1 and 1.8 times higher, respectively) [28].

Procedural cost and reduced hospital stay favor ES but subsequent follow-up has shown adjunctive costs for reintervention. Stent migration and tumor in- or overgrowth may lead to recurrent duodenal obstruction in up to 25% of patients, who then need a second stent, thus decreasing the cost benefits of ES [25, 29]. However, even after stent replacement, ES is less costly than surgical procedures, with significantly less morbidity and mortality [30].

The choice of a palliation method depends on several factors including the patient's age and clinical condition, the site of the lesion and the specific cause of the GOO, as well as the clinician's skill and type of stent. In gastric cancer, the extension of the stenosis over the pylorus is less frequent than in pancreatic cancer. Rarely, the stent causes obstructive jaundice due to closure of the access to the common bile duct. Here, a non-covered stent is easily implanted and allows placement of a biliary stent in the same session. Non-covered stents also reduce the incidence of migration (6 vs. 19% with covered stents) [25]. Contraindications to ES are: high migration risk due to easy endoscope passage through the stricture, presence of multiple sites of stenosis not bridged by a single or two overlapping stents, severity of obstruction preventing passage of a guide-wire, and perforations. On the other hand, limitations for OGJ or LGJ are related to the position of the anastomosis at the greater curvature, which causes difficulty in oral intake.

In patients with pancreatic cancer, who have a very poor median survival, good results have been obtained with ES while in patients with gastric cancer, who have a relatively longer life expectancy, LGJ is preferred because of its more durable effects and fewer recurrent obstructive symptoms. In either case, OGJ or LGJ has to be considered in the absence of local skill in stent positioning or when ES fails to relieve duodenal obstruction

The use of stents 2–4 cm longer than the stenosis and with the largest diameter (20 or 22 mm) is recommended to prevent migration. A prospective multicenter clinical trial showed that WallFlex Nitinol (nickel titanium alloy) stents better conform to the duodenum than stents made of stainless steel or other alloys, allowing the resumption of solid foods within 7 days in 56% of patients, with 48% of them remaining on solid food until death or last follow-up [31].

There is no need to pass the endoscope through the stricture; rather, the stent, through the operative channel of the endoscope, may be deployed under radioscopic and direct visual control. Recurrent obstructive symptoms are classified based on timing and etiology: unrecognized multiple obstructions distal to the stent or poor gastrointestinal motility due to medications or infiltrations of the muscular layers or celiac plexus produce immediate symptoms. Stents that are too short may result in the need for reintervention (with a second, longer stent); this problem typically becomes apparent 1–2 weeks after the initial procedure. Delayed (weeks to months) recurrent symptoms are usually due to tumor in- or overgrowth and may be treated endoscopically [32].

Several chemotherapeutic agents have demonstrated activity against AGC and may be used after stent implantation to prolong the patient's survival. Shimura et al. compared 15 patients who received chemotherapy after surgery with 11 patients who received a stent followed by chemotherapy. No significant differences were reported in terms of survival and time to treatment failure [33].

A specific problem may arise from the gastric cancer infiltrating the esophago-gastric junction. In these cases, the angled position may produce severe stent complications, such as perforation or bleeding due to posterior gastric wall erosions or erosions of the proximal esophageal mucosa. Gastroesophageal reflux is reported in 5–7% of cases. Several authors have used stents with an anti-reflux valve. This has led to a reduction in the reflux symptom score but with similar effects on dysphagia as obtained with standard stents [34, 35].

References

1. Ohtsu A (2008) Chemotherapy for metastatic gastric cancer: past, present, and future. J Gastroenterol 43:256-264
2. Gencer D, Kästle-Larralde N, Oliz LR et al (2009) Presentation, treatment, and analysis of prognostic factors of terminally ill patients with gastrointestinal tumors. Onkologie 32:380-386
3. Oken MM, Creech RH, Tormey DC et al (1982) Toxixity and response criteria of the Eastern Cooperative Oncology Group. Am J Clin Oncol 5:649-655
4. Sarela AI, Miner TJ, Karpeh MS et al (2006) Clinical outcomes with laparoscopic M1 unresected gastric adenocarcinoma. Ann Surg 243:189-195
5. Kikuchi S, Tsutsumi O, Kobayashi N et al (1999) Does gastrojejunostomy for unresectable cancer of the gastric antrum offer satisfactory palliation? Hepatogastroenterology 46:584-587
6. Maltoni M, Caraceni A, Brunelli C et al (2005) Prognostic factors in advanced cancer patients: evidence-based clinical recommendations – A study by the Steering Committee of the European Association for Palliative Care. J Clin Oncol 23:6240-6248
7. Park JM, Chi KC (2010) Unresectable gastric cancer with gastric outlet obstruction and distant metastasis responding to intraperitoneal and folfox chemotherapy after palliative laparoscopic gastrojejunostomy: report of a case. World J Surg Oncol 8:109
8. Ohashi M, Kanda T, Hirota M et al (2008) Gastrojejunostomy as induction treatment for S-1-based chemotherapy in patients with incurable gastric cancer. Surg Today 38:1102-1107
9. Jeurnink SM, Steyerberg EW, van Hooft JE et al (2010) Surgical gastrojejunostomy or endoscopic stent placement for the palliation of malignant gastric outlet obstruction (SUSTENT study): a multicenter randomised trial. Gastrointest Endosc 71:490-499
10. de Rooij PD, Rogatko A, Brenna MF (1991) Evaluation of palliative surgical procedures in unresectable pancreatic cancer. Br J Surg 78:1053-1058
11. Neuberger TJ, Wade TP, Swope TJ et al (1993) Palliative operation for pancreatic cancer in the hospitals of the US Department of Veterans Affairs from 1987 to 1991. Am J Surg 166:632-637
12. Choi YB (2002) Laparoscopic gastrojejunostomy for palliation of gastric outlet obstruction in unresectable gastric cancer. Surg Endosc 16:1620-1626
13. Kaminishi M, Yamaguchi H, Shimizu N et al (1997) Stomach-partitioning gastrojejunostomy for unresectable gastric carcinoma. Arch Surg 132:184-187
14. Kubota K, Kuroda J, Origuchi N et al (2007) Stomach-partitioning gastrojejunostomy for gastroduodenal outlet obstruction. Arch Surg 142:607-611
15. Mimatsu K, Oida T, Kawasaki A et al (2009) Laparoscopic-assisted stomach-partitioning gastrojejunostomy for the palliation of gastric outlet obstruction from antral gastric cancer. Surg Laparosc Endosc Percutan Tech 19:e76-e79
16. Suzuki O, Shichinohe T, Yano T et al (2008) Laparoscopic

modified Devine exclusion gastrostomy as a palliative surgery to relieve malignant pyloroduodenal obstruction. Am J Surg 191:428-432
17. de Liaño AD, Yarnoz C, Aguilar R et al (2008) Surgical treatment of recurrent gastric cancer. Gastric Cancer 11:10-14
18. Badgwell B, Cormier N, Xing Y et al (2009) Attempted salvage resection for recurrent gastric or gastroesophageal cancer. Ann Surg Oncol 16:42-50
19. Song KY, Park SM, Kim SN, Park CH (2008) The role of surgery in the treatment of recurrent gastric cancer. Am J Surg 196:19-22
20. Cho YK, Kim SW, Nam KW et al (2009) Clinical outcomes of self-expandable metal stents in palliation of malignant anastomotic strictures caused by recurrent gastric cancer. World J Gastroenterol 28:3523-3527
21. Kim HJ, Park JY, Bang S et al (2009) Self-expandable metal stents for recurrent malignant obstruction after gastric surgery. Hepatogastroenterology 56:914-917
22. Kim J, Choi IJ, Kim CG et al (2011) Self-expandable metallic stent placement for malignant obstruction in patients with locally recurrent gastric cancer. Surg Endosc 25:1506-15013
23. Ly J, O'Grady G, Mittal A et al (2010) A systematic review of methods to palliate gastric outlet obstruction. Surg Endosc 24:290-297
24. Hosono S, Ohtani H, Arimoto Y, Kanamiya Y (2007) Endoscopic stenting versus surgical gastroenterostomy for palliation of malignant gastroduodenal obstruction: a meta-analysis. J Gastroenterol 42:283-290
25. Jeurnink SM, van Eijck CHJ, Steyerberg EW et al (2007) Stent versus gastro-jejunostomy for the palliation of gastric outlet obstruction: a systematic review. BMC Gastroenterology 7:18
26. Mehta S, Hindmarsh A, Cheong E et al (2006) Prospective randomized trial of laparoscopic gastrojejunostomy versus duodenal stenting for malignant gastric outflow obstruction. Surg Endosc 20:239-242
27. Mittal A, Windsor J, Woodfield J et al (2004) Matched study of three methods for palliation of malignant pyloroduodenal obstruction. Br J Surg 91:205-209
28. Siddiqui A, Spechler SJ, Huerta S (2007) Surgical bypass versus endoscopic stenting for malignant gastroduodenal obstruction: a decision analysis. Dig Dis Sci 52:276-281
29. Ely CA, Arregui ME (2003) The use of enteral stents in colonic and gastric outlet obstruction. Surg Endosc 17:89-94
30. Raikar GV, Melin MM, Ress A et al (1996) Cost-effective analysis of surgical palliation versus endoscopic stenting in the management of unresectable pancreatic cancer. Ann Surg Oncol 3:470-475
31. Piesman M, Kozarek RA, Brandabur JJ et al (2009) Improved oral intake after palliative duodenal stenting for malignant obstruction: a prospective multicenter clinical trial. Am J Gastroenterol 104:2404-2411
32. Carr-Locke DL, Alshalabi SM (2001) Expandable metal stents for malignant gastroduodenal and intestinal obstruction. Tech Gastrointest Endosc 3:85-92
33. Shimura T, Kataoka H, Sasami M et al (2009) Feasibility of self-expandable metallic stent plus chemotherapy for metastatic gastric cancer with pyloric stenosis. J Gastroenterol Hepatol 24:1358-1364
34. Shim CS, Jung IS, Cheon YK et al (2005) Management of malignant stricture of the esophagogastric junction with a newly designed self-expanding metal stent with an anti-reflux mechanism. Endoscopy 37:335-339
35. Power C, Byrne PJ, Lim K et al (2007) Superiority of anti-reflux stent compared with conventional stent in the palliative management of patients with cancer of the lower esophagus and esophago-gastric junction; results of a randomized clinical trial. Dis Esoph 20:466-470

Palliative Treatment

27

Mario Scartozzi, Walter Siquini, Alessandro Bittoni,
Luca Faloppi, and Stefano Cascinu

Abstract

Palliative care, defined as active total care of the patient, is a crucial concern in advanced gastric cancer. In the last few years, supportive treatment of cancer patients has considerably improved, mainly as a result of a multimodal approach involving surgery, endoscopic treatment, nutritional support, medical therapy, and nursing care. The main problems to be addressed by palliative care are ascites, intestinal obstruction, anorexia, and cachexia.

Keywords

Supportive care • Peritoneal carcinosis • Ascites • Catumaxomab • Pain management

27.1 Ascites

27.1.1 Introduction

Ascites is the abnormal build-up of excess fluid in the abdominal (peritoneal) cavity. It can be a sign of disease relapse or a mode of presentation for gastrointestinal tumors, particularly of the stomach, colon, and pancreas. [1–3]. Malignant ascites may be a manifestation of end-stage events in a variety of cancers and is associated with significant morbidity. About 50% of patients with malignant ascites present with ascites at the initial diagnosis of their cancer [4, 5]. Its onset and progression are associated with a deterioration in the quality of life and a poor prognosis [6]. Indeed, the median survival of patients with gastrointestinal cancer and malignant ascites is 1–4 months and is < 1% at 1 year [7].

M. Scartozzi (✉)
Dept. of Medical Oncology,
"Ospedali Riuniti" University Hospital,
Polytechnic University of Marche,
Ancona, Italy

27.1.2 Pathogenesis of Malignant Ascites

The pathogenesis of malignant ascites is multifactorial [8]: (1) Neoplastic colonization of the visceral or parietal peritoneum results in irritation and the blockage of fluid reabsorption; (2) decreased serum protein levels reflect malnutrition, liver damage, etc.; (3) hepatic invasion by the tumor causes portal venous system compression, leading to increased venous pressure, which in turn forces fluid out of the blood vessels and into the abdominal cavity. Invasion of the abdominal lymphatic vessels results in the inability of the lymphatic system to drain off excess fluid from the body.

G. de Manzoni, F. Roviello, W. Siquini (eds.), *Surgery in the Multimodal Management of Gastric Cancer*,

Table 27.1 Symptoms associated with ascites

• Swollen stomach and distended abdomen
• Abdominal pain, discomfort, and bloating
• Lethargy
• Breathlessness due to increased pressure on the diaphragm
• Dyspnea
• Nausea or vomiting
• Indigestion
• Reduced appetite
• Weight gain due to fluid accumulation
• Sense of fullness or bloating
• Ankle and feet swelling
• Constipation
• Hemorrhoids

27.1.3 Symptoms of Ascites

Mild ascites is usually asymptomatic, but as it progresses an increase in abdominal size is commonly seen. Other symptoms associated with ascites in advanced gastric cancer and other diseases are listed in Table 27.1.

27.1.4 Diagnosis

In the absence of clear clinical signs of an abdominal effusion, an ultrasound examination may be useful and can be added to an evaluation of ascites by paracentesis cytology. In fact, the cytologic examination may be particularly important if ascites is the first sign of neoplastic disease and the primary site of the cancer is not yet known. Indeed, the primary cause of malignant ascites is not clearly identifiable at presentation in approximately 20% of patients [2, 9].

27.1.5 Management of Ascites

Malignant ascites is in itself not a disease but merely a symptom; therefore, the best therapy is to treat the cancer directly. However, in many cases, malignant ascites occurs in a very advanced stage of disease. In these cases, the only treatment is palliative care, with the goal of reducing the associated symptoms.

Several studies have shown that paracentesis and the use of diuretics are the most common procedures in the management of patients with ascites, followed by the installation of a peritoneal-venous shunt and systemic or intraperitoneal chemotherapy [10]. However, very few prospective randomized trials have been conducted to compare the efficacy of the different treatment options.

27.1.6 Palliative Treatment

There are no data from prospective randomized trials to support the effectiveness of diuretics in patients with malignant ascites. Overall, in such cases, diuretics have an efficiency of 43% [10]. Some diuretics, such as spironolactone and furosemide, can be prescribed to reduce blood pressure, promote urination, and thus slow the accumulation of ascites. Reducing the patient's intake of sodium and fluid intake are also suggested.

However, the most frequent cause of ascites in advanced gastric cancer is blockage by peritoneal deposits. In these cases, diuretics or other drugs are usually of no help, since the malignant ascites is not caused by increased venous pressure. Although diuretics improve the condition of some patients, the risk of severe dehydration due to the use of these drugs in palliative care patients often exceeds the benefit. Thus, the only effective solution is palliative paracentesis [11], i.e., the removal of large amounts of liquids by aseptic puncture of the abdominal wall using a cannula connected to a drain. The ascitic fluid then drains out of the abdomen and into a drainage bag.

The potential complications of paracentesis are: (1) the risk of infection, especially peritonitis; (2) perforation of the bowel, other visceral organs, or tumor mass because of insufficient data on the location, type, and volume of the ascitic fluid; and (3) fluid volume depletion and protein loss. About 90% of patients receive good but temporary relief of symptoms with paracentesis. In patients with mild ascites that does not cause any discomfort, treatment may not be necessary.

There is currently no consensus either on the amount of liquid to be drained or on supportive actions aimed at preventing the complications of paracentesis [10]. The results of a prospective study of 44 patients treated with 48 paracentesis procedures suggested that a significant improvement in symptoms is achieved by removing a few liters of ascites (mean 5.3 L, median 4.9 L) [12]. Paracentesis, as already mentioned, can reduce the symptoms caused by ascites only temporarily, and several repeat procedures are necessary. Consequently, in patients who require frequent paracentesis and in whom life expectancy is more than 4 weeks, a permanent exterior peritoneal catheter may be a reasonable option.

In rare instances, surgery may be needed to control ascites associated with advanced gastric cancer and other types of ascites. The procedure involves placing a permanent shunt into an appropriate location to reduce portal pressure or to drain the ascitic fluid directly from the abdomen into a large vein. Initially used for intractable ascites due to liver cirrhosis, this device has since been applied in the treatment of cancer. The main systems used are the shunts of LeVeen and Denver [13, 14]. The main contraindications to shunt use are the presence of hemorrhagic ascites and ascitic fluid with a protein content > 4.5 g/l, due to the risk of occlusion associated with these conditions. Other contraindications are the presence of loculated ascites, portal hypertension, bleeding disorders, and cardiac and renal failure. Although the data may as yet be incomplete, the use of shunts does not appear to increase the risk of metastasis [15].

The response rate in patients with ascites from cancer of the gastrointestinal (GI) tract in whom a shunt device was placed is very low (10–15%). According to many authors, given the poor prognosis of these patients, the insertion of a peritoneal venous shunt is contraindicated [10]. In general, the placement of a peritoneal-venous shunt should be reserved for patients with ascites from non-GI tumors and who have a life expectancy > 3 months.

27.1.7 Medical Therapy with New Pharmacological Agents

Catumaxomab (Removab) is a trifunctional antibody that simultaneously activates T cells and accessory immune cells to destroy target tumor cells possessing the surface antigen epithelial cell adhesion molecule (Ep-CAM). It has been submitted for approval by the European authorities for the treatment of malignant ascites caused by Ep-CAM-positive metastatic epithelial-derived tumors, and is in phase II trials for the treatment of ovarian and gastric cancers.

A recent randomized phase II/III trial [16] showed that treatment with four intraperitoneal doses of catumaxumab yielded clinically relevant benefits in patients with recurrent malignant ascites due to carcinomas of different origin. As concluded by the authors of that study "Positive trends in OS together with its demonstrated efficacy against tumor cells in the peritoneal cavity support the antitumor activity of catumaxomab and suggest that it could be even more effective if used at an earlier stage in the treatment of epithelial cancers. Catumaxomab showed a typical pattern of adverse events that are mainly related to its immunologic mode of action. However, these are both, manageable and generally reversible. The [intraperitoneal] administration of catumaxomab can be regarded as a promising new therapy for malignant ascites." [16].

It also has been demonstrated that the release of vascular endothelial growth factor (VEGF) by tumor cells is a major factor promoting the secretion of intraperitoneal fluid. Consequently, recent studies have shown that targeting VEGF may stop the production of ascites caused by peritoneal metastases. Intraperitoneal administration of the anti-VEGF antibody bevacizumab (Avastin), which is already in use as an intravenous therapeutic drug for a variety of tumors, could be an effective way to prevent the local accumulation of fluid. Future clinical studies should rigorously assess the effectiveness of this targeted therapy for the treatment of malignant ascites [17].

27.2 Intestinal Obstruction

Complete or partial obstruction of the GI tract is a common occurrence in patients with advanced gastric cancer. Gastric cancer can cause upper-GI obstruction, as may occur in carcinoma of the gastric antrum with gastric outlet obstruction, or small-bowel obstruction, due to intra-abdominal metastasis and peritoneal carcinomatosis. Symptoms in upper-GI obstruction include postprandial pain, vomiting, and epigastric fullness while small-bowel obstruction can cause crampy abdominal pain, distension, and vomiting. Physical examination usually reveals percussion tympanism, and high-pitched bowel sounds. There may also be palpable masses and abdominal distension due to ascites. An abdominal X-ray with the patient in the supine and standing positions and contrast studies help to establish the site of occlusion and whether it is partial or complete. Endoscopy is useful to determine the site and cause of proximal-GI obstruction [18].

27.2.1 Treatment

The management of intestinal obstruction in patients with advanced gastric cancer includes surgery, endoscopic treatment, and palliative medical treatment. The patient should be carefully evaluated in order to determine the most appropriate and least distressing treatment for symptom management. In upper-GI obstruction, palliative surgery with the creation of gastrojejunostomy can be considered for bypassing the obstruction and maintaining gastrointestinal continuity. Nevertheless, some patients with advanced disease or those who are in generally poor condition, with a short life expectancy, are unfit for surgery and require alternative approaches to relieve distressing symptoms [18]. In accordance with the literature data, there are a number of absolute and relative contraindications to surgery in advanced cancer patients suffering from intestinal obstruction (Table 27.2).

Another option in the treatment of gastric outlet obstruction is the insertion of a bare or covered self-expanding metallic stent. These endoscopic, mini-invasive procedures are useful in patients with advanced disease who are not fit for surgery. High success rates (about 90%) in terms of symptom resolution and increased dietary intake following stent insertion have recently been reported. Severe complications are rare and include stent collapse (8–11%), intestinal perforation (1%), and stent migration (1%) (see Chap. 26) [19, 20].

Nasogastric suction and intravenous hydration comprise the usual initial hospital treatment of bowel obstruction; they are aimed at reducing secretions, vomiting, pain, and abdominal distension and at avoiding dehydration. The long-term use of a nasogastric tube is usually not indicated: in fact, it is often very uncomfortable for the patient and may cause complications. Medical treatment is an effective option for managing symptoms of inoperable bowel obstruction, the most useful agents being analgesics, anti-secretory drugs, and anti-emetics. The recommended route of drug administration in patients with intestinal obstruction is intravenously. Opioid analgesics, such as morphine, are the treatment of choice to control pain, with anti-cholinergics an option to better control colic pain. Vomiting can be managed through the use of anti-emetics, such as metoclopramide, and drugs that reduce gastrointestinal secretions, such as scopolamine butylbromide and octreotide. Octreotide is a synthetic analogue of somatostatin with the same biological effects but greater specificity and longer action (about 12 h). Octreotide decreases the secretion of water, sodium, and chloride by the intestinal epithelium, suppresses gas-

Table 27.2 Contraindications to surgery in intestinal obstruction (Modified from [18])

Absolute contraindications	Relative contraindications
1. Recent laparotomy demonstrating that further corrective surgery is not possible	1. Extra-abdominal metastases producing symptoms that are difficult to control, e.g., dyspnea
2. Previous abdominal surgery that confirmed diffuse metastatic cancer	2. Non-symptomatic extensive extra-abdominal malignant disease, e.g., widespread metastases, pleural effusion
3. Involvement of the proximal stomach	3. Poor general performance status
4. Intra-abdominal carcinomatosis demonstrated radiologically with a contrast study and revealing a severe motility problem	4. Poor nutritional status, e.g., marked weight loss/cachexia, marked hypo-albuminemia, low lymphocyte count
5. Diffuse palpable intra-abdominal masses	5. Advanced age in association with cachexia
6. Massive ascites that rapidly recurs after drainage	6. Previous radiotherapy of the abdomen or pelvis

trointestinal and pancreatic secretion, reduces mesenteric flow and pressure, and inhibits intestinal motility. It can be administered by subcutaneous bolus injection or intravenous infusion. The starting dose is 0.3 mg/day but the dose can be titrated until symptom control is reached. Two randomized studies compared octreotide 0.3 mg/day and scopolamine butylbromide 60 mg/day in patients with inoperable malignant bowel obstruction. Octreotide was shown to be more effective and faster than scopolamine butylbromide in reducing GI secretions, nausea, and number of vomiting episodes [21, 22]. Corticosteroids, such as dexamethasone, may be combined with other anti-emetics drugs to reduce peritumoral and perineural edema in order to improve vomiting control. Intravenous hydration is important to avoid dehydration. The administration of 1000–1500 ml/day is effective to reduce symptoms such as nausea and drowsiness. If a central catheter is not available, fluid administration via hypodermoclysis is a valid alternative.

27.3 Anorexia and Cachexia

In patients with gastric cancer, the disease course includes a progressive under-nutrition. Essentially, this is the result of two main mechanisms: anorexia, in which there is a reduced nutritional intake due to symptoms linked to the primary disease or to the side effects of treatment, and cachexia, a complex metabolic syndrome caused by the release of endogenous transmitters and cytokines by tumor cells.

Anorexia is quite usual in gastric cancer patients for several reasons. The primary tumor can be responsible for anorexia by causing both stenosis of the GI tract and dysphagia, such as frequently occurs in esophago-gastric junctions tumors. In addition, patients with peritoneal metastasis may have alterations of intestinal motility, with subsequent nausea and vomiting and therefore reduced nutritional intake. The side effects of systemic treatment such as chemotherapy also can be responsible for anorexia, due to the common toxicities of nausea, vomiting, and taste alterations, which lead to reduced nutrition.

Cachexia is a syndrome characterized by loss of body weight (> 10%), negative energetic balance, and loss of skeletal muscle. In these patients, there are important metabolic and hormonal alterations as well as a change in body composition. Cytokines such as tumor necrosis factor (TNF)-α, interleukin (IL)-6, and interferon (IFN)-y are possible mediators of the enhanced protein catabolism. The clinical features of cachexia include weight loss, with a very low subcutaneous fat mass and reduced muscle mass but normal levels of serum proteins. Hormonal alterations include an increase in serum insulin and cortisol, with subsequent alterations in carbohydrate metabolism, such as glucose intolerance and an increase in gluconeogenesis (see Chap. 28).

Anorexia and cancer cachexia may have synergistic negative effects on patients' status, in terms of quality of life, morbidity, and survival. Nutritional support is thus an essential component of the palliative treatment of patients with advanced gastric cancer. A preliminary assessment of nutritional status and energy intake should be performed at the beginning of the disease. If a low energy intake for a long period of time is expected, nutritional therapy is indicated. Usually, energy intake should be about 1.2–1.5 times higher than the resting energy expenditure. To counteract cachexia, the lipid proportion of nutrition should account for 40–60% of total energy intake. Also, protein intake should be higher than in healthy people. High-calorie and high-protein dietary supplements, with the use of sip feeding, are recommended as a first step in the nutritional support of cancer patients. Tube feeding is indicated when adequate energy and nutrient uptake is not possible through oral strategies for a long period of time (more than 7–10 days). Naso-gastric or naso-jejunal tubes can be used if nutrition is necessary only for short periods, as they are very uncomfortable for patients, while percutaneous endoscopic gastrostomy is useful in cases of upper-GI obstruction or when nutritional support is necessary for longer periods. Parenteral nutrition (PN) is indicated when enteral nutrition is not possible, as often occurs in bowel obstruction or bowel disease with impaired digestion. PN can help to stabilize the patient's weight, attenuate deterioration of nutritional status, and improve quality of life [23]. However, the use of PN in patients with advanced cancer who are receiving palliative treatment and have a low life expectancy (< 3 months and Karnofsky performance status < 50%) is very controversial [24] and should be discussed with the patient and his or her family. In the very last phase of life, hydration with 1000–1500 ml of isotonic saline is generally sufficient.

References

1. Runyon BA (1994) Care of patients with ascites. N Engl J Med 330:337-342
2. Parsons SL, Watson SA, Steele RJC (1996) Malignant ascites. Br J Surg 83:6-4
3. Runyon BA, Hoefs JC, Morgan TR (1988) Ascitic fluid analysis in malignancy-related ascites. Hepatology 8:1104-1109
4. Garrison RN, Kaelin LD, Galloway RH, Heuser LS (1986) Malignant ascites: clinical and experimental observations. Ann Surg 203:644-651
5. Parsons SL, Lang MW, Steele RJC (1996) Malignant ascites: a 2 year review from a teaching hospital. Eur J Surg Oncol 22:237-239
6. Ayantude AA, Parsons SL (2007) Pattern and prognostic factors in patients with malignant ascites: a retrospective study. Ann Oncol 18:945-949
7. Runyon BA (1994) Care of patients with ascites. N Engl J Med 330:337-342
8. Rosemberg SM (2006) Palliation of malignant ascites. Gastroenterol Clin N Am 35:189-199
9. Ringenberg QS, Doll DC, Loy TS et al (1989) Malignant ascites of unknown origin. Cancer 64:753-755
10. Becker G, Galand D, Blum HE (2006) Malignant ascites: systematic review and guidelines for treatment. Eur J Cancer 42:589-597
11. Pockros PJ, Esrason KT, Nguyen C et al (1992) Mobilization of malignant ascites with diuretics is dependent on ascitic fluid characteristics. Gastroenterology 103:1203-1306
12. McNamara P (2000) Paracentesis - an effective method of symptom control in the palliative care setting? Palliative Med 14:62-64
13. LeVeen HH, Cristoudias G, Ip M et al (1974) Peritoneovenous shunting for ascites. Ann Surg 180:580-590
14. Lund RH, Newkirk JB (1979) Peritoneovenous shunting system for surgical management of ascites. Vol Surg 14:31-45
15. Adam RA, Adam YG (2004) Malignant ascites: past, present, and future. J Amer Coll Surg 198:999-1011
16. Heiss MM, Murawa P, Koralewski P et al (2010) The trifunctional antibody catumaxomab for the treatment of malignant ascites due to epithelial cancer: results of a prospective randomized phase II/III trial. Int J Cancer 127:2209-2221
17. Kobold S, Hegewisch-Becker S, Oechsle K et al (2009) Intraperitoneal VEGF inhibition using bevacizumab: a potential approach for the symptomatic treatment of malignant ascites? Oncologist 14:1242-1251
18. Ripamonti C, Twycross R, Baines M et al (2001 Clinical-practice recommendations for the management of bowel obstruction in patients with end-stage cancer. Support Care Cancer 9:223-233
19. Lowe AS, Beckett CG, Jowett S et al (2007) Self-expandable metal stent placement for the palliation of malignant gastroduodenal obstruction: experience in a large, single, UK centre. Clin Radiol 62:738-744
20. Kim JH, Song HY, Shin JH et al (2009) Metallic stent placement in the palliative treatment of malignant gastric outlet obstructions: primary gastric carcinoma versus pancreatic carcinoma. AJR Am J Roentgenol 193:241-247
21. Ripamonti C, Mercadante S, Groff L et al (2000) Role of octreotide, scopolamine butylbromide, and hydration in symptom control of patients with inoperable bowel obstruction and nasogastric tubes: a prospective randomized trial. Pain Symptom Manag 19:23-34
22. Mercadante S, Ripamonti C, Casuccio A et al (2000) Comparison of octreotide and hyoscine butylbromide in controlling gastrointestinal symptoms due to malignant inoperable bowel obstruction. Support Care Cancer 8:188-191
23. Ockenga J, Valentini L (2005) Review article: anorexia and cachexia in gastrointestinal cancer. Aliment Pharmacol Ther 22:583-594
24. Bozzetti F, Cozzaglio L, Biganzoli E et al (2002) Quality of life and length of survival in advanced cancer patients on home parenteral nutrition. Clin Nutr 21:281-288

Gastric Cancer: a Model to Study Skeletal Muscle Wasting of Cachexia

28

Maurizio Bossola, Fabio Pacelli, Fausto Rosa, Giacomo Cusumano, Antonio Tortorelli, and Giovan Battista Doglietto

Abstract

Cancer cachexia is a multifactorial paraneoplastic syndrome characterized by anorexia, decreased body weight, and loss of adipose tissue and skeletal muscle. It accounts for at least 20% of deaths in neoplastic patients. Cancer cachexia significantly impairs the quality of life and the response to anti-neoplastic therapies, thereby increasing morbidity and mortality of cancer patients. Muscle wasting is the most important phenotypic feature of cancer cachexia and the principal cause of function impairment, fatigue, and respiratory complications, mainly related to the hyperactivation of muscle proteolytic pathways. Most therapeutic strategies aimed at preventing cancer cachexia have proven to be only partially effective. The inhibition of catabolic processes in muscle has been attempted pharmacologically, with encouraging results in animal models. However, data in the clinical setting are scant and contradictory. Stimulation of muscle anabolism could represent a promising and valid therapeutic alternative for cancer-related muscle wasting.

Keywords

Cancer cachexia • Muscle wasting • Anabolic mechanisms • Gene-therapy

28.1 Introduction

Each year, approximately 2 million people die worldwide due to the consequences of cancer-related cachexia [1, 2]. This debilitating and life-threatening syndrome is present in about 50% of cancer patients, with a higher prevalence in patients with tumors of the gastrointestinal tract and the lung, than in those with other solid neoplasms, such as breast and thyroid cancer, and hematological malignancies. The clinical features that characterize cancer cachexia are progressive weight loss, anorexia, metabolic alterations, asthenia, depletion of lipid stores, and severe loss of skeletal muscle protein.

Cachexia occurs in most terminally ill cancer patients, accounting for about 20% of all cancer deaths [1, 2]. However, 80% of patients with cancers of the upper gastrointestinal tract and 60% of those with lung cancer will, upon diagnosis, have already experienced some degree of weight loss [1, 2]. Moreover, several of the metabolic, biochemi-

M. Bossola (✉)
Digestive Surgery Unit, Dept. of Surgical Sciences,
Catholic University of Rome,
"A. Gemelli" Hospital,
Rome, Italy

G. de Manzoni, F. Roviello, W. Siquini (eds.), *Surgery in the Multimodal Management of Gastric Cancer*,

cal, and molecular alterations currently believed to be responsible for the phenotypic features of cachexia are already present upon first cancer diagnosis, even in the absence of a significant reduction in body weight [3, 4]. Cancer cachexia negatively affects mortality, surgical risk, response to first- and second-line chemo-/radiotherapy, and quality of life [1, 2]. Unfortunately, the progressive loss of muscle mass and function that is the predominant feature of cancer cachexia is only minimally reversible with the currently available nutritional, metabolic, and pharmacological therapies [1, 2]. Consequently, the development of early and effective interventions aimed at preventing rather than reversing the metabolic perturbations ultimately leading to muscle wasting and cachexia is urgently needed and as such has fostered intensive basic and clinical research efforts.

28.2 Pathogenesis

The pathogenesis of cancer cachexia is multifactorial and includes reduced food intake, alterations in energy and substrate metabolism, and accelerated fat and muscle loss [5]. These are discussed in detail in the following sections.

28.2.1 Anorexia and Reduced Food Intake

Many cancer patients experience a substantial reduction in nutrient intake that certainly contributes to weight loss [6]. Insufficient energy and protein intakes may be secondary to mechanical obstruction in the gastrointestinal tract, mucositis, vomiting, malabsorption, pain, depression, anti-neoplastic treatments and, importantly, anorexia, i.e., the decreased desire to eat [7]. The pathogenesis of cancer-related anorexia is complex and multifactorial and implies a disruption of the central and peripheral messages physiologically regulating eating behavior [8].

28.2.2 Altered Energy and Substrate Metabolism

Together with reduced food intake, increased resting energy expenditure (REE), secondary to the imbalance between pro-inflammatory and anti-inflammatory cytokines, has been long considered an essential factor in the pathogenesis of cancer cachexia. However, this view has been recently reconsidered because the metabolic response to cancer may be extremely heterogeneous, with some patients showing hypermetabolism and others hypometabolism, the latter as a consequence of reduced physical activity [9-13]. Glucose intolerance, insulin resistance, increased gluconeogenesis from amino acids and lactate, increased fat oxidation, and reduced lipogenesis are the prominent disturbances in energy substrate metabolism [3]. Protein metabolism is also affected as there is an increase in whole-body protein turnover in the majority of patients with advanced-stage cancer [12]. Loss of fat mass, frequently severe, also commonly occurs in cachectic cancer patients [13].

28.2.3 Muscle Wasting

The loss of muscle mass is the most prominent phenotypic feature of cancer cachexia. It causes functional impairment with consequent deterioration of the quality of life. Muscle mass is the result of the balance between the rates of muscle-protein synthesis and breakdown. Cancer-related muscle atrophy may result from increased protein degradation, reduced protein synthesis, or both [14]. Muscle hypercatabolism is secondary to the hyperactivation of the calcium-dependent and the ATP-ubiquitin-dependent proteolytic pathways [15, 16]. Activation of calcium-dependent proteases (calpains), which have been demonstrated in the muscle of tumor-bearing rats, seems to be essential for the initial degradation of myofibrillar proteins, thus releasing actin and myosin, and for rendering them available for further degradative steps [15]. ATP-ubiquitin-dependent protein degradation is made up of two main steps: First, through an enzymatic cascade (ubiquitin-activating, ubiquitin-conjugating, and ubiquitin-ligating enzymes), multiple ubiquitin molecules are covalently attached to the protein substrate. Second, the polyubiquitinated protein is degraded by the 26S proteasome complex, whose catalytic core, the 20S proteasome, is characterized by five peptidase activities, namely, trypsin-like (TL), chymotrypsin-like (CTL), peptidyl-glutamyl peptidase (PGP), branched-chain amino acid-preferring, and small neutral-amino-acid-preferring activities [17]. Up-regulation of components of the ATP-ubiquitin-dependent pathway has been reported in experimental models of wasting conditions, such as sepsis, trauma, burns, renal failure, acidosis, and cancer [18-22]. Three intracytoplasmic ubiquitin-ligating enzymes, namely, E3α and ligases encoded by the genes *MURF-1* (muscle ring finger protein 1) and *MAFbx* (muscle atrophy F-box protein, also called atrogin-1), play significant roles in the onset of muscle atrophy [23].

28.3 Gastric Cancer: A Model to Study Skeletal Muscle Wasting of Cachexia

Patients with gastric cancer suffer anorexia, weight loss, and metabolic alterations suggestive of cachexia. This frequently happens in advanced stages of the disease but it may occur also in early-stage gastric cancer. For many years, our group has studied the cellular mechanisms underlying the loss of muscle mass in these patients. These studies are based on the resection and analysis of a small fragment of the rectus abdominis muscle in gastric cancer patients undergoing surgery at the Division of Digestive Surgery of the Catholic University of Rome. The results of these studies are summarized below:

28.3.1 Calpains

Samples were obtained from 15 gastric cancer patients with weight loss < 5% and from 15 patients who underwent abdominal surgery for benign disease (cholelithiasis) [24]. The biopsy samples were analyzed in the Department of Surgery, Beth Israel Deaconess Medical Center, Boston, MA. Muscle calpain activity was approximately 70% higher in the samples from cancer patients than in those from control patients. Expression of the μ- and m-calpain genes as well as the endogenous calpain inhibitor calpastatin was similar in muscle from control and cancer patients. Although there was a trend towards higher mRNA levels for atrogin-1 and MuRF1 in cancer patients, these differences did not reach statistical significance. Taken together, our results suggest that increased calpain activity in skeletal muscle is an early response to cancer, occurring before activation of the ubiqutin-proteasome pathway and loss of muscle mass have become evident.

Various authors have proposed a model of muscle wasting in which calpain-dependent cleavage of myofilaments and proteins anchoring myofilaments to the Z disk result in the release of myofilaments from the sarcomere followed by ubiquitination and proteasome-dependent degradation of the myofilaments [25-28]. Although the present results support such a model, that support needs to be interpreted with great caution, since we did not measure myofilament release from the sarcomere or the ubiquitination and proteasome-dependent degradation of the myofibrillar proteins. In addition, other mechanisms have been proposed for the release of myofilaments from the sarcomere, most importantly, increased caspase-3 activity [29]. Indeed, a recent study by our laboratory could not confirm caspase-3 activation in muscle from cancer patients [30].

28.3.2 NF-κB

The expression of NF-κB and IκB was assessed in muscle from 10 control patients and 14 gastric cancer patients in collaboration with the Department of Health Sciences of the University of Boston. The nuclear levels of p50 or Bcl-3 were similar to those of controls; there was no change in nuclear p65 levels, although a moderate increase in phospho-p65 was noted; and the expression of IκB (25%) was significantly decreased [31]. This observation was independent of the stage of cancer or the degree of cachexia, suggesting that IκB degradation and thus NF-κB activation are early and sustained events in gastric cancer muscle cells. NF-κB represents a family of five transcription factors (p65 (Rel A), Rel B, c-Rel, p52 and p50) that mediate a variety of processes depending on cell type and upstream trigger. All of these transcription factors are expressed in skeletal muscle [32]. The activation of NF-κB is achieved by nuclear transport of heterodimers of NF-κB family members and often occurs by the ubiquitination and degradation of the inhibitory protein IκB. The observation that IκB protein expression is decreased by 25% in the skeletal muscle of cancer patients is in agreement with data obtained in rodent disuse muscle atrophy [33] and in muscle from patients with chronic obstructive pulmonary disease [34].

28.3.3 Ubiquitin-proteasome

Consistent with experimental observations, we found that ubiquitin (Ub) mRNA expression was markedly and significantly increased in muscle biopsies obtained preoperatively in 20 patients undergoing surgery for gastric cancer [35]. Northern blot analysis of the skeletal muscle revealed two-fold higher Ub mRNA levels in gastric cancer patients than in controls (2345 ± 195 vs. 1162 ± 132, p = 0.0005). The levels of Ub mRNA did not correlate with age, percent weight loss, or total lymphocyte count nor with serum cortisol, fT3, sTNFR, serum albumin, or BMI. The levels of Ub mRNA and serum sTNF-receptor were not influenced by the magnitude of weight loss. Ub levels were higher in samples obtained from patients with stage IV disease (3,799±66) than in those with stages I and II disease (1945 ± 786; p = 0.009) and stage III disease (2480 ± 650; p = 0.026). The Spearman rank test revealed a direct correlation between Ub mRNA levels and disease stage (p = 0.005). Further confirmatory evidence of the involvement of ATP-ubiquitin-dependent proteolysis in cancer-related muscle degradation comes from the finding that proteasome activity is significantly increased in the muscle of gastric cancer patients (5-fold increase in CTL activity, and a 2-fold increase in TL and PGP activities) and that these changes are paralleled by concomitant overexpression of muscle Ub mRNA. The observation that both Ub mRNA overexpression and increased proteasome proteolytic activities occur even in patients with insignificant or no weight loss strongly suggests that the causative mechanisms of cancer cachexia are functionally present early during the clinical course of human neoplastic disease, underscoring the need for early preventive/therapeutic interventions.

28.3.4 Apoptosis

Apoptosis is a tightly regulated process in which cell death is mediated by a programmed sequence of events [36]. In mononucleated cells, apoptosis leads directly to cell death while in multinucleated cells such as the myocyte it causes cell atrophy [36]. Recent experimental studies have reported that skeletal muscle apotosis is increased in cancer [37], burns [38], hindlimb unweighting [39], denervation [40], and aging [41], suggesting that apoptosis is an alternative mechanism by which the loss of muscle tissue can be initiated by perturbations such as ischemia, direct injury, heat shock, growth factor withdrawal, or toxins and cytokines. Evidence of enhanced muscular apoptosis has been demonstrated in humans with chronic heart failure [42], chronic alcoholic skeletal myopathy [43], thyroid myopathies [44], sporadic amyotrophic lateral sclerosis [45], and polyneuropathy spinal muscular atrophy [46]. A study conducted by our group [30] was aimed at verifying enhanced apoptosis in the skeletal muscle of 16 patients with gastric cancer with respect to controls. A biopsy specimen was obtained from the rectus abdominis muscle of subjects in each group. The occurrence of apoptosis in muscle biopsies was determined morphologically by the fluorescent transferase-mediated dUTP nick end.labeling assay and by immunohistochemistry for caspase-3 and caspase-1. The percentage of apoptotic myonuclei was found to be similar in cancer patients and in controls (1.5 ± 0.3 vs. 1.4 ± 0.2, respectively; p = ns), in gastric cancer patients with mild (1.6 ± 0.4) or moderate-severe weight loss (1.4 ± 0.5; p = ns), and in the different stages of disease (stages I–II: 1.5 ± 0.7; stage III: 1.3 ± 0.4; stage IV: 1.6 ± 0.3; p = ns). Immunohistochemistry showed the absence of caspase-1- and caspase-3-positive fibers in controls and in neoplastic patients. Poly-ADP-ribosyl polymerase, a typical caspase-3 substrate whose processing is indicative of caspase-3 activation, was not cleaved in muscle biopsies of cancer patients. These data suggest that skeletal muscle apoptosis is not increased in neoplastic patients with mild-moderate weight loss and argue against the hypotheses that caspase-3 activation is an essential step of myofibrillar proteolysis in cancer-related muscle wasting.

28.3.5 Muscle Regeneration

Another factor potentially contributing to the loss of muscle mass is a decrease in skeletal muscle regeneration. Skeletal muscle tissue, upon certain physiological stimuli or in pathological conditions, undergoes extensive repair processes aimed at preventing the loss of muscle mass [47]. The key cells in these processes are satellite cells [48]. During the perinatal phases of muscle growth and following any form of muscle injury, satellite cells are activated, initiate proliferation, and express Myf5 and MyoD, while Pax7 expression is progressively reduced; at this stage satellite cells are often referred to as myogenic precursor cells [47]. Subsequently, the expression of myogenin and MRF4 (both being MRF members) is up-regulated in cells beginning their terminal differentiation program, followed by permanent exit from the cell cycle, activation of muscle-specific proteins, such as sarcomeric myosin, and fusion with damaged muscle fibers or with themselves to produce new fibers that replace the dead ones. Defective skeletal muscle regeneration secondary to the potent inhibiting action of tumor necrosis factor-a was shown to contribute to muscle wasting in a mouse model of cachexia [49, 50]. Indeed, we demonstrated that necdin, a member of the MAGE family that plays an important role in skeletal muscle growth and repair in vivo, is selectively expressed in muscles of cachetic mice and that its expression is causally linked to a protective response of the tissue against tumor-induced wasting, inhibition of myogenic differentiation, and fiber regeneration [51]. In a recent study carried out in collaboration with the Department of Experimental Medicine of the University of Milano-Bicocca [52], we compared a group of gastric cancer patients with a group made up of similar age- and gender-matched controls. Gastric cancer patients showed a significantly higher percentage of weight loss and lower serum albumin levels. Pax7 expression was significantly higher in the muscle of gastric cancer patients than in controls. Expression of this protein was determined in stages IA–IB and in stages II and III. MyoD expression also was higher in cancer patients than in controls but only in stages IA–IB and not in more advanced stages of the disease. Myf5 expression did not differ significantly between cancer patients and controls nor did expression of the neonatal isoform of myosin heavy chain. Necdin expression was negligible in healthy adult muscles and significantly up-regulated in the muscle of gastric cancer patients, being highly increased in stages IA-IB but similar to control levels in stages II and III. The increased expression of genes involved in muscle regeneration in the skeletal muscle of gastric cancer patients suggests that, in contrast to what is commonly held, muscle regeneration is not impaired in cancer cachexia.

28.4 Conclusions

Cancer cachexia still represents a frustrating condition for both the patient and the physician. To date, very few therapies have been "approved" for the prevention and treatment of cancer-related anorexia and cachexia. However, in the last decade, various drugs have been tested in experimental animal models and in preliminary human trials, with promising results. The development of early and effective interventions aimed at preventing and reversing the metabolic perturbations ultimately leading to muscle wasting and cachexia is urgently needed and is currently the focus of intensive basic and clinical research efforts.

References

1. Inui A (2002) Cancer anorexia-cachexia syndrome: current issues in research and management. CA Cancer J Clin 52:72-91
2. MacDonald N, Easson AM, Mazurak VC et al (2003) Understanding and managing cancer cachexia. J Am Coll Surg 197:143-161
3. Rossi Fanelli F, Cangiano C, Muscaritoli M et al (1995) Tumour-induced changes in host metabolism: a possible marker of neoplastic disease. Nutrition 11:595-600
4. Bossola M, Muscaritoli M, Costelli P et al (2003) Increased muscle proteasome activity correlates with disease severity in gastric cancer patients. Ann Surg 237:384-389
5. Tisdale MJ (2003) Pathogenesis of cancer cachexia. J Support Oncol 1:159-168
6. Stepp L, Pakiz TS (2001) Anorexia and cachexia in advanced cancer. Nurs Clin North Am 36:735-744
7. Barber MD, Ross JA, Fearon KC (1999) Cancer cachexia. Surg Oncol 8:133-141
8. Laviano A, Meguid MM, Rossi Fanelli F (2003) Cancer anorexia: clinical implications, pathogenesis, and therapeutic strategies. Lancet Oncol 4:686-694

9. Dempsey DT, Knox L.S, Mullen JL et al (1996) Energy expenditure in malnourished patients with colorectal cancer. Arch Surg 121:789-795
10. Gibney E, Elia M, Jebb SA et al (1997) Total energy expenditure in patients with non small-cell lung cancer: results of a validated study using the bicarbonate-urea method. Metabolism 46:1412-1417
11. Falconer JS, Fearon KC, Plester CE et al (1994) Cytokines, the acute-phase response, and resting energy expenditure in cachectic patients with pancreatic cancer. Ann Surg 219:325-331
12. Jeevanandam M, Horowitz GD, Lowry SF et al (1984) Cancer cachexia and protein metabolism. Lancet 1:1423-1426
13. Fearon KCH (1992) The mechanisms and treatment of weight loss in cancer. Proc Nutr Soc 51:251-265
14. Bossola M, Pacelli F, Tortorelli A et al (2008) Skeletal muscle in cancer cachexia: the ideal target of drug therapy. Curr Cancer Drug Targets 8:285-298
15. Costelli P, Baccino FM (2003) Mechanisms of skeletal muscle depletion in wasting syndromes: role of ATP-ubiquitin-dependent proteolysis. Curr Opin Clin Nutr Metab Care 6:407-412
16. Costelli P, Tullio RD, Baccino FM et al (2001) Activation of Ca (2+)-dependent proteolysis in skeletal muscle and heart in cancer cachexia. Br J Cancer 84:946-950
17. Ciechanover A (1994) The ubiquitin-proteasome proteolytic pathway. Cell 79:13-21
18. Tiao G, Hobler S, Wang JJ et al (1997) Sepsis is associated with increased mRNAs of the ubiquitin-proteasome proteolytic pathway in human skeletal muscle. J Clin Invest 99:163-168
19. Fang CH, Li BG, Fischer DR et al (2000) Burn injury upregulates the activity and gene expression of the 20S proteasome in rat skeletal muscle. Clin Sci 99:181-187
20. Bailey JL, Wang X, England BK et al (1996) The acidosis of chronic renal failure activates muscle proteolysis in rats by augmenting transcription of genes encoding proteins of the ATP-dependent ubiquitin-proteasome pathway. J Clin Invest 97:1447-1453
21. Costelli P, Carbó N, Tessitore L et al (1993) Tumour necrosis factor-alpha mediates changes in tissue protein turnover in a rat cancer cachexia model. J Clin Invest 92:2783-2789
22. Baracos VE, DeVivo C, Hoyle DH, et al (1995) Activation of the ATP-ubiquitin-proteasome pathway in skeletal muscle of cachectic rats bearing a hepatoma. Am J Physiol 268:E996-E1006
23. Bodine SC, Latres E, Baumhueter S et al (2001) Identification of ubiquitin ligases required for skeletal muscle atrophy. Science 294:1704-1708
24. Smith I, Aversa Z, Hasselgren PO et al (2010) Calpain activity is increased in skeletal muscle from gastric cancer patients with no or minimal weight loss. Muscle Nerve 43:410-414
25. Williams AB, DeCourten-Myers GM, Fischer JE et al (1999) Sepsis stimulates release of myofilaments in skeletal muscle by a calcium-dependent mechanism. FASEB J 13:1435-1443
26. Goll DE, Thompson VF, Li H et al (2003) The calpain system. Physiol Rev 83:731-801
27. Hasselgren PO, Fischer JE (2001) Muscle cachexia: current concepts of intracellular mechanisms and molecular regulation. Ann Surg 233:9-17
28. Jackman RW, Kandarian SC (2004) The molecular basis of skeletal muscle atrophy. Am J Physiol Cell Physiol 287:C834-C843
29. Du J, Wang X, Miereles C et al (2004) Activation of caspase-3 is an initial step triggering accelerated muscle proteolysis in catabolic conditions. J Clin Invest 113:115-123
30. Bossola M, Mirabella M, Ricci E, et al (2006) Skeletal muscle apoptosis is not increased in gastric cancer patients with mild-moderate weight loss. Int J Biochem Cell Biol 38:1561-1570
31. Rhoads MG, Kandarian SC, Pacelli F et al (2010) Expression of NF-kappaB and IkappaB proteins in skeletal muscle of gastric cancer patients. Eur J Cancer 46:191-197
32. Hunter RB, Stevenson E, Koncarevic A et al (2002) Activation of an alternative NF-kappaB pathway in skeletal muscle during disuse atrophy. Faseb J 16:529-538
33. Judge AR, Koncarevic A, Hunter RB et al (2007) Role for I{kappa}B{alpha}, but not c-Rel, in skeletal muscle atrophy. Am J Physiol Cell Physiol 292:C372-C382
34. Agusti A, Morla M, Sauleda J et al (2004) NF-KappaB activation and iNOS upregulation in skeletal mucle of patients with COPD and low body weight. Thorax 59:483-487
35. Bossola M, Muscaritoli M, Costelli P et al (2001) Increased muscle ubiquitin mRNA levels in gastric cancer patients. Am J Physiol Regul Integr Comp Physiol 280:R1518-R1523
36. Sandri M (2002) Apoptotic signaling in skeletal muscle fibers during atrophy. Curr Opin Clin Nutr Metab Care 5:249-253
37. Ishiko O, Yoshida H, Sumi T et al (2001) Expression of skeletal muscle cells apoptosis regulatory proteins in plasma-perfused VX2 carcinoma bearing rabbits. Anticancer Res 21:2363-2368
38. Fujita T, Jeevendra Martyn JA (2000) Skeletal muscle apoptosis after burns is associated with activation of proapoptotic signals. Am J Physiol Endocrinol Metab 279:E1114-E1121
39. Allen DL, Linderman JK, Roy RR et al (1997) Apoptosis: a mechanism contributing to remodelling skeletal muscle in response to hindlimb suspension. Am J Physiol Cell Physiol 273:C579-C587
40. Rodrigues AC, Schmalbruch H (1995) Satellite cells and myonuclei in long-term denervated rat muscles. Anat Rec 243:430-437
41. Dirks A, Leeuwenburgh C (2002) Apoptosis in skeletal muscle with aging. Am J Physiol Regulatory Integrative Comparative Physiology 282:R519-R527
42. Adams V, Jiang H, Yu L et al (1999) Apoptosis in skeletal muscle of myocytes of patients with chronic heart failure is associated with exercise intolerance. J Am Coll Cardiol 33:959-965
43. Tews DS (2002) Apoptosis and muscle fibre loss in neuromuscular disorders. Neuromuscul Disord 12:613-622
44. Vescovo G, Volterrani M, Zennaro R (2000) Apoptosis in the skeletal muscle of patients with heart failure: Investigation of clinical and biochemical changes. Heart 84:431-437
45. Schoser BGH, Wehling S, Blottner D (2001) Cell death and apoptosis-related protein in muscle biopsies of sporadic amyotrophic lateral sclerosis and polyneuropathy. Muscle Nerve 24:1083-1089
46. Tews DS, Goebel HH (1996) DNA-fragmentation and bcl-2 expression in infantile spinal muscular atrophy. Neuromus-

cul Disord 6:265-273
47. Zammit PS, Golding JP, Nagata Y et al (2008) Muscle satellite cells adopt divergent fates: a mechanism for self-renewal? J Cell Biol 166:347-357
48. Cossu G, Biressi S (2005) Satellite cells, myoblasts and other occasional myogenic progenitors: possible origin, phenotypic features and role in muscle regeneration. Semin Cell Dev Biol 16:623-631
49. Coletti D, Moresi V, Adamo S (2005) Tumor necrosis factor-alpha gene transfer induces cachexia and inhibits muscle regeneration. Genesis 43:120-128
50. Moresi V, Pristerà A, Scicchitano B et al (2008) TNF inhibition of skeletal muscle regeneration is mediated by a caspase dependent stem cell response. Stem Cells 6:997-1008
51. Sciorati C, Touvier T, Buono R et al (2009) Necdin is expressed in cachectic skeletal muscle to protect fibers from tumor-induced wasting. J Cell Sci 122:1119-1125
52. Pessina P, Conti V, Pacelli F et al (2010) Skeletal mucle of gastric cancer patients expresses genes involved in muscle regeneration. Oncol Rep 24:741-745

Quality of Life After Gastrectomy

29

Natale Di Martino and Francesco Torelli

Abstract

The prognosis for gastric cancer patients in the Western world is poor, with an overall curability rate seldom exceeding 20%. Worldwide, however, thousands of "cured" patients will suffer from the consequences imposed by the surgical procedure. After total gastrectomy, many patients develop a variety of symptoms that are collectively referred to as the "postgastrectomy syndrome." Roux-en-Y esophago-jejunostomy is the preferred reconstructive method after total gastrectomy. Although the customary 50-cm-long Roux limb usually prevents alkaline-reflux esophagitis, other postoperative symptoms and malnutrition are still common problems. Some authors have suggested that malabsorption is responsible for postoperative malnutrition after total gastrectomy, whereas others hold the major cause to be inadequate caloric intake; however, it is most likely to be a multifactorial problem. Defining "quality of life" for gastrectomy patients is a complex matter, and there is no universally accepted definition. Functional effects, whether physiological, psychological, or social, are clearly an important consideration.

Keywords

Gastric cancer • Gastrectomy • Quality of life • Nutritional status • Food intake • Surgery • Malnutrition

29.1 Introduction

The prognosis for gastric cancer patients in the Western world is poor, with an overall curability rate seldom exceeding 20%. World-wide, however, thousands of "cured" patients will suffer from the consequences imposed by the surgical procedure [1, 2].

N. Di Martino (✉)
VIII Unit of General Surgery and Gastrointestinal Physiophatology,
Second University of Naples,
Naples, Italy

After total gastrectomy, many patients develop a variety of symptoms that are collectively referred to as the "postgastrectomy syndrome." These include early and late dumping, alkaline reflux, maldigestion, malabsorption, diarrhea, flatulence, tenesmus, and lack of appetite. Several hypotheses have been proposed to explain these symptoms, such as hypocaloric food intake, loss of duodenal passage, loss of the gastric absorption surface, lack of peptic digestion, bacterial intestinal overgrowth, and the development of exocrine and endocrine pancreatic insufficiencies. After total gastrectomy, most patients suffer from malnutrition and from weight loss (5–10 kg, or 2 BMI units), the majority of which takes place within the

G. de Manzoni, F. Roviello, W. Siquini (eds.), *Surgery in the Multimodal Management of Gastric Cancer*,

first 3 months postoperatively. If the patient remains without tumor recurrence, his or her weight then stabilizes and slowly recovers to nearly the preoperative level [1, 2].

Roux-en-Y esophago-jejunostomy is the preferred reconstructive method after total gastrectomy [3, 4]. Although the customary 50-cm-long Roux limb usually prevents alkaline-reflux esophagitis, other postoperative symptoms [5] and malnutrition are still common problems after total gastrectomy. The Roux-en-Y reconstruction bypasses the physiological route through the duodenum and may therefore result in disturbances in digestion and absorption mechanisms. The reservoir function of the stomach is lost after total gastrectomy as well—one of the many reasons that gastrointestinal surgeons are actively searching for an optimal reconstructive method for patients undergoing total gastrectomy [6].

In addition to curative resection of the cancer, postoperative quality of life is of vital importance for the patient [7]. Bacterial overgrowth may be an important pathophysiologic mechanism underlying the malnutrition that characteristically follows total gastrectomy, but results concerning the incidence of bacterial overgrowth are conflicting.

29.2 Historical Trends

The history of the treatment of gastric carcinoma can be said to start with Theodor Billroth's first successful gastric resection for carcinoma, in 1881 [8]. This was the first Billroth I operation; the Billroth II operation, i.e., gastric resection with gastrojejunostomy, was introduced in 1883. Total gastrectomy was first successfully performed by Schlatter in Switzerland in 1897 [9]. The patient was a 56-year-old woman who lived nearly 14 months after the operation. Her death was a consequence of secondary tumor implants in the liver.

Initially, intestinal reconstruction after total gastrectomy was for the most part performed by suturing the esophagus to the duodenum or to a loop of jejunum. The inevitable problem of regurgitation was solved with the adoption of the Roux-en-Y esophago-jejunostomy, in 1909 [10]. The concept of end-to-side esophago-jejunostomy was introduced in 1947 [3]; this procedure is now the standard method of reconstruction after total gastrectomy. The main objective in choosing the Roux-en-Y method after total gastrectomy is to prevent bile from refluxing into the esophagus. Bile may cause mucosal damage to the esophageal mucosa, i.e., alkaline esophagitis [11]. The great majority of experienced surgeons today use limb lengths of 40–60 cm.

29.3 Consequences of Total Gastrectomy

Malnutrition, assessed in terms of weight loss, is regarded as the most frequent complication after total gastrectomy. On the one hand, postgastrectomy postoperative symptoms, including early satiety, dumping, and anorexia, may reduce the amount of ingested food and thus cause malnutrition [12]. On the other hand, total gastrectomy causes many defects and disorders in digestive physiology. Nutrient digestion and absorption are altered by many different mechanisms. The grinding of foodstuffs and their mixing with digestive enzymes are changed, as is the timing of bile and digestive-enzyme secretion; gastric reservoir function is lost and hormonal and nervous regulation of the gastrointestinal canal is disturbed. Intestinal motility is frequently altered, as is the normal bacteriology of the small intestine. The pathophysiological mechanisms of malnutrition after total gastrectomy are listed in Table 29.1.

29.3.1 Malnutrition

29.3.1.1 Lost Gastric Function

After total gastrectomy, over and above the lost reservoir function of stomach, the mixing and the step-by-step delivery of chyme to the small intestine may be impaired. In addition, subsequent to a Roux-en-Y reconstruction the duodenum is bypassed and the output and mixing of bile and pancreatic enzymes with ingested food are delayed beyond the time necessary for proper digestion [13].

Intrinsic factor, which is delivered from the parietal cells of the stomach, is necessary for the absorption of vitamin B12. Consequently, vitamin B12 substitution is necessary after total gastrectomy.

Table 29.1 Pathophysiological mechanisms of malnutrition after total gastrectomy

Decreased intake	Lost reservoir function Postoperative symptoms Decreased appetite		
Maldigestion and malabsorption	Fat malabsorption	Inadequate mixing Inadequate micelle formation Inappropriate pancreas Stimulation	Loss of antrum Bacterial overgrowth Duodenal bypass (Roux-en-y) Vagotomy
	Increased motility Mucosal lesions Lack of gastric acid Lack of gastric lipase Lack of intrinsic factor Calcium, vitamin D, Fe Malabsorption	Lactose intolerance Villus atrophy	

29.3.1.2 Weight Loss

Malnutrition and weight loss characteristically occur in most patients after total gastrectomy. Significant weight loss after total gastrectomy has been reported [12, 14, 15], but both the frequency of weight loss and the opinions as to the cause of postoperative malnutrition are discussed controversially. Contrary to most other reports, Cristallo et al. [16] did not find weight loss in patients studied 1–3 years after total gastrectomy with Roux-en-Y reconstruction. They concluded that malnutrition is uncommon if adequate dietary intake is maintained.

29.3.1.3 Decreased Food Intake

Bradley [17] has shown that when patients are cared for under controlled hospital conditions after total gastrectomy, they are able to take in a well-balanced diet of carbohydrates, fats, proteins, vitamins, and minerals that is sufficient to maintain proper nutrition. These and similar results suggest that malnutrition is not an inevitable consequence of total gastrectomy and can be prevented by adequate calorie intake [15].

29.3.1.4 Maldigestion and Malabsorption

Proper nutrition initially requires the availability of the five essential foodstuffs: proteins, fats, carbohydrates, vitamins, and minerals. While access to these nutrients is necessary after total gastrectomy, it is equally important that the proper amounts of these foodstuffs be ingested, that digestion and absorption proceed in a normal fashion, and that the incorporation and conversion of these foodstuffs into tissue and energy sources occur.

Fat, rather than carbohydrate or protein, malabsorption is the most common malabsorptive disorder after total gastrectomy. Related to fat malabsortion, deficiencies in the absorption of fat-soluble vitamins (vitamin D, A, E, and K) may be possible after total gastrectomy. In particular, a deficiency of vitamin D together with calcium malabsorption may result in bone disorders in gastrectomized patients [18].

29.3.1.5 Mechanism of Maldigestion and Malabsorption After Total Gastrectomy

Fat malabsorption in post-gastrectomy patients has been explained by pancreatic insufficiency and pancreatico-cibal dyssynchrony. Pancreatic insufficiency is probably due to truncal vagotomy, which always accompanies total gastrectomy. Truncal vagotomy has been shown to disrupt enteropancreatic reflexes and to reduce the mucosal release of cholecystokinin [18].

Bypass of the duodenal passage, as is the case after Roux-en-Y reconstruction, may result in decreased pancreatic and bile excretion by diminished hormonal stimulation. Pancreatico-cibal dyssynchrony [18, 19] means that the timing of pancreatic juice excretion during digestion is too late to be effective for the proper absorption of fats. Both inadequate mixing of digestive enzymes with the ingested fat and diminished micelle formation due to bacterial overgrowth have also been suggested [17, 19].

Lack of gastric lipase is an inevitable consequence of total gastrectomy and likewise may alter fat absorption. Shortened small-bowel transit times after total gastrectomy have been described [5, 20] and lead to the inadequate absorption of nutrients.

29.3.2 Heartburn, Alkaline Reflux, and Regurgitation

Esophagitis after total gastrectomy would appear to be secondary to duodeno-esophageal reflux. In patients who have undergone subtotal or total gastrectomy, Stein et al. [21] found intestino-esophageal reflux to occur particularly during the postprandial period and in the early morning hours. Roux-en-Y esophago-jejunostomy has been the preferred reconstructive procedure after total gastrectomy because it prevents postoperative alkaline-reflux esophagitis [22].

A 35- to 50-cm length of small intestine between the esophago-jejunal and entero-entero anastomosis is considered necessary to prevent bile reflux into the esophagus [4, 23].

29.3.3 Roux-en-Y Stasis Syndrome and Early Satiety

The Roux-en-Y procedure may itself be partially responsible for the post-prandial fullness experienced by most patients after subtotal gastrectomy. This "Roux-en-Y syndrome" is characterized by chronic abdominal pain, persistent nausea, intermittent vomiting of food and bile, and weight loss, all in the absence of mechanical obstruction [24, 25].

29.3.4 Dumping and Diarrhea

The term "dumping" was coined by Mix in 1922 in reference to the rapid emptying of gastric content seen on barium radiography in patients with this condition [14]. Breakfast, which typically consists of high-carbohydrate liquids, is often associated with early postprandial dumping symptoms. Vasomotor and cardiovascular symptoms usually predominate, sometimes without gastrointestinal symptoms. The patient notes a rather rapid onset of weakness, faintness, and dizziness and will have an immediate urgent desire to adopt a reclining position. The late postprandial or hypoglycemic dumping syndrome is much less common.

After total gastrectomy, the primary mechanisms leading to dumping are obvious: lost reservoir function of the stomach and rapid emptying of hyperosmolar carbohydrates into the small intestine. However, after total gastrectomy, not every patient suffers from dumping; the disorder has been reported to occur in 29% of cases [26]. The most popular theory on the pathogenesis of dumping is the hyperosmolar load theory, according to which the rapid passage of a hyperosmolar meal into the small intestine results in a marked shift of extracellular fluid into the lumen [27]. This causes hypovolemia and hemoconcentration as well as dumping symptoms early after the meal. Late dumping is associated with hypoglycemia, as insulinotrophic factors from the small intestine are thought to be involved in the pathogenesis. It has been proposed that the exaggerated plasma levels of immunoreactive glucagon are due to the abnormal exposure of the distal intestinal mucosa (where the glucagon gene is expressed) to unabsorbed nutrients [28].

All types of gastric surgery may result in diarrhea postoperatively, but the incidence is higher in patients who have undergone vagotomy. Indeed, truncal vagotomy is associated with the highest incidence of postoperative diarrhea, around 20% [29].

29.3.5 Intestinal Dismotility

Surgical interruption of the vagus nerve, always a product of total gastrectomy, may alter co-ordination of the complex mechanisms of intestinal motility. Although truncal vagotomy has no dramatic effect on the gastrointestinal motor pattern per se, it may cause severe dysmotility when associated with a surgical repositioning of intestinal loops [30].

29.3.6 Bacterial Overgrowth

There are three main factors preventing the growth and accumulation of enteric bacteria in the upper intestinal lumen in a healthy person: intestinal motility, gastric acid, and immunologic or bacteriostatic intestinal secretions [31]. All of these defense mechanisms may be compromised after total gastrectomy. Bacterial overgrowth of the small intestine can result in bacterial overgrowth syndrome, with malabsorption of fat, carbohydrate, protein, and micronutrients, and clinical manifestations such as abdominal pain, diarrhea, and malnutrition. Fat malabsorption may be due to bile-acid deconjugation and intestinal mucosal damage caused by the overgrowing bacteria. Interestingly, bacterial overgrowth caused by atrophic gastritis or omeprazole treatment has not been associated with clinically significant fat or carbohydrate malabsorption [32].

29.4 Quality of Life After Total Gastrectomy

Defining quality of life (QoL) is a complex matter, and a universally accepted definition does not exist. Schipper et al. proposed "the functional effect of an illness and its consequent therapy upon a patient, as perceived by the patient" [33]. Functional effects usually are separated into three categories: physiological, psychological, and social. QoL, therefore, is a multidimensional construct. In a patient with gastric cancer, a physiological effect might be nausea or problems with swallowing, a psychological effect could be depression, and a social effect might be withdrawal due to embarrassment about being ill. Sometimes economic consequences are included in the functional effects of illness. There is also discussion of the spiritual effect of illness. In general, however, the triad of physiological, psychological, and social effects is considered to represent the QoL [34].

In gastric cancer specifically, the topic of QoL is virtually unexplored. Recent reviews of gastric cancer in major journals do not mention QoL at all, let alone discuss QoL in the context of one of the outcome measures. This is in sharp contrast, for instance, to breast cancer, in which QoL is assessed using well-developed and validated measures. Indeed, QoL is a major outcome variable that also influences the choice of medical management.

The number of long-term survivors after surgical resection for gastric cancer has been increasing as a result of early detection and the improved surgical techniques. Although survivors may be rendered free of disease by surgery, they often suffer from postoperative symptoms and functional losses. Thus, it is imperative to give more attention to the QoL of surgically treated patients with gastric cancer [35].

The QoL of patients with gastric cancer can be determined by assessing patient health perceptions

Table 29.2 Korenaga score of treatment-specific symptoms

Assessments	Score
1. Appetite	Good 2 Fair 1 Poor 0
2. Consistency of food	Normal 2 Soft 1 Liquid 0
3. Volume of food	Increased 2 Unchanged 1 Decreased 0
4. Frequency of eating	3 Times 2 4–5 Times 1 >6 Times 0
5. Eating time	<30 minutes 2 30–60 minutes 1 >60 minutes 0
6. Postprandial abdominal fullness	Never 2 Sometimes 1 Often 0
7. Heartburn	Never 2 Sometimes 1 Often 0
8. Diarrhea	Never 2 Sometimes 1 Often 0
9. Constipation	Never 2 Sometimes 1 Often 0
10. Insomnia	Never 2 Sometimes 1 Often 0
11. Body weight	Increased or unchanged 3 Decreased <5 kg 2 5–10 kg 1 > 10 kg 0
12. Swallowing problem	Never 2 Sometimes 1 Often 0
13. Vomiting	Never 2 Sometimes 1 Often 0
14. Dizziness	Never 2 Sometimes 1 Often 0

Table 29.3 Spitzer index scores after radical gastrectomy

Assessment Score
Activity
Working or studying full time or nearly so 2
Requires major assistance or reduced hours of work 1
Not working or studying 0
Daily living
Self-reliant for daily activities including transport 2
Requires assistance for daily activities 1
Not managing personal care or light tasks 0
Health
Appears to feel well most of time 2
Lacks energy more than just occasionally 1
Feels very ill, seems weak 0
Support
Good relationships and strong support from other(s) 2
Support limited by patient's condition 1
Support only when absolutely necessary 0
Outlook
Calm, positive outlook 2
Periods of anxiety or depression 1
Consistently anxious and depressed 0

Table 29.4 Post-gastrectomy diet

1. Meals are divided into six small feedings.
2. Avoid temperature extremes, not too hot or too cold.
3. Sugars and sweets are avoided.
4. Fluids are restricted to 5–6 glasses per day and offered 30–45 min after a meal.
5. Milk is eliminated in the beginning and gradually reintroduced (may never be tolerated with total gastrectomy).
6. The meal pattern is strict at first then liberalized as tolerated.
7. Eat slowly. A reclining position may be beneficial.
8. Increase portion sizes of foods gradually.
9. Avoid smoking, drinking alcoholic beverages.
10. Do not drink carbonated beverages.

according to the Spitzer index and by measuring treatment-specific symptoms according to the method of Korenaga et al., with some modifications [36]. Table 29.2 provides a 14-item survey designed to assess primary gastrointestinal function. The Spitzer index includes the following five items rated on a three-point scale: activity, daily living, health, support of family and friends, and outlook (Table 29.3). High scores reflect a better QoL [37].

Surgeons often recommend small, frequent meals after total gastrectomy. Carbohydrate-rich liquids should be avoided and solids should be eaten separately. Dietary short-chain fructo-oligosaccharides increase iron absorption and were shown to completely prevent subsequent anemia in rats subjected to total gastrectomy (Table 29.4).

The follow-up examination should include hematological and biochemistry tests of peripheral blood: red blood cell count, hemoglobin level, hematocrit, mean corpuscular volume of red blood cells, total protein level, albumin level, globulin level, iron, total iron binding capacity, calcium, phosphorus, magnesium, alkaline phosphatase, and vitamin B12 levels. Finally, a QoL assessment with, e.g., Korenaga score/Spitzer-index questionnaires, should be conducted.

References

1. Tyrvainen T, Sand J, Sintonen H, Nordback I (2008) Quality of life in the long-term survivors after total gastrectomy for gastric carcinoma. Journal of Surgical Oncology 97:121-124
2. Murawa D, Murawa P, Oszkinis G, Biczysko W (2006) Long-term consequences of total gastrectomy: quality of life, nutritional status, bacterial overgrowth and adaptive changes in esophagojejunostomic mucosa. Tumori 92:26-33
3. Orr TG (1947) A modified technique for total gastrectomy. Arch Surg 54:279-286
4. Donovan IA, Fielding JW, Bradby H et al (1982) Bile diversion after total gastrectomy. Br J Surg 69:389-390
5. Brägelmann R, Armbrecht U, Rosemeyer D et al (1996) Nutrient malassimilation following total gastrectomy. Scand J Gastroenterol 218:26-33
6. Nakane Y, Okumura S, Akehira K et al (1995) Jejunal pouch reconstruction after total gastrectomy for cancer. A randomized controlled trial. Ann Surg 222:27-35.
7. Liedman B, Svelund J, Sullivan M et al (2001) Symptom control may improve food intake, body composition, and aspect of quality life after gastrectomy in cancer patients. Dig Dis Sci 2001 Vol 46 N.12 pp 2673-2680
8. Billroth T, Offenes Schraiben an Herr Dr. L. Wittelshofer (1881) Wien. Med Wochenschrift 1:31-161
9. Schlatter CA (1897) A unique case of complete removal of the stomach – successful esophago-enterostomy recovery. Med Res 52:909-914
10. Ikard RW (1989) Collective reviews. The Y anastomoses of César Roux. Surg Gyn Obstet 169:559-567
11. Liedman B, Andersson H, Berglund B et al (1996) Food intake after gastrectomy for gastric carcinoma:the role of a gastric reservoir. Br J Surg 83:1138-1143
12. Ryu SW, Kim IH (2010) Comparison of different nutritional assessments in detecting malnutrition among gastric cancer patients. World J Gastroenterol 16:3310-3317
13. Olbe L, Lundell L (1987) Intestinal function after total gastrectomy and possible consequences of gastric replacement.

World J Surg 11:713-719
14. Eagon JC, Brent WM, Kelly K (1992) Postgastrectomy syndromes. Surg Clin North Am 72:446-465
15. Braga M, Zuliani W, Foppa L et al (1988) Food intake and nutritional status after total gastrectomy:results of a nutritional follow-up. Br J Surg 75:477-480
16. Cristallo M, Braga M, Agape D et al (1986) Nutritional status, function of the small intestine and jejunal morphology after total gastrectomy for carcinoma of the stomach. Surg Gyn Obstet 163:125-230
17. Bradley EL, Isaacs J, Hersh T et al (1975) Nutritional consequences of total gastrectomy. Ann Surg 182:415-427
18. Bae J-M, Park J-W, Yang H-K, Kim J-P (1998) Nutritional status of gastric cancer patients after total gastrectomy. World J Surg 22:254-261
19. Armbrecht U, Brägelmann R, Baumgart I, Stockbrügger RW (1994) Fecal chymotrypsin output in relation to fecal fat after partial and total gastrectomy. Gastroenterology 106:A219
20. Armbrecht U, Lundell L, Lindstedt G, Stockbrügger RW (1988) Causes of malabsorption after total gastrectomy with Roux-en-Y reconstruction. Acta Chir Scand 154:37-41
21. Stier A, Hölscher AH, Schwaiger M and Siewert JR (1994): Jejunumpouch nach totaler Gastrectomie - klinische und szintigraphisch Untersuchungen zu Funktion und Befindlichkeit. Zentralbl Chir 119:838-844
22. Matikainen M, Laatikainen T, Kalima T, Kivilaakso E (1982) Bile composition and esophagitis after total gastrectomy. Am J Surg 143:196-198
23. Hubens A, van Hee R, van Vooren W, Peeters R (1989): Reconstruction of digestive tract after total gastrectomy. Hepato-Gastroenterol 36:18-22
24. Fich A, Neri M, Camilleri M et al (1990) Stasis syndromes following gastric surgery: clinical and motility features of 60 symptomatic patients. Clin Gastroenterol 12:505-512
25. Mathias JR, Fernandez A, Sninski CA et al (1985) Nausea, vomiting and abdominal pain after Roux-en-Y anastomosis. Motility of the jejunal limb. Gastroenterology 88:101-107
26. Gustavsson S, Ilstrup MD, Morrison P, Kelly KA (1988) Roux-Y stasis syndrome after gastrectomy. Am J Surg 155:490-494
27. Geer RJ, Richards WO, O`Dorisio TM et al (1990) Efficacy of octreotide acetate in treatment of severe postgastrectomy dumping syndrome. Ann Surg 212:678-687
28. Miholic J, Ørskov C, Holst JJ et al (1991) Emptying of the gastric substitute, glucagon-like peptide-1 (GLP-1), and reactive hypeglycemia after total gastrectomy. Dig Dis Sci 36:1361-1370
29. Storer EH (1976) Postvagotomy diarrhea. Surg Clin North Am 56:1561-1568
30. Altomare DF, Rubini D, Pilot M-A et al (1997) Oral erythromycin improves gastrointestinal motility and transit after subtotal but not total gastrectomy for cancer. Br J Surg 84:1017-1021
31. Haboudi N, Montgomery R (1992) Small-bowel bacterial overgrowth in elderly people: clinical significance and response to treatment. Age Ageing 21:13-19
32. Saltzman JR, Kowdley KV, Pedrosa MC et al (1994): Bacterial overgrowth without clinical malabsorption in elderly hypochlorhydric subjects. Gastroenterology 106:615-623
33. Schipper H, Clinch J, Olweny LM (1996) Definitions and conceptual issues. In: Spilker B, ed. Quality of life and pharmacoeconomics in clinical trials. Philadelphia: Lippincott-Raven, pp 11-24
34. Kaptein A, Morita S, Sakamoto J (2005) Quality of life in gastric cancer. World J Gastroenterol 11:3189-3196
35. Lee SS, HY Chung, W Yu (2010) Quality of Life of Long-Term Survivors after a Distal Subtotal Gastrectomy. Cancer Res Treat 42:130-134
36. Korenaga D, Orita H, Okuyama T et al (1992) Quality of life after gastrectomy in patients with carcinoma of stomach. Br J Surg 79:248-250
37. Spitzer WO, Dobson AJ, Hall J et al (1981) Measuring the quality of life of cancer patients. A concise QL-index for use by physicians. J Chronic Dis 34:585-597

Total and Subtotal Gastrectomy with D2 Lymphadenectomy: Technical Notes

30

Walter Siquini, Pierpaolo Stortoni, Emilio Feliciotti, Raffaella Ridolfo, Sonia Maurizi, Alessandro Cardinali, Cristina Marmorale, Aroldo Fianchini, and Edoardo Landi †

Abstract

R0 resection remains the only potentially curative treatment for gastric cancer. The extent of the operation depends on tumor location and disease stage. The options for candidates for gastric resection include total, proximal, and distal subtotal gastrectomy. This chapter describes the technical performance of total and distal subtotal gastrectomy by providing a detailed step-by-step guide to both mechanical and manual procedures. Total gastrectomy is a major operation even in the hands of the experienced gastric surgeon. In those patients in whom adequate margins can be obtained, distal subtotal gastrectomy is associated with the same survival as total resection, diminishes perioperative morbidity, and improves quality of life. Since, in our opinion, both total and subtotal gastrectomy should be performed in association with extended lymphadenectomy (D2), we also provide an accurate description of this procedure.

Keywords

Total gastrectomy • Manual subtotal gastrectomy • D2 lymphadenectomy • Stapled subtotal gastrectomy • Roux-en-Y end-to-side esophagojejunostomy • Jejunal loop • Roux limb • Enteroenterostomy • Gastric stump • Gastrojejunostomy

30.1 Patient Preparation

Patients with severe malnutrition (i.e. > 10% loss of habitual body weight in the previous 6 months and/or serum albumin < 3 mg/dl without liver disease) are at greater risk of postoperative complications and mortality and require perioperative enteral or parenteral nutritional support. Parenteral feeding involves placing a central venous catheter (CVC).

The day before the operation, the patient is administered 2 L of an oral electrolyte solution for bowel preparation in the afternoon, and antithrombotic prophylaxis with low-molecular-weight heparin (SC enoxaparin sodium 4000 IU, 1 pre-filled syringe) approximately 12 h prior to surgery.

W. Siquini (✉)
Surgical Clinic, Dept. of Medical and Surgical Sciences,
"Ospedali Riuniti" University Hospital,
Polytechnic University of Marche,
Ancona, Italy

G. de Manzoni, F. Roviello, W. Siquini (eds.), *Surgery in the Multimodal Management of Gastric Cancer*,

Before the patient is transported to the operating theater, body hair extending from the intermammary line to the pubis vertically and between the midaxillary lines laterally is removed with electric shaver.

A CVC, a peridural catheter for post-operative analgesia, and a radial arterial line for arterial-pressure evaluation are placed in the operating room.

Antibiotic prophylaxis (2 g IV piperacillin) is administered together with the general balanced anesthesia and again after 3 h, if the operation has not been completed.

A vescical catheter and a nasogastric tube (NGT) are placed after induction of anesthesia.

30.2 Positioning the Patient on the Table

The patient is placed supine, with the left arm abducted, as required by the anesthetist, and the right arm adducted to leave sufficient room for the surgeon and the assistant standing on the surgeon's left. A heating mat is placed between the patient and the surgical table; further heating is provided by placing a warm air blanket on the patient's legs.

Optimal exposure of the operating field is obtained by raising the operating table at the base of the patient's chest. If a multisection table is not available, a bolster or an inflatable pillow is placed under the patient's back at the same level.

30.3 Positioning of the Operating Team

The surgeon stands on the patient's right side, opposite the first assistant. Two further assistants stand, respectively, on the surgeon's left and on the first assistant's right. The scrub nurse stands on the surgeon's right.

30.4 Start of the Surgical Procedure

30.4.1 Steps Shared by Total and Subtotal Gastrectomy

Incision

The operative field is disinfected by passing in succession two gauze pads soaked in povidone-iodine, or benzalkonium chloride if the patient is allergic to iodine. The disinfectant is allowed to act for 1-2 min.

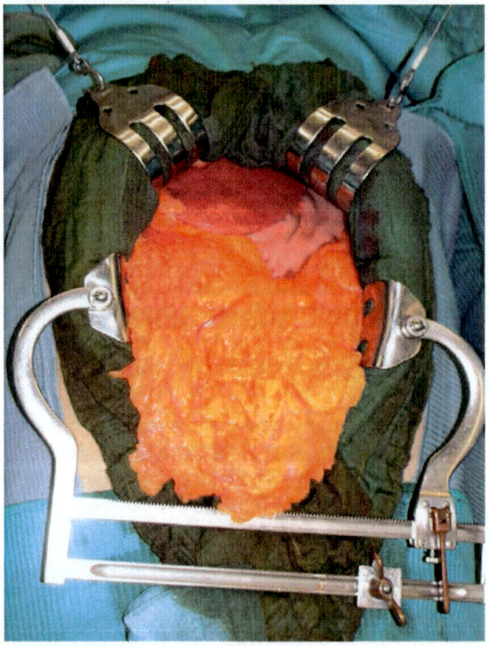

Fig. 30.1 The operative field is exposed

A midline incision from the xiphoid process to below the umbilicus is the most common approach for total and subtotal gastrectomy in patients with normal stature and weight. A bilateral subcostal incision provides better exposure of the esophagocardial region in short and obese patients; however, comparable exposure is afforded by a median incision using Kent or Rochard retractors (Fig. 30.1).

To minimize the risk of operation site infection, we secure a gauze laparotomy pad soaked in povidone iodine or benzalkonium chloride to either side of the incision with three full-thickness sutures, to protect those tissue layers in direct contact with the operating field (Fig. 30.1).

Exploration of the Abdominal Cavity

After the peritoneal cavity has been opened, the round and falciform ligaments are resected to expose the stomach and anterior surface of the liver. The left lateral portion of the liver usually covers the cardial region and the medial portion of the gastric fundus. For this reason, we prefer to resect the left triangular ligament completely and mobilize segments II and III medially, holding them back with a gauze-padded Mikulicz retractor. This affords optimal exposure of the cardia and the gastric fundus. The supra- and inframesocolic spaces are explored for nodules of omental or peritoneal carcinosis. In female patients the ovaries are inspected to exclude metastatic disease (Krukenberg tumor). The liver is also inspected, palpated, and subjected to ultrasound examination, thereby ruling out any metastases not documented on pre-operative computed tomography (CT) or magnetic resonance imaging (MRI).

Lavage Cytology

If free fluid is found in the supramesocolic space, a sample is collected and submitted for intraoperative cytology; otherwise, peritoneal lavage is performed with ca. 100 ml of saline poured upstream of the gastric wall involved by the neoplasm. The fluid is then recovered for intraoperative cytology.

Complete Detachment of the Greater Omentum from the Transverse Colon

The transverse colon is gently pulled caudalad by the first assistant and the omentum folded back and held cephalad by the second assistant. This allows the surgeon to identify the avascular embryonic fusion plane between the greater omentum and the anterior layer of the transverse mesocolon, and divides it from right to left. On the right side, the right posterior attachment of the transverse mesocolon is mobilized downward, to free the avascular plane and reach and expose the anterior surface of the duodenum and the pancreas. On the left side, it is essential to avoid excessive traction, resecting the phrenocolic and splenocolic ligaments early on and mobilizing the splenic flexure of the colon downward, to avoid splenic bleeding from accidental tear of the splenic capsule by some fibers of these ligaments. Complete detachment of the greater omentum from the transverse colon provides access to the lesser sac and exposure of the posterior wall of the stomach, anterior surface of the pancreas, right gastroepiploic vascular pedicle, and first and second portions of the duodenum. This leaves the right and left gastroepiploic arcade and the omentum attached to the stomach, allowing their en bloc removal.

Lavage of the Lesser Sac for Intraoperative Cytology

Exploration of the lesser sac after complete detachment of the greater omentum from the transverse colon enables assessment of the possible involvement of the serosa of the stomach by the posterior portion of the neoplasm. If the neoplasm infiltrates the serosa of the posterior portion of the stomach the exploration may show peritoneal carcinosis involving exclusively the lesser sac. In the absence of carcinosis more accurate staging is provided by sampling the fluid that may be found in the lesser sac. If no fluid is found, the neoplasm is flushed with saline and the solution is recovered for intraoperative cytology.

Kocherization and Para-aortic Lymph Node Dissection

If the para-aortic lymph nodes are enlarged on preoperative CT, these node stations should be removed (D3 lymphadenectomy) before the duodenal resection. Kocher's maneuver is executed with gentle duodenopancreatic mobilization and exposure of the inferior vena cava and aorta. The para-aortic lymphatic and adipose tissue between the left renal vein and the origin of the inferior mesenteric artery is removed and submitted for intraoperative consultation (Fig. 30.2). Positivity of these nodes is a highly unfavorable prognostic factor.

Division of the Pyloric Vessels

Detachment of the greater omentum from the transverse colon allows exposure of the right gastroepiploic pedicle, which is isolated and divided at its origin between double ligatures, leaving the infrapyloric lymph nodes (station 6) attached to the stomach. Subsequently the right gastric vessels are divided, allowing anterior and posterior dissection of the pylorus and the duodenal bulb for at least 3–4 cm.

Duodenal Transection and Oversewing

The duodenum is transected with a mechanical linear stapler (GIA 55) placed 2–3 cm below the

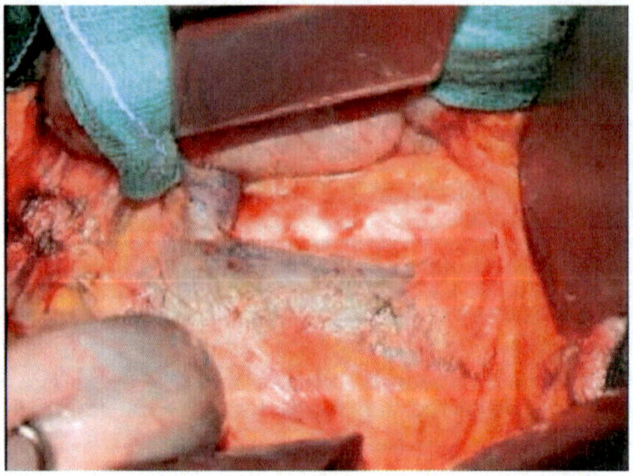

Fig. 30.2 The para-aortic lymphatic and adipose tissue between the left renal vein and the origin of the inferior mesenteric artery is removed and submitted for intraoperative consultation (D3 lymphadenectomy)

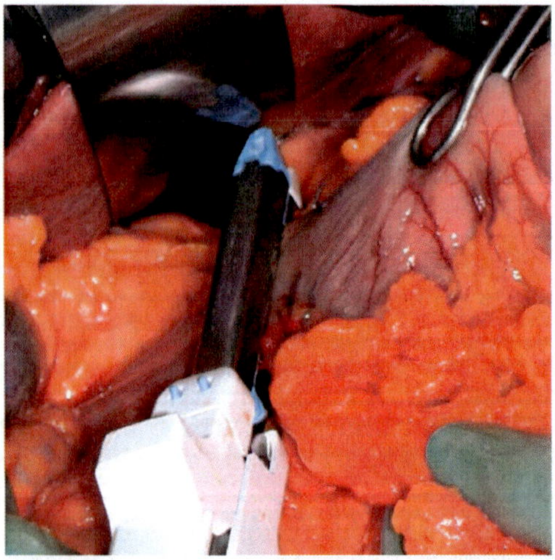

Fig. 30.3 After identification of the ideal resection level, the stapler's jaws are locked

pylorus, leaving an inferior margin of duodenal wall of at least 1 cm to allow subsequent oversewing. After identification of the ideal resection level, the stapler's jaws are locked (Fig. 30.3) and the duodenum is closed and resected. Unlike the TA 55, the GIA 55 closes both stumps, preventing contamination of the operative field by gastroduodenal secretions. A tampon soaked in povidone iodine is, however, passed on both stumps to minimize microcontamination. We then oversew the stapler line of the duodenal stump with interrupted seromuscular sutures using absorbable (polyglactin 910) braided 3–0 thread, to reduce the risk of leakage.

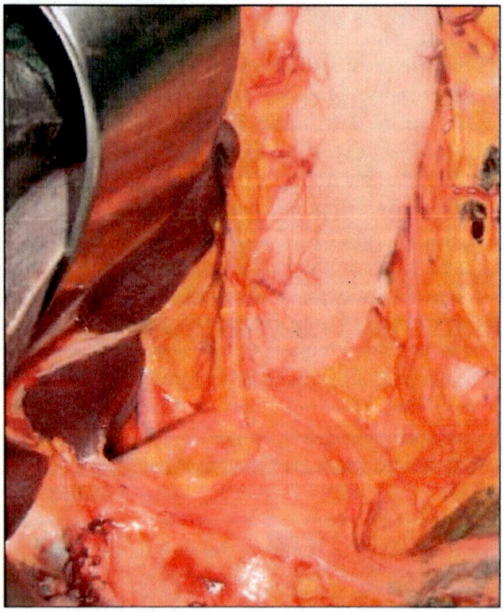

Fig. 30.4 The left gastric artery and vein are prepared for division

Ligature at the Origin of the Left Gastric Artery and Vein

After duodenal resection, the stomach is elevated and retracted over the subcostal retractor, slightly tensioning its posterior wall and, consequently, the left gastric pedicle, which is thus easily identified and prepared for division (Fig. 30.4). With the stomach elevated and retracted upward, the left gastric vein is usually seen anterior to the artery; the vein is dissected first and ligated at its origin, then the artery, which is found immediately behind it, is resected at its origin with double ligature. The lymph nodes found at the origin of this vascular pedicle (station 7) are collected and sent separately for the final histological examination.

30.5 Total Gastrectomy

30.5.1 Division of the Lesser Omentum

On the medial side, if tumor site and oncological guidelines mandate total gastrectomy, the inferior (pars flaccida) and superior (pars condensa) portions of the lesser omentum close to the liver are resected, so that they can be removed en bloc with the stomach. If the lesser omentum is divided up to the right crus of the diaphragm and the right esophageal wall, the lymphatic and adipose tissue of the lesser curvature and the right paracardial lymph nodes will remain attached to the stomach. The latter nodes (station 1) should be collected and sent separately for final histological examination.

30.5.2 Resection of the Gastrosplenic Ligament

On the side of the greater curvature, the gastrosplenic ligament is identified on the plane of the dissection of the greater omentum from the transverse colon and resected, proceeding from low to high, carefully ligating its 4–6 short gastric vessels. After ligation of short gastric vessels, the spleen is definitively freed from the stomach and access is gained to the left paracardial region and crus of the diaphragm. Both crura of the diaphragm are now free, and the posterior right and left portions of the intra-abdominal esophagus are completely mobilized. Only the tumor's close relationship to the spleen, or the presence of multiple, macroscopically enlarged splenic hilar lymph nodes warrant splenectomy en bloc with the gastric specimen.

30.5.3 Division of the Phrenoesophageal Membrane and Vagus Nerves

Resection of the phrenoesophageal membrane releases the anterior esophageal wall and allows complete dissection of the intra-abdominal esophagus. Division of the two vagus nerves, which are easily identified because they are strung longitudinally at the level of the external portion of the esophageal wall, allows further mobilization of the intra-abdominal esophagus. The right vagus nerve courses posteriorly, whereas the left runs along the anterior wall, owing to the 90° clockwise rotation around its longitudinal axis undergone by the stomach during organogenesis. Their division after dissection results in a greater mobility of the intra-abdominal esophagus.

30.5.4 Preparation of the Purse-string Suture

The surgeon firmly holds the stomach at the esophagogastric junction with the left hand and uses the right hand to close the rake clamp at the center of the intra-abdominal esophagus on macroscopically healthy tissue, 1–2 cm upstream of the cardia, carefully avoiding trapping the NGT. Two straight needles are inserted through the rake clamp jaws to execute a purse-string suture in the distal esophagus with non-absorbable monofilament suture 2-0.

30.5.5 Esophageal Resection, and Insertion of the Stapler Anvil in the Distal Esophagus

A Resano forceps is placed on the cardia, to avoid operating field contamination. As the first assistant holds the ends of the purse-string suture, to prevent their accidental resection, the surgeon cuts the distal esophagus with curved scissors close to the rake clamp, thus freeing the specimen, which consists of the whole stomach, the omentum, and all first-level perigastric lymph nodes (stations 1–6). The specimen is submitted for intraoperative consultation to establish the tumor's distance from the proximal and distal margins and exclude microscopic positivity. Ideally, the surgeon and the pathologist should dissect the perigastric lymphatic and adipose tissue, separating the six first-level lymph node stations.

With the rake clamp still in place, the resected esophageal stump is disinfected with a tampon soaked in povidone iodine. The surgeon opens the

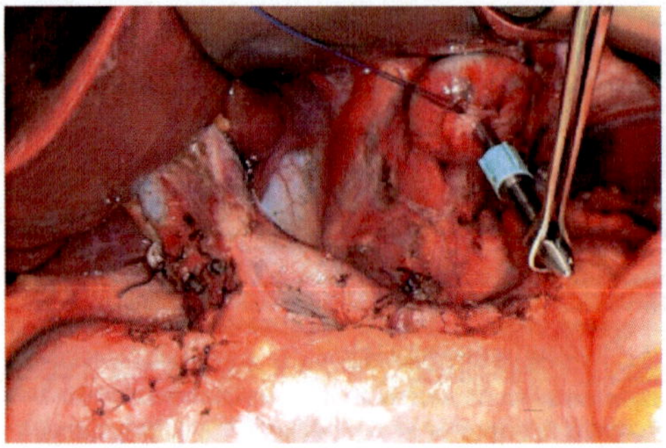

Fig. 30.5 The purse-string suture is tied at the base of the anvil's shaft; the esophageal stump is now ready for the anastomosis

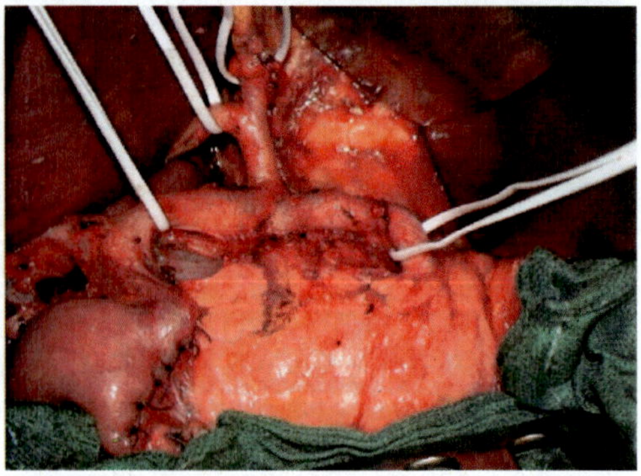

Fig. 30.6 Complete lymphadenectomy involving the left gastric artery (station 7), the common hepatic artery (station 8), and the celiac trunk (station 9). This patient has an anatomical variant, the left hepatic artery originating from the left gastric artery

rake jaws with the right hand to remove it while tightening the purse-string suture with the left hand, to close the esophageal stump and avoid operative field contamination. Any leakage from the esophagus is, however, removed with the aspirator, held close to the stump by the first assistant. At this point the purse-string suture is released and three Allis forceps are placed 120° apart along of the esophageal stump, grasping the entire thickness of the wall. While the first and the second assistants open the esophageal stump by gently pulling the Allis clamps, the surgeon introduces a Carmalt or a ring clamp into the lumen, gently distending the wall to avoid mucosal tears, to establish the caliber of the circular mechanical stapler required for the esophagojejunal anastomosis.

A 25-mm stapler or, less commonly, a 21-mm stapler, is used in most cases. The surgeon introduces the oiled anvil of the stapler into the esophagus with the right hand, tightening the purse-strings with the left hand as the first and the second assistant remove the Allis clamps. The purse-string suture is then tied at the base of the anvil's shaft, and the esophageal stump is ready for the anastomosis (Fig. 30.5). To prevent stump retraction into the chest, a right-angled clamp can be placed on the distal esophagus upstream of the anvil. We prefer to leave it free, with the two ends of the purse-string suture on the anvil held together by a Pean clamp. At the time of the anastomosis, gentle pulling of the strings will allow safe and easy recovery.

30.5.6 D2 Lymphadenectomy

After removal of the stomach and prior to reconstruction, D2 lymphadenectomy is performed according to Japanese Gastric Cancer Association (JGCA) criteria. The arterial-phase CT scans show the course of the arterial branches of the celiac trunk and any anatomical variation, which need to be identified to avoid possible errors (Fig. 30.6). Recognition of any abnormalities prior to the operation provides for safe and correct execution of D2 lymphadenectomy. We prefer to begin the lymph node dissection by identifying—medial to the duodenal stump—the gastroduodenal artery, which is dissected backward until its origin in the common hepatic artery. Vascular tape is then placed around this pedicle; the pedicle is dissected in the direction of the celiac trunk, which is now completely exposed, enabling recovery of the stump of the previously divided left gastric artery. Complete lymphadenectomy involving the left gastric artery (station 7), the common hepatic artery (station 8), and the celiac trunk (station 9) is then performed (Fig. 30.6). Along the course of the common hepatic artery, the right and left branches of the proper hepatic artery and the common bile duct are identified and the anterior lymph nodes of the hepatoduodenal ligament are removed (station 12a). If enlarged nodes are found at this station, lymphadenectomy of the common bile duct (12c), and

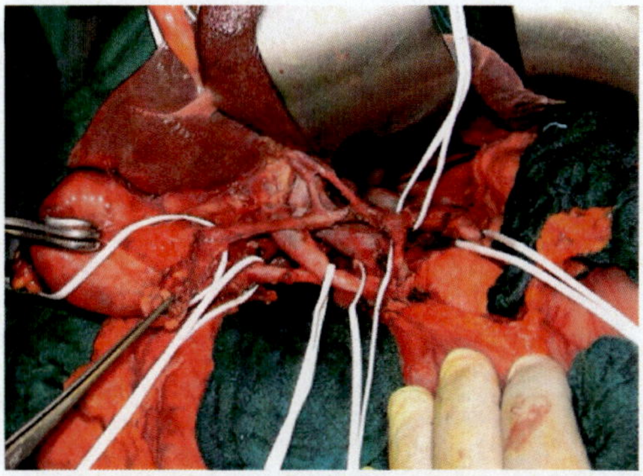

Fig. 30.7 Lymphadenectomy of the arterial (12a), common bile duct (12c), and portal (12p) portions of the hepatoduodenal ligament is performed after preparing and placing these structures in a vascular tape

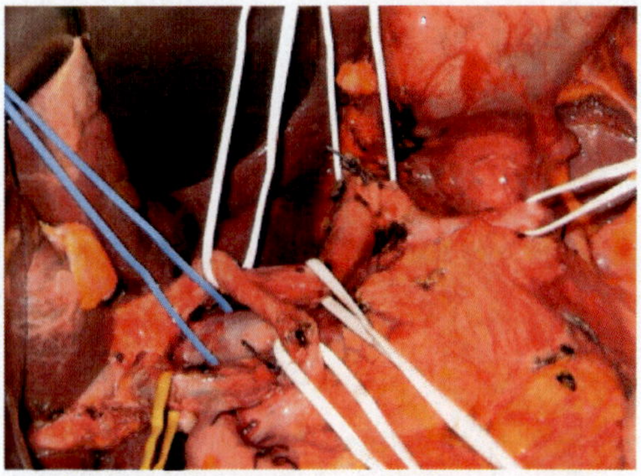

Fig. 30.8 View of the operating field after D2 lymphadenectomy with removal of the node stations of the splenic artery and splenic hilum (stations 11 and 10)

portal (12p) portions is performed after preparation and placement of these structures in a vascular tape (Fig. 30.7). Tumors of the middle and proximal third also entail removal of the node stations of the splenic artery and splenic hilum (stations 11d and 10) (Fig. 30.8). Distant third entails removal of the nodes of proximal splenic artery (station 11p). Radical removal of these nodes cannot be performed by distal splenopancreatectomy, because this procedure is indicated only in the presence of macroscopic pancreas infiltration by the tumor.

30.6 Reconstruction After Total Gastrectomy: Roux-en-Y End-to-Side Esophagojejunostomy

30.6.1 Preparation of the Jejunal Loop

With the transverse colon gently retracted, the second jejunal loop is spread to examine the anatomy of the arterial arcades by transillumination. The arcades are then divided nearly up to the base of the mesentery, to mobilize the jejunum and gain tension-free access to the cardial region. After two non-crushing intestinal clamps have been placed upstream and downstream of the resection site, the jejunal loop is resected and the two stumps are disinfected. The afferent loop, closed with a non-crushing intestinal clamp and covered with gauze, is abandoned in the abdomen. With the transverse mesocolon still gently retracted, an avascular area in its left inferior paramedian portion is identified by transillumination and excised, to allow transposition of the efferent jejunal limb to the supramesocolic compartment through the transverse mesocolon.

30.6.2 Stapled End-to-Side Esophagojejunostomy

Three Allis clamps are placed 120° apart to keep the jejunal limb open; while the first assistant applies gentle countertraction, the surgeon inserts the oiled circular stapler 10–15 cm into the Roux limb. The site of the jejunal limb to be perforated with the spike is identified. There must be no mechanical tension between the esophageal stump and the jejunal limb itself. The jejunal wall is perforated. Than, after recovery of the anvil and the distal esophageal stump by pulling the ends of the purse-string suture, the anvil is joined to the stapler. The two stumps are approximated by screwing the stapler shut; correct approximation of the margins is signaled by the stapler, authorizing firing (Fig. 30.9). The integrity of the two anastomotic rings is checked and the esophageal ring sent for histology. The anastomosis must be supple and tension-free.

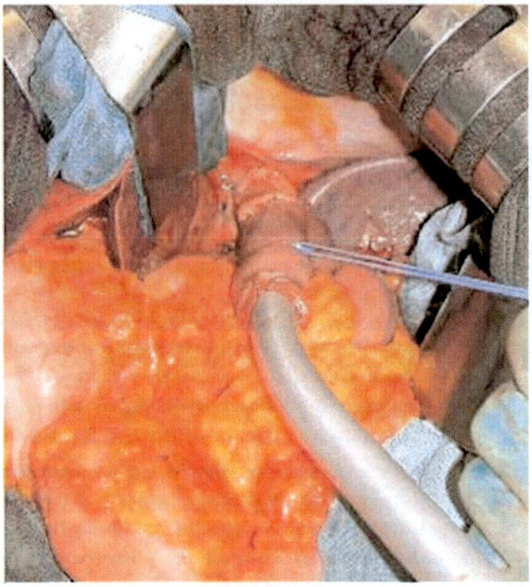

Fig. 30.9 Stapled end-to-side esophagojejunostomy

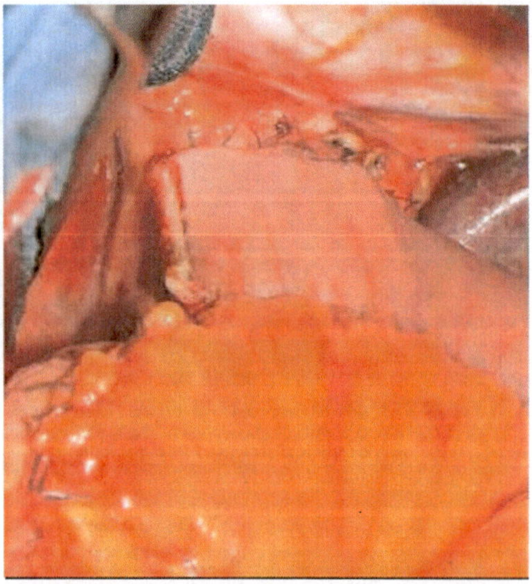

Fig. 30.10 The jejunal stump is closed with the TA 30 stapler 2-3 cm lateral to the esophagojejunal anastomosis

30.6.3 Closure of the Jejunal Stump and Reinforcement of the Esophagojejunal Anastomosis

The gentle traction exerted by the three Allis clamps placed on the edge of the jejunal loop allows its spread as well as the identification of the ideal site for closing the jejunal stump. The mesentery of the redundant jejunal loop is then resected; after closing the Roux limb 2–3 cm lateral to the esophagojejunal anastomosis with the TA 30, the visceral wall is resected with a blade (Fig. 30.10). The closed jejunal stump is disinfected and oversewn using interrupted slowly absorbable braided 3-0 sutures to obtain a short jejunal stump that does not disturb the esophagojejunal transit (Fig. 30.11).

To minimize the risk of leakage of the esophagojejunal anastomosis, which is associated with considerable postoperative mortality, we apply slowly absorbable interrupted seromuscular 3-0 sutures all around the anastomosis (360°) to avoid staple line tension and reinforce the anastomosis. Care should be taken to avoid any traction on the esophagus while tightening the knot (Fig. 30.11).

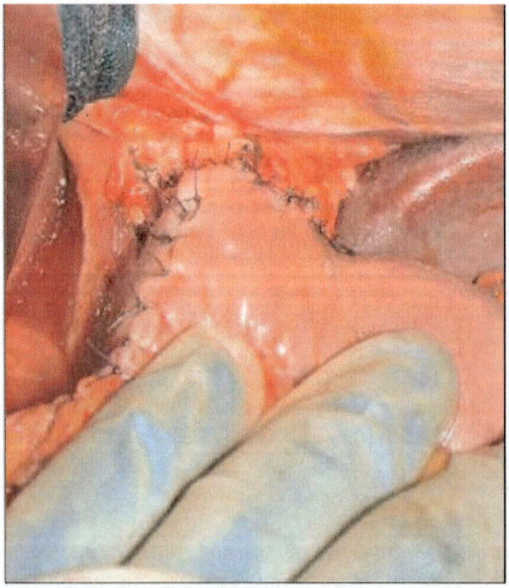

Fig. 30.11 The esophagojejunal anastomosis is reinforced with slowly absorbable interrupted seromuscular 3-0 sutures all around the anastomosis. The lateral jejunal stump is also oversewn

The transmesocolic wound is closed with one or two interrupted slowly absorbable 3-0 sutures, to minimize the risk of internal herniation.

30.6.4 Intraoperative Testing of Anastomotic Integrity

A non-crushing intestinal clamp is placed on the jejunal loop 10 cm downstream of the anastomosis; the NGT is then gently advanced ca. 5 cm past the suture and injected with 40–60 ml of saline added with methylene blue for anastomotic leak testing. The solution distends and tensions the anastomosis, demonstrating any leaks.

The solution is then pumped out through the NGT, the clamp is removed, and the NGT recovered, since it does not help to reduce the incidence of esophagojejunal fistulas. In patients with severe malnutrition requiring postoperative enteral feeding, the NGT is advanced 30–40 cm past the esophagojejunal anastomosis to administer the nutritional support.

30.6.5 Creation of the Enteroenterostomy

To re-establish intestinal continuity, the afferent jejunal stump is recovered and a two-layer, end-to-side jejunojejunal anastomosis is performed on the efferent jejunal loop 60 cm from the esophagojejunal anastomosis using interrupted slowly absorbable 3-0 sutures. The mesenteries are closed with interrupted slowly absorbable 3-0 sutures to minimize the risk of internal herniation.

30.6.6 Drainage and Wound Closure

Once hemostasis has been established, two abdominal drains are placed, the right one coursing posterior to the anastomosis below the hepatoduodenal ligament, also draining the duodenal stump, and the left one running anterior to the anastomosis, also draining the left hypochondrium.

The peritoneum is then closed with a continuous slowly absorbable 2-0 suture, the fascia and subcutis with interrupted sutures, and the cutis with staples.

30.7 Manual Subtotal Gastrectomy

30.7.1 Dissection of the Upper Portion of the Lesser Curvature

If the site of the tumor allows subtotal gastrectomy sparing the gastric fundus, the transection line affording both macroscopically correct margins and removal of antral G cells (thus avoiding retained antrum syndrome) is identified. To achieve the latter objective, the angle of the transection line through the lesser and greater curvature must measure 120–130° with respect to the lesser curvature.

Complete removal of lymphatic and adipose tissue of the proximal portion of the lesser curvature up to the right wall of the cardia exposes the medial wall of the stomach and the esophagogastric junction, ensuring optimal exposure and safe closure of the medial portion of the gastric stump. The right paracardial (station 1) and proximal lymphatic and adipose tissue of the lesser curvature (station 3) is thus dissected and sent for definitive histology. The arteriovenous branches of the left gastric pedicle, which penetrate the gastric wall, also need to be ligated close to the gastric wall.

30.7.2 Preservation of Gastric Stump Vascularity

After identification of the transection point on the greater curvature, the gastric wall is dissected at this level, carefully preserving two or more short gastric vessels and the posterior gastric artery to ensure viability and trophism of the gastric stump.

30.7.3 D2 Lymphadenectomy

After upward retraction of the stomach, D2 lymphadenectomy is performed as described above.

30.8 Reconstruction After Subtotal Gastrectomy: Gastrojejunostomy on a Roux Limb

The reconstruction method we prefer after subtotal gastrectomy is antiperistaltic, manual, end-to-side, two-layer, partial inferior gastrojejunostomy on a defunctionalized Roux limb. The main reasons that have led us to abandon the Billroth II technique are:(i) despite the safety and low rate of fistulas of the gastrojejunal anastomosis, any anastomotic leakage does not significantly affect the mortality rate of patients undergoing Roux limb reconstruction, because in this case bile does not pass through the stomach, unlike in the Billroth II procedure; and (ii) enteroenterostomy 60 cm from the gastrojejunal anastomosis prevents bile reflux and alkaline gastritis, which are associated with an incidence of ca. 5% of stump carcinoma at 20 years after Billroth II gastrojejunostomy. For this reason, the latter procedure should be performed only in patients older than 70 years, as needed.

30.8.1 Preparation of the Roux Limb and Supramesocolic Transposition

With the transverse colon gently retracted, the second jejunal loop and the associated mesentery are spread to examine the anatomy of its arterial arcades by transillumination. The arcades are then divided nearly up to the base of the mesentery, to mobilize the jejunum and gain tension-free access to the gastric stump.

The section site on the jejunum is then identified and the jejunum is closed with a TA 30 linear stapler; after placement of a non-crushing intestinal clamp, the afferent portion is also sectioned with a traditional blade and remains open. The stapled efferent portion is oversewn with interrupted slowly absorbable 3-0 sutures. With the transverse colon still gently retracted, an avascular area in its left inferior paramedian portion is identified by transillumination and incised to allow transposition of the efferent jejunal limb to the supramesocolic compartment through the transverse mesocolon.

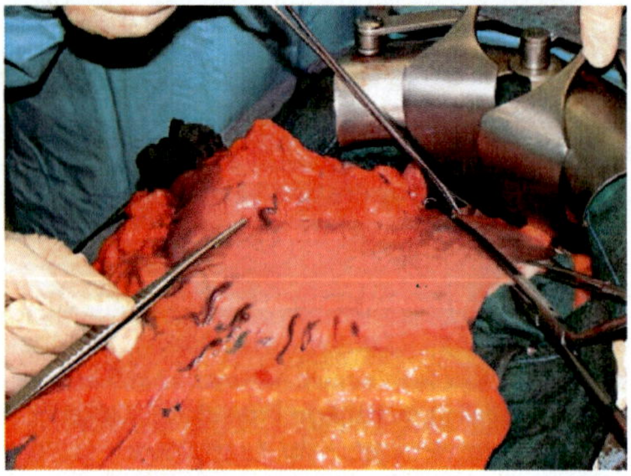

Fig. 30.12 The gastric tool of the Haberer intestinal and stomach clamp is applied to the gastric fundus at an obtuse angle (120-130°) with respect to the lesser curvature and at an adequate distance between proximal tumor pole and resection line

30.8.2 Placement of the Haberer Intestinal and Stomach Clamp

After the stomach has been replaced, the gastric tool of the Haberer intestinal and stomach clamp is applied to the gastric fundus at an obtuse angle, which entails that the anastomosis is performed ca. 2 cm below it (Fig. 30.12). This allows objective measurement of the distance between the proximal tumor pole and the resection line, hence accurate margin evaluation. The NGT is withdrawn before closing the clamp, to avoid its entrapment.

Now the stomach is again elevated and retracted upward, to expose its posterior wall which is held in slight tension by the second assistant. The first assistant raises the previously prepared closed Roux limb with two forceps, while the surgeon gently tightens the jejunal tool of the clamp at the level of the mesenteric edge (Fig. 30.13). The gastric and jejunal clamps are then brought close together and blocked with the third clamp. The latter is locked when the gastric and the jejunal wall are approximated on the lateral side of the greater curvature. Three laparotomy pads, one behind the stomach, another in front of the Roux limb, and the third above the three clamps, are applied prior to execution of the anastomosis, to prevent contamination of the operating field and trapping of the suture threads in the clamp jaws.

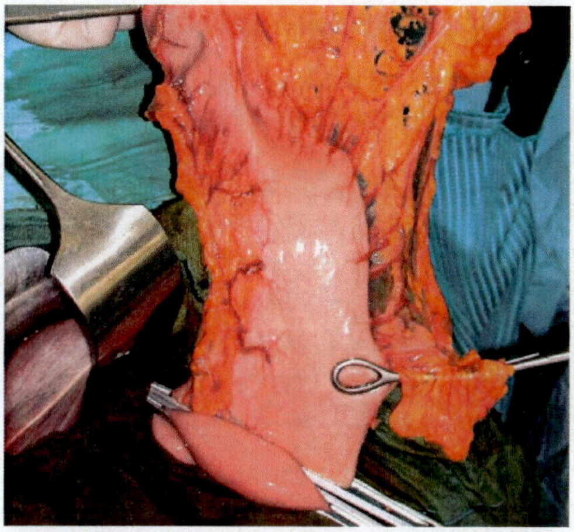

Fig. 30.13 The jejunal tool of the Haberer clamp is tightened at the level of the mesenteric edge; the gastric and jejunal clamps are then approximated and blocked with the third clamp

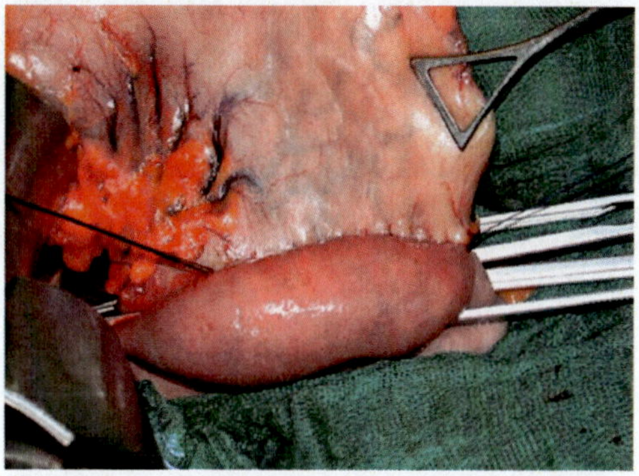

Fig. 30.14 First layer of the posterior wall. A continuous seromuscular slowly absorbable 2-0 suture is passed from the lateral portion of the greater curvature toward the lesser curvature for a length of ca. 6 cm

30.8.3 Creation of the Gastrojejunostomy

First Layer of the Posterior Wall

The first layer of the posterior wall is realized from the lateral portion of the greater curvature, where the gastric and the jejunal walls have been approximated, toward the lesser curvature using a continuous seromuscular slowly absorbable suture (2-0) and a 30-mm needle. The needle is passed at closely spaced (5–7 mm) intervals through the walls at a 45° angle with respect to the major axis of the suture, taking an abundant portion of the gastric seromuscular layer. The first assistant tightens the continuous suture, closely approximating the two walls, carefully avoiding tearing the tissue. Inability to see the suture commonly indicates that the correct amount of tension has been applied (Fig. 30.14). The mouth of the partial inferior anastomosis that we prefer measures ca. 6 cm, or the width of three fingers. Mosquito forceps are placed at either end of the suture.

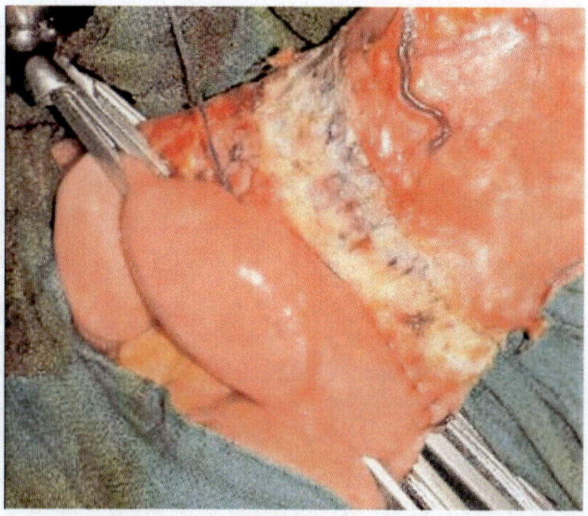

Fig. 30.15 The posterior gastric wall is resected first, 1 cm from the suture on the side of the greater curvature and 1.5–2 cm on the side of the lesser curvature

Resection of the Stomach and Intraoperative Consultation

A long clamp encompassing the whole stomach is placed upstream of the suture, to avoid operative field contamination; then the posterior gastric wall is resected first, at a distance of 1 cm from the suture on the side of the greater curvature, and of 1.5–2 cm on the side of the lesser curvature. The seromuscular layer is excised with electrocautery (Fig. 30.15) and the vessels of the rich submucosal venous plexus are coagulated tangent to the section margin, to avoid leaving excess mucosa, which would complicate execution of the internal layer of the anastomosis. The mucosal and submucosal layers of the posterior gastric wall are then excised with electrocautery. The open gastric stump is disinfected and a gauze soaked in povidone iodine is

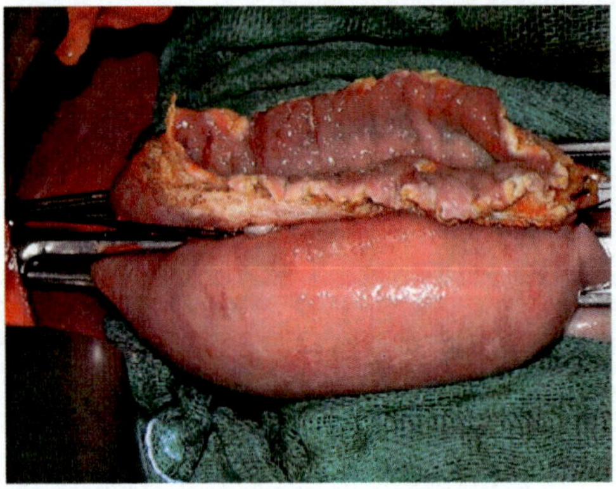

Fig. 30.16 The anterior wall is excised as described for the posterior wall, enabling removal of the specimen

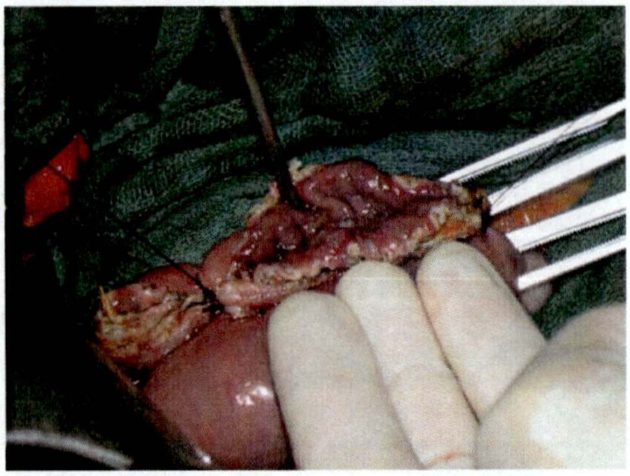

Fig. 30.17 Closure of the medial portion of the gastric stump not sutured to the jejunal limb. The first stitch is close to the knot of the first layer of the posterior wall of the anastomosis. This ensures that the mouth of the partial inferior anastomosis is the size of the width of three fingers

applied; the stomach is resected, excising the anterior wall as described for the posterior wall. The resection line on the anterior wall should be made 2 cm from the suture on the side of the greater curvature and 3 cm from it on the side of the lesser curvature, to facilitate creation of the anastomosis and oversewing of the medial portion of the gastric stump.

After resection of the anterior wall the specimen is removed (Fig. 30.16) and submitted for frozen section assessment of the margins and microscopic evaluation of their negativity. Finally, the gastric stump is disinfected with povidone iodine.

Closure of the Medial Gastric Stump

The medial portion of the gastric stump not sutured to the jejunal limb is closed with a continuous slowly absorbable 2-0 suture according to O'Connell. The first stitch is full-thickness, straddling the anterior and posterior gastric walls close to the knot of the first layer of the posterior wall of the anastomosis (Fig. 30.17). The loose ends of these sutures are tied together and cut. The surgeon passes the needle through the full thickness of the two gastric walls (in-out-in) at 5- to 7-mm intervals as far as the medial corner of the gastric stump (Fig. 30.18) while the first assistant tucks in the mucosa and approximates the seromuscular layer, carefully avoiding tearing it.

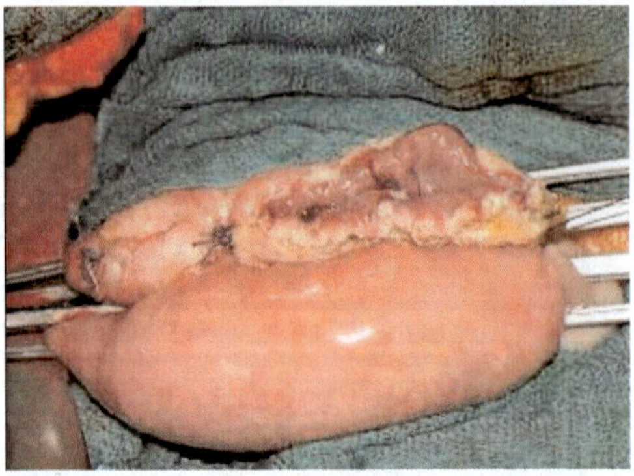

Fig. 30.18 The medial gastric stump is closed with a continuous slowly absorbable 2-0 suture according to O'Connell

Incision of the Jejunal Loop and Execution of the Second Layer of the Posterior Wall and of the First Layer of the Anterior Wall

The jejunum is incised approximately 1 cm from the posterior suture line for a length corresponding to the width of the anastomosis (Fig. 30.19).

After disinfection of the jejunal mucosa the second layer of the posterior wall is begun with a continuous running locked slowly absorbable suture (2-0) from the lesser to the greater curvature. The first stitch is inside-out, passing first through the gastric

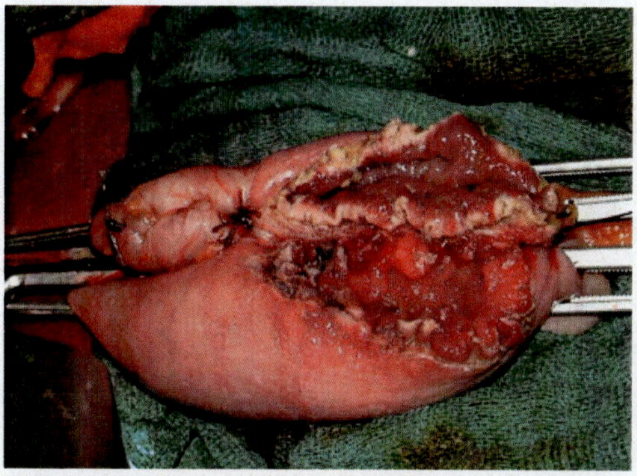

Fig. 30.19 The jejunum is incised approximately 1 cm from the posterior suture line for a length corresponding to the width of the anastomosis

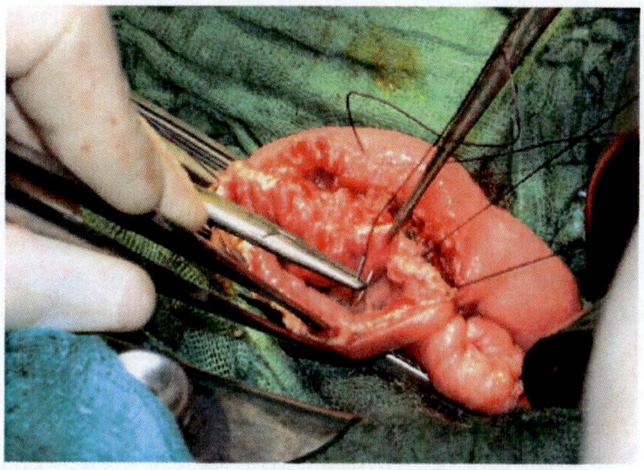

Fig. 30.20 The second layer of the posterior wall is begun with a continuous running locked slowly absorbable suture (2-0) from the lesser to the greater curvature

wall and then through the medial side of the jejunal wall. While the surgeon tightens the knot, pushing it posteriorly, the first assistant tucks in the excess mucosa using two forceps so as to close and seal the medial corner of the anastomosis. The loose end of this suture is knotted with the thread of the continuous suture of the first layer of the posterior wall and cut. The surgeon passes the needle through the gastric wall and then through the jejunal wall at intervals of 5- to 7-mm above the first seromuscular suture, executing a running locked suture with help from the first assistant, thus ensuring hemostasis and sealing the inner layer (Fig. 30.20).

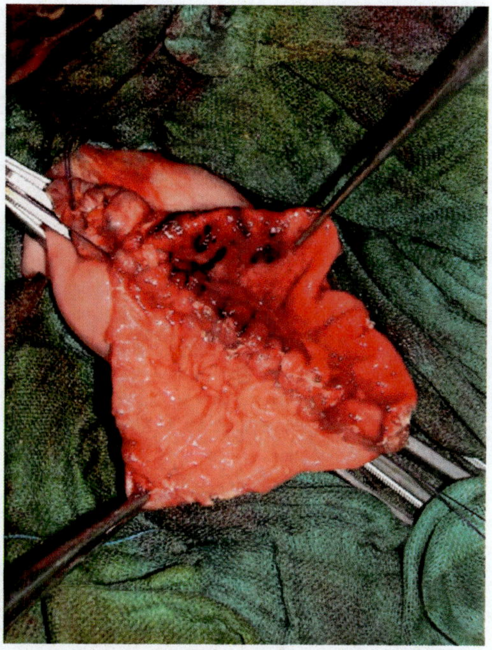

Fig. 30.21 The running locked suture of the second layer of the posterior wall ensures hemostasis and seals the inner layer

After completion of the second layer of the posterior wall (Fig. 30.21), the needle exits through the jejunal wall and is reintroduced through the end of the anastomosis on the side of the greater curvature. From here the suture is begun again, proceeding from the greater to the lesser curvature, using the same thread; the first layer of the anterior wall is performed from the gastric to the jejunal wall at 5-7 mm intervals with a full-thickness suture, according to O'Connell. The first assistant sutures the two tissue walls to close and seal the medial end of the anastomosis, carefully avoiding tearing the tissue (Fig. 30.22). The end of this suture is knotted with the one of the first layer.

Oversewing of the Medial Gastric Stump

The non-anastomosed gastric stump, which has been closed with a continuous suture, forms an acute angle that needs to be straightened (Fig. 30.23). This is accomplished by passing a semi-pouch suture through the seromuscular layer on the

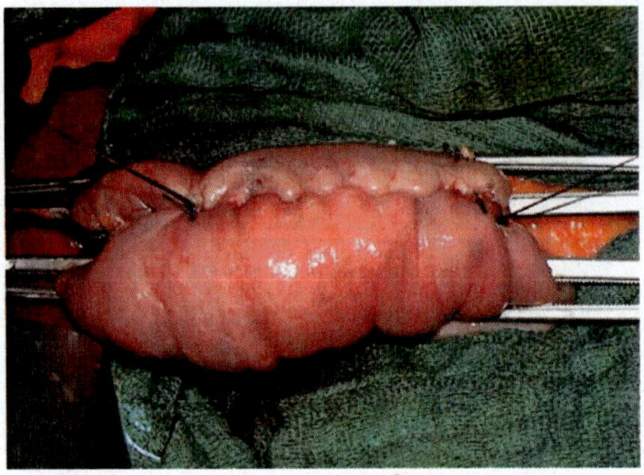

Fig. 30.22 The first layer of the anterior wall is performed from the gastric to the jejunal wall at 5- to 7-mm intervals with a full-thickness suture, according to O'Connell

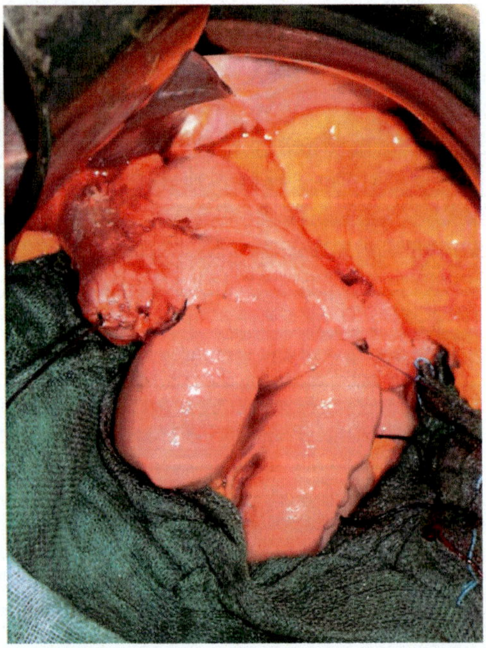

Fig. 30.23 The non-anastomosed gastric stump, which has been closed with a continuous suture, forms an acute angle that needs to be straightened

anterior gastric wall, 2–3 cm from the angle, through the angle itself, and through the seromuscular layer of the posterior gastric wall. The first

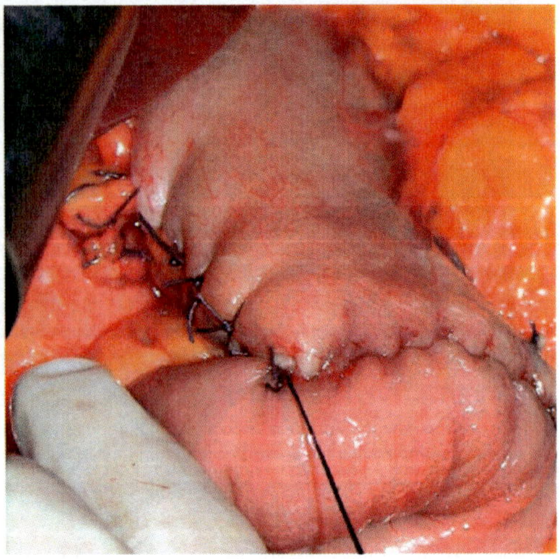

Fig. 30.24 The entire second layer of the non-anastomosed gastric stump is finally achieved; the stump is straightened and reduced to the size of the anastomosis

assistant oversews then tucks in the angle of the gastric stump, thus straightening the wall and reducing the gastric stump to the size of the anastomosis. Two or three interrupted, slowly absorbable seromuscular sutures (2-0) are placed upstream of the semipouch suture as far as the right subcardial region; one or two additional interrupted stitches are placed downstream to oversew the lower portion of the medial gastric stump nearly to the medial corner of the gastrojejunal anastomosis. This procedure allows achievement of the whole second layer of the non-anastomosed gastric stump (Fig. 30.24).

Second Layer of the Anterior Wall

The second layer of the anterior wall is performed starting laterally from the continuous suture of the first layer of the posterior wall, using a continuous slowly absorbable 2-0 suture, proceeding from the greater to the lesser curvature with seromuscular sutures placed 5- to 7-mm apart. The first assistant tightens the suture of the second layer of the anterior wall, carefully avoiding tearing the tissue. The thread of the first continuous suture is met and overcome close to the medial corner, which is sealed using a triple stitch encompassing the sero-

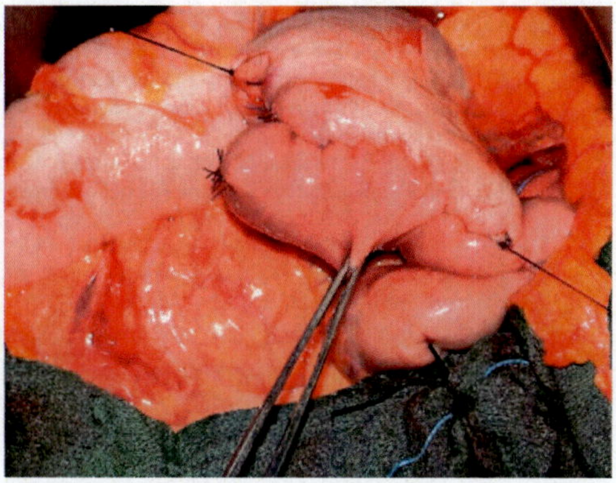

Fig. 30.25 Final appearance of the gastrojejunal anastomosis

muscular layer of the anterior wall of the non-anastomosed gastric stump, its posterior wall, and the jejunal seromuscular layer (Fig. 30.25). Once the anastomosis has been realized, a NGT is placed to drain the gastric stump, taking care that its tip does not rest on the suture line.

30.8.4 Creation of the Enteroenterostomy

The afferent jejunal stump is recovered. Intestinal continuity is re-established by creating a two-layer, end-to-side jejunojejunal anastomosis on the efferent jejunal loop 60 cm from the gastrojejunal anastomosis. The mesenteries are carefully closed with interrupted slowly absorbable 3-0 sutures to avoid internal herniation.

30.8.5 Drainage and Wound Closure

Once hemostasis has been established, a right abdominal drain is placed behind the anastomosis and under the hepatoduodenal ligament, also draining the duodenal stump.

The wound is closed as described above

30.9 Stapled Subtotal Gastrectomy

There are several techniques to be chosen when performing a stapled subtotal gastrectomy: total or partial inferior anastomosis, side-to-side anastomosis using a linear stapler (GIA), and circular anastomosis after closure and transection of the gastric stump with a GIA. We prefer to close the gastric stump completely with a GIA 90, then create a stapled end-to-side gastrojejunal circular anastomosis on defunctionalized Roux limb on the low lateral portion of the greater curvature. Preparation and transposition of the jejunal loop to the supramesocolic compartment are as described above.

30.9.1 Stomach Resection with the GIA Stapler

A GIA 90 linear mechanical stapler allows closure and transection of the stomach, usually by a single firing, along the transection line passing through the lesser and greater curvature and forming a 120–130° angle to the lesser curvature. This angle ensures adequate margins and removal of antral G cells. Before the stapler jaws are locked, the NGT needs to be drawn back, to avoid inclusion in the staple line.

30.9.2 Creation of the Stapled End-to-Side Gastrojejunal Anastomosis

A rake is placed on the acute angle formed by the suture line and the greater curvature, then a non-absorbable monofilament 2-0 purse-string suture is performed. Excess gastric tissue is removed and a 25 or 31 mm anvil of a circular mechanical stapler is inserted into the gastric stump. The stapler is introduced into the previously prepared Roux limb to create the end-to-side gastrojejunal anastomosis. The lateral jejunal stump is closed with a TA 30 stapler and oversewn with interrupted slowly absorbable 3-0 sutures. The same thread is passed to reinforce the anastomosis using interrupted sutures. The staple line closing the whole gastric stump is also strengthened by oversewing with interrupted sutures or with a continuous slowly absorbable 2-0 suture. The surgical procedure ends with the execution of the end-to-side enteroenterostomy, suturing of the mesenteries and placement of a drain, as in the manual procedure.

Suggested Readings

Brennan MF (2006) Total gastrectomy for carcinoma. In: Fischer J E (ed) Mastery of surgery, 5th edn., vol 1. Lippincott Williams & Wilkins, Philadelphia, PA, pp 916-926

Mullen JT, Pisters PWT (2006) Subtotal gastrectomy for gastric cancer. In: Fischer JE (ed) Mastery of surgery, 5th edn., vol 1. Lippincott Williams & Wilkins, Philadelphia, PA, pp 927-937

Sasako M (2007) Total gastrectomy with radical systemic lymphadenectomy (Japanese procedure). In: Clavien PA, Sarr MG, Fong Y (eds) Atlas of upper gastrointestinal and hepato-pancreato-biliary surgery. Springer, Berlin Heidelberg New York, pp 179-188

Staley CA (2010) Subtotal gastrectomy. In: Wood CW, Staley CA, Skandalakis JE (eds) Anatomic basis of tumor surgery. Springer, Berlin Heidelberg New York, pp 317-328

Staley CA (2010) Total gastrectomy. In: Wood CW, Staley CA, Skandalakis JE (eds) Anatomic basis of tumor surgery. Springer, Berlin Heidelberg New York, pp 328-334

Proximal Gastrectomy: Technical Notes

31

Claudio Cordiano, Gerardo Mangiante, Simone Giacopuzzi, and Giovanni de Manzoni

Abstract

A new technique for recostruction after proximal gastrectomy for EGJ adenocarcinoma (Siewert II with < 2 cm esophageal invasion and Siewert III) and upper-third early gastric cancer is presented. Since January 2000, 50 patients have been treated with this new technique. Postoperative morbidity and mortality were respectively, 25% and 2%, with a leak rate of 8%. At 6 and 12 months, reflux rates were 30% and 33% and stricture rates 20% and 6.7%, respectively. The data show that this technique is feasible, with good results in terms of morbidity and mortality as well as functional outcome.

Keywords

Proximal gastrectomy • Esophagogastric junction adenocarcinoma • Upper-third early gastric cancer • End-to-end anastomosis

31.1 Background

Total gastrectomy with Roux-en-Y reconstruction is considered the standard operation for early gastric cancer of the esophago-gastric junction (EGJ) and of the upper third of the stomach. To avoid the problems of food tolerance and performance status experienced by patients undergoing total gastrectomy, the use of a proximal gastrectomy reconstructed by jejunal interposition has been proposed [1, 2]. However, this procedure is complicated, time-consuming, and risky due to the three anastomoses that are needed. An alternative approach consists of a proximal gastrectomy with gastric tube reconstruction. This simple and useful technique is the subject of this chapter.

As shown in Fig. 31.1, the procedure allows the removal of all first- and second-tier lymph nodes, except those along the right gastro-epiploic artery and the infrapyloric nodes, which are not involved in the T1 and T2 stages of gastric cancer [3].

31.2 Surgical Technique

Access to the abdominal cavity is obtained by laparotomy with median approach. Separation of the greater omentum from a transverse colon mobilizing downward right and left colon flexure; after completion of the Kocher maneuver, the left gastroepiploic and short gastric vessels are ligated.

G. de Manzoni (✉)
Dept. of Surgery,
Upper G.I. Surgery Division,
University of Verona,
Verona, Italy

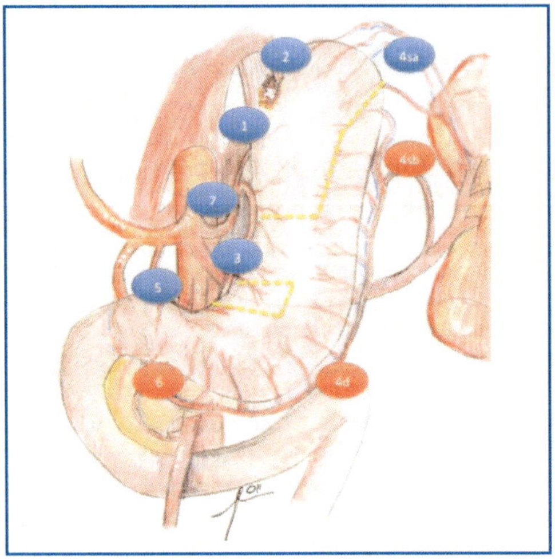

Fig. 31.1 Lymph node dissected during proximal gastrectomy with gastric tube reconstruction (*blue oval*) and lymph nodes not removed (*red oval*)

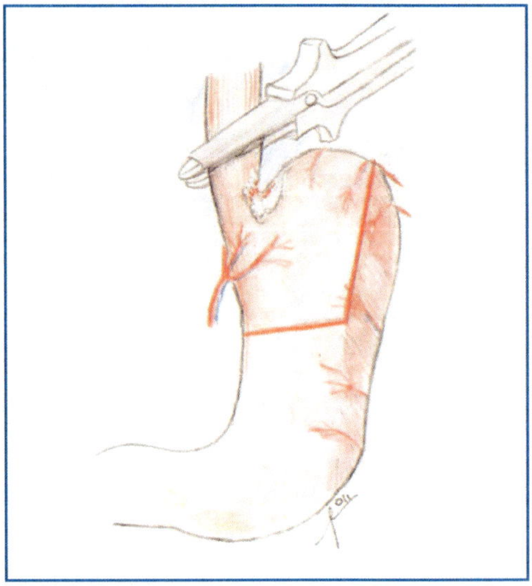

Fig. 31.2 Division of the esophagus, 2 cm above the tumor edge

Once the greater curvature of the stomach has been mobilized, the abdominal portion of the esophagus is completely exposed, with sectioning of the anterior and posterior trunks of the vagus nerve. The esophagus is divided using a GIA 60 linear surgical stapler above the level of the EGJ or at least 2 cm above the tumor in case of early-stage cancer of the EGJ (Fig. 31.2). The surgeon then constructs the gastric tube along the greater curvature using multiple serial firings of linear staplers (GIA 60 and 80). In the first step, we start from the fundus, dividing the stomach for 5–6 cm parallel to the greater curvature and then in the direction of the lesser curvature (Fig. 31.3). In the second step, the sectioning is conducted starting at the distal part of the lesser curvature parallel to the greater curvature and finishing up to 5 cm away from the upper section. This results in a gastric tube about 20 cm in length and 4 cm in width, with an access pouch that will be used for entry of the circular stapler (Fig. 31.4).

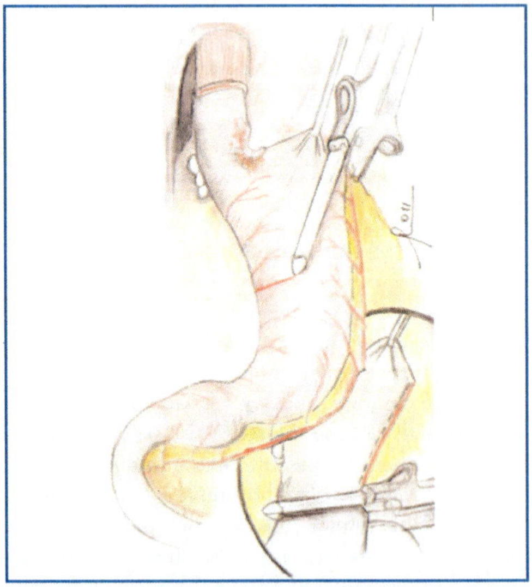

Fig. 31.3 Gastric-conduit construction, starting from the fundus and using a linear stapler, moving parallel to the greater curvature for 5–6 cm and then toward the lesser curvature

Extramucosal pyloroplasty is performed and the esophageal hiatus is opened to free the lower esophagus and to complete lower mediastinal node dissection. A 25-mm anvil is placed in the esophageal stump, secured with a purse-string suture, and a second purse-string suture is created at the top of the conduit (Fig. 31.5). The circular stapler is inserted through a gastrotomy performed

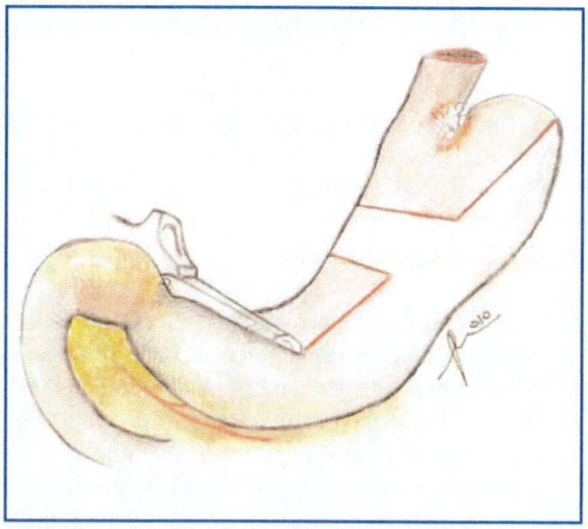

Fig. 31.4 To complete the conduit, the section starts above the pylorus, creating a pouch on the lesser curvature

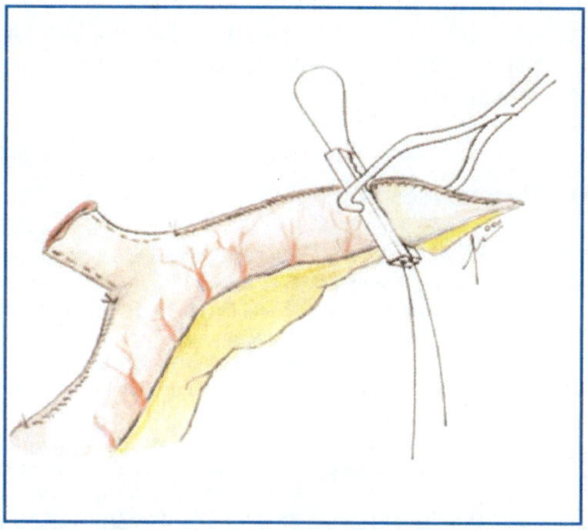

Fig. 31.5 A second purse-string is created at the top of the conduit

on the access pouch and advanced along the gastric conduit until the tip emerges from the purse-string at the top of the tube.

The cartridge on the circular stapler is attached to the anvil placed in the esophageal stump and a circular stapled end-to-end anastomosis is created (Fig. 31.6). The access pouch is closed with a linear GIA 60 stapler and the anastomosis is oversewn with a running suture (Fig. 31.7). A naso-gastric tube is positioned through the anastomosis under direct visualization, with the distal end immediately upstream of the pyloroplasty.

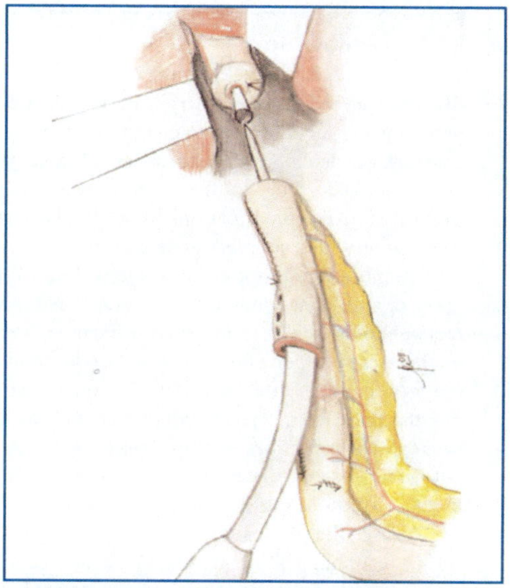

Fig. 31.6 Creation of the anastomosis by introduction of the circular stapler through the access pouch

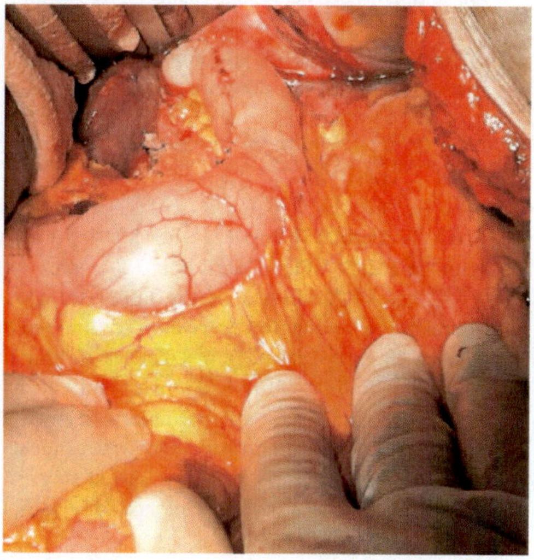

Fig. 31.7 Final overview of the intramediastinic esophago-gastro-anastomosi

31.3 Follow-up

Six days after surgery, we routinely evaluate the patient using a contrast esophagogram to check for anastomotic leakage. The presence of leakage is classified according to the system proposed by Lerut [4]. All complications directly associated with surgery are recorded, as is mortality.

Patients are required to adhere to a strict follow-up program consisting of outpatient visits, thoracic/abdominal CT scan, measurement of cancer markers, and upper gastrointestinal endoscopy initially 4 months after surgery and then every 6 months thereafter. Reflux symptoms such as pharyngeal regurgitation, retrosternal/cervical heartburn, pain, throat disturbance, or nocturnal cough are also assessed during the examination.

During the endoscopic procedure, signs of reflux esophagitis or anastomotic stenosis are recorded. We define stenosis as the difficult passage of a 9.8-mm diagnostic endoscope. Patients who clinically present with dysphagia or anastomotic narrowing at the endoscopic control undergo dilatation. Delayed presentation of reflux is diagnosed on the basis of signs of esophagitis during the endoscopic examination.

31.4 Results

From January 2000 to December 2010, 50 patients with EGJ early adenocarcinoma (24 patients) and T1–T2 adenocarcinoma of the upper third of the stomach (26 patients) underwent proximal gastrectomy with gastric tube reconstruction. Among these 50 patients, four (8%) had postoperative anastomotic leakage: three patients underwent medically conservative treatment together with endoscopic clipping [5] while one patient required surgery.

During follow-up, the incidence of anastomotic stricture was 20% after 4 months, decreasing to 6.7% after 1 year. All patients were treated conservatively with pneumatic dilatation. After 1 year, reflux esophagitis grade I was present in 33% of the patients.

31.5 Conclusions

The technique of proximal gastrectomy with end-to-end stapled esophagogastric anastomosis, performed as described herein, has several advantages. First, it is safe, requiring just one anastomosis, and the operation time is shorter. Second, it is a true end-to-end anastomosis that allows preservation of the entire vascularization at the end of the tube without cutting the vessels coming from the greater curvature; this is in contrast to the esophagogastric anastomoses presently performed in esophageal surgery. Third, food tolerance is good and the rate of reflux esophagitis is only slightly higher than in patients treated by total gastrectomy and Roux-en-Y reconstruction.

References

1. Stein J (2005) Surgery for early stage esophageal adenocarcinoma. J Surg Oncol 92:210-217
2. Takeshita K, Saito N, Saeki I et al (1997) Proximal gastrectomy and jejunal pouch interposition for the treatment of early gastric cancer of the upper third of the stomach: surgical techniques and evaluation of postoperative function. Surgery 121:278-286
3. Di Leo A, Marrelli D, Roviello F, de Manzoni G (2007) Lymph node involvement in gastric cancer for different tumor sites and T stage. Italian Research Group for Gastric Cancer (IRGGC) Experience. J Gastroint Surgery 11(9):1146-1145
4. Lerut T, Coosemans G, Deker P et al (2002) Anastomotic complications after esophagectomy. Dig Surg 19:92-98
5. Rodella L, Laterza E, de Manzoni G et al (1998) Endoscopic clipping of anastomotic leakages in esophagogastric surgery. Endoscopy 30:453-456

Total and Subtotal Minimally Invasive Gastrectomy: Technical Notes

32

Raffaele Pugliese, Dario Maggioni, Giovanni C. Ferrari, Andrea Costanzi, and Monica Gualtierotti

Abstract

JGCA Gastric Cancer Treatment Guidelines (2010) include Laparoscopic Assisted Distal Gastrectomy (LADG) within the chapter of modified surgery. A metanalysis published in 2010 shows that LADG seems superior to Open Distal Gastrectomy (ODG) if comparing short term outcomes. Oncologic results prove to be comparable to ODG by one RCT and two retrospective studies. Little evidence is available on Laparoscopic Total Gastrectomy and concerns are raised about long-term oncologic outcomes.

Laparoscopic Subtotal Gastrectomy is carried out with 4 trocars in a semicircular shape from left to right upper quadrants, the laparoscope being placed in the periumbilical port. After exploration of the abdominal cavity surgical steps include coloepiploic detachment, omentectomy, dissection of the gastrocolic ligament, division of the left gastroepiploic vessels, division of right gastroepiploic vessels, division of pyloric vessels. The duodenum is transected with a linear stapler. Incision of the lesser omentum and dissection of the hepatoduodenal ligament allows completion of D2 lymphadenectomy. The 4/5ths of the stomach are transected starting from the greater curve at the junction of left and right gastro-epiploic arcades by linear stapler. Roux-en-Y loop reconstruction is performed through a stapled side-to–side gastro-jejunal anastomosis and a side-to-side jejuno-jejunal anastomosis. Reconstruction after Laparoscopic Total Gastrectomy is performed preferably by a side-to-side esophago-jejunal anastomosis according to Orringer.

A robotic assisted approach adds precision on lymphadenectomy and reconstructive techniques.

Keywords

Minimally Invasive Gastrectomy • Laparoscopic Subtotal Gastrectomy • Robotic surgery

R. Pugliese (✉)
Minimally Invasive and Oncology Surgery,
Niguarda Hospital "Ca'-Granda";
AIMS Academy,
Milan, Italy

32.1 Introduction

32.1.1 History of Laparoscopic Gastric Surgery

The official history of laparoscopic gastric surgery dates back to 1992, when Goh reported the first entirely laparoscopic Billroth II distal gastrectomy in a patient with a chronic gastric ulcer [1]. In the same year, Kitano performed the first laparoscopic distal gastrectomy with Billroth I reconstruction for carcinoma [2]. Successful laparoscopy-assisted total gastrectomy for gastric cancer was first reported by Azagra in 1999 [3]. Simultaneously, Uyama reported the first laparoscopic total gastrectomy with D2 lymphadenectomy for gastric cancer [4].

32.1.2 Evidence and Indications

The most recent edition of the JGCA Gastric Cancer Treatment Guidelines (2004) includes laparoscopically assisted gastrectomy (LADG) within the chapter on modified surgery [5]. It suggests that LADG could be performed for stage Ib distal tumors (T1N1, T2N0) only within the framework of clinical studies. According to the American National Comprehensive Cancer Network Guidelines of 2010, "the role of laparoscopic resection in gastric cancer requires further investigation in large randomized clinical trials" [6].

A meta-analysis published in 2010 showed that LADG seems superior to open distal gastrectomy (ODG) and results in less blood loss, shorter hospital stay, less pain, and lower risk of complications [7]. There was no significant difference in the 5-year survival rate between patients treated with LADG vs. ODG in one randomized controlled study [8] and two retrospective studies [9, 10]. Our retrospective experience confirms the same data [11].

However, concern remains regarding laparoscopically assisted total gastrectomy (LATG). Few studies are available on the outcomes of LATG with D2 lymphadenectomy for gastric cancer because of the technical difficulty in completing the procedures and questions about long-term oncologic outcomes. A number of small series advocating LATG for gastric cancer have appeared in the literature [12, 13]. In a retrospective multicenter study by Kitano of 1294 patients with early gastric cancer (EGC), 55 LATGs with D1-D2 lymphadenectomy were performed, with good short- and long-term outcomes [14].

32.1.3 Critical Issues in Standardization

Reconstruction after LADG is open to different solutions, from the modern Roux-en-Y gastro-jejunal anastomosis to the standard Billroth I, often preferred in the large case series published in Japan and Korea for EGC [15-17].

The use of LATG with D2 lymphadenectomy for gastric cancer has two problems: whether to perform a concomitant splenectomy to completely retrieve station 10 lymph nodes and how to achieve an intracorporeal anastomosis. The former is still a matter of debate for open surgery, while different solutions have been proposed for the latter since as yet there is no standard procedure [3, 4, 17-20].

Our technique for laparoscopic total gastrectomy complies with the previously described indications for EGC of the proximal or middle portion of the stomach and a D2 lymph node dissection (lymph node stations 7, 8a, 9, 11p, and 12a.

32.2 Laparoscopic Set-up

32.2.1 Patient and Team Placement

The patient is placed under general anesthesia in the lithotomy position with 20° head-up tilt (reverse Trendelenburg's position), legs parted, left arm abducted. A central venous line, naso-gastric tube, and urinary catheter are inserted.

The operating surgeon stands between the patient's legs, the surgeon holding the camera stands at the operating surgeon's left side, and a second assistant on the right side. The monitor is placed to the right of the patient's head; a second monitor on the left side is useful.

32.2.2 Laparosocopic Instrumentation

The instrumentation required for the procedure consists of one 12-mm Hasson trocar, three single-use 10- to 12-mm trocars, and, optionally, a 5-mm trocar. A 30° HD laparoscope is used through the umbilical port.

All dissecting maneuvers are conducted by ultrasonic scalpel with a 5-mm shaft (Harmonic Ace, Ethicon Endo-Surgery, Cincinnati, OH). Organ retraction is carried out by means of 10-mm shaft Babcock forceps and 5-mm shaft Johann forceps. A liver retractor is inserted through the right hypochondrium port (fan-type foldable retractor).

Additional laparoscopic instruments that are required include bipolar forceps, needle-holders, suction-irrigation cannula, endoscopic linear stapler, and clip applicator.

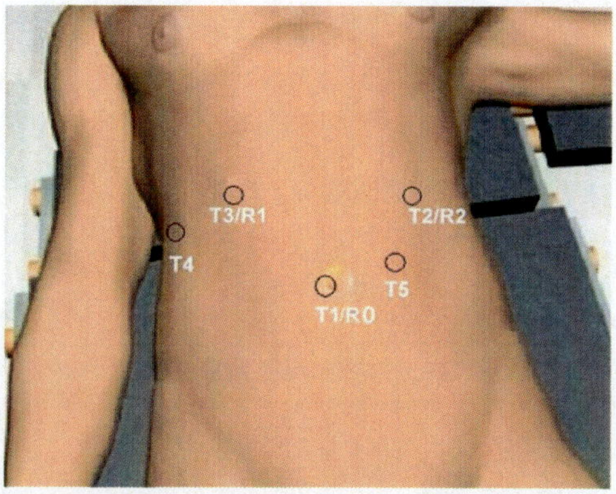

Fig. 32.1 Trocar placement

32.2.3 Trocar Placement

A CO_2 pneumoperitoneum is induced at 12 mmHg through a 12-mm right peri-umbilical port for open laparoscopy (T1 in Fig. 32.1). Three more 10- to 12-mm trocars are then inserted, in a semicircular shape, in the left (T2) and right (T3) upper quadrants on the midclavicular line 3 cm above the trans-umbilical line and in the right subcostal space (T4) for liver retraction through a fan-type foldable retractor. One optional 5-mm trocar for retraction is inserted in the left hypochondrium.

32.3 Laparoscopic Subtotal Gastrectomy (LSG)

32.3.1 Technical Notes

The procedure begins with an exploration of the abdominal cavity. Once it has been found to be free of metastatic disease, the first surgical steps are coloepiploic detachment and omentectomy, followed by dissection of the gastrocolic ligament. The left gastroepiploic vessels are divided. All of these maneuvers are performed by means of ultrasonic shears.

Entering the lesser sac allows adhesions to be sectioned between the pancreas and the posterior wall of the stomach.

After lowering the right colonic flexure and exposing the anterior surface of both the duodenum and the pancreatic head, the Henle trunk is identified and the affluent right gastroepiploic vessels are isolated (Fig. 32.2) and divided separately between absorbable clips. The right gastroepiploic artery is sectioned at its origin from the gastroduodenal artery, just above the pancreatic head. This allows clearance of station 6 and of Fredet's area, where lymph node station 14v is removed.

By following the hepatic and gastroduodenal arteries, the right gastric arcade is identified and divided. The pyloric vessels are sectioned, the pylorus is freed, and station 5 nodes are resected.

The duodenum is transected (Fig. 32.3) with a 45-mm cartridge linear stapler (blue reloads, with triple-staggered rows of staples). We use a linear endostapler reload reinforced by a bioabsorbable polycarbonate membrane (Seamguard, W.L. Gore & Associates); as an alternative, it is advisable to oversew the staple line [21]. The stomach can now be lifted in the left hypochondrium and the patient is rotated onto the left side in order to facilitate lymphadenectomy.

The lesser omentum is incised, the hepatoduodenal ligament cleared from station 12a nodes, followed by dissection of nodes associated with the common hepatic artery (station 8), nodes of the celiac axis (station 9), and nodes of station 11p, proximal to the splenic artery (Fig. 32.4). The left

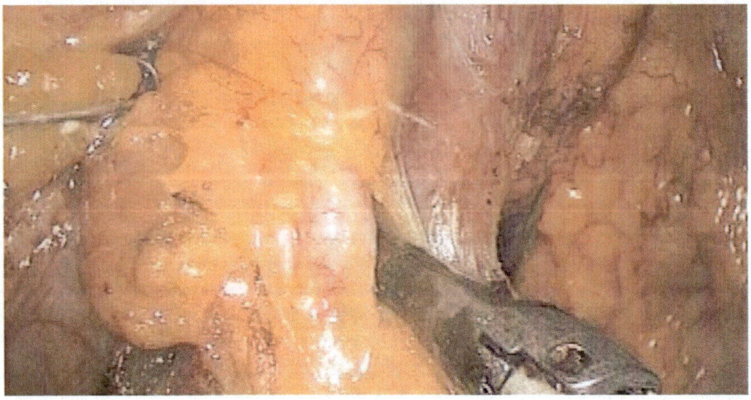

Fig. 32.2 Isolation of the gastroepiploic artery

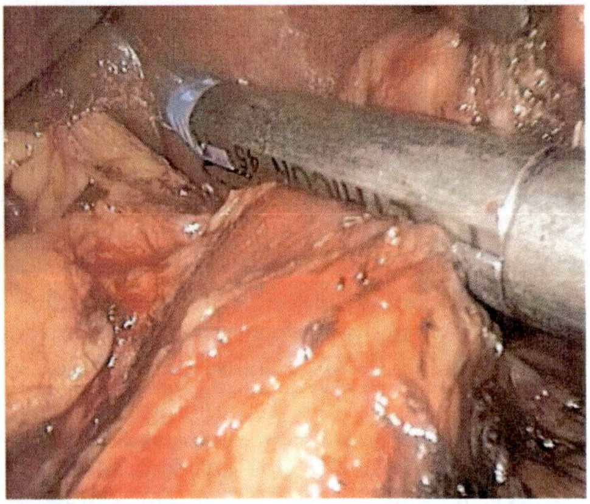

Fig. 32.3 Duodenal section with 4-mm endolinear stapler

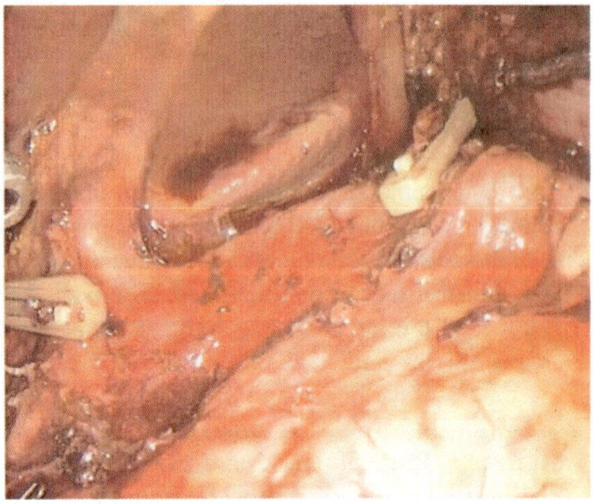

Fig. 32.4 The celiac region after lymphadenctomy of lymph node stations 7–9 and sectioning of the right and left gastric arteries (clips)

gastric artery is sectioned using a linear endostapler or between clips, with removal of station 7 nodes. Lifting of the gastric remnant allows excision of the perigastric lymph nodes along the lesser curvature (station 3) up to the esophago-gastric region (station 1) and completion of the lymphadenectomy.

Four-fifths of the stomach are transected (Fig. 32.5), starting from the greater curve at the junction of the left and right gastroepiploic arcades, by a 45-mm linear stapler (3–5 blue reloads). The specimen is collected into an endo bag and temporarily placed on the liver surface.

32.3.2 Gastro-jejunal Anastomosis

The second jejunal loop is chosen to prepare a 70-cm Roux-en-Y transmesocolic loop. The gastric remnant is set close to the jejunal loop and two openings are created through which a 45-mm cartridge stapler is inserted to fashion a side-to–side gastro-jejunal anastomosis (Fig. 32.6). Suture of the openings by running suture closes access to the gastric stump and jejunal limb. The side-to-side jejunojejunal anastomosis at the foot of the Roux-en-Y loop is created with a 45-mm endostapler. The endobag containing the specimen is retrieved

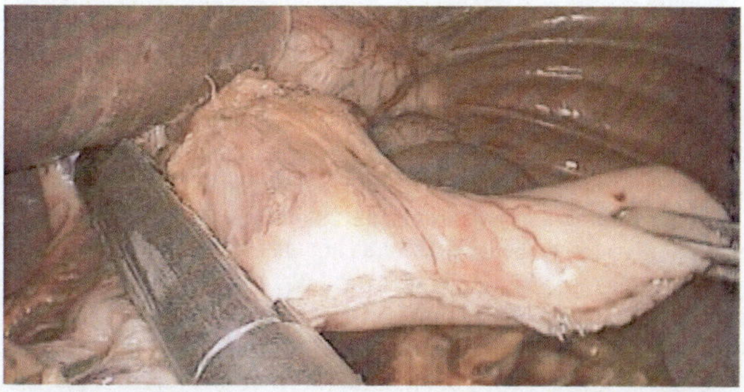

Fig. 32.5 Subtotal resection of four-fifths of the stomach

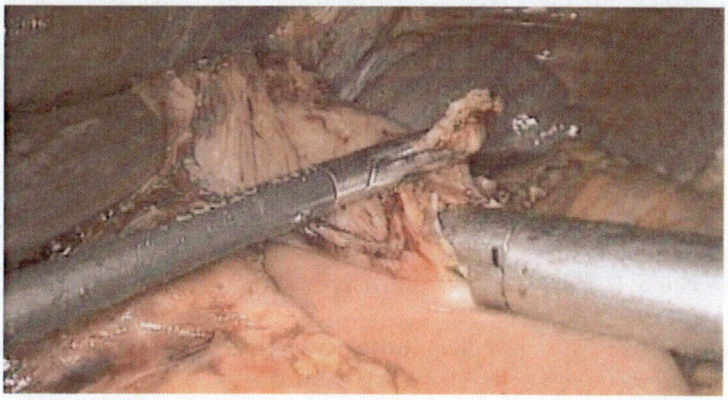

Fig. 32.6 Side-to-side gastro-jejunal stapled anastomosis

through the umbilical port. Minimal enlargement of the incision (3–4 cm) may be necessary in some instances. A drain, inserted through the right trocar, is placed near the duodenal stump. Closure of port incisions ends the procedure.

32.4 Laparoscopic Total Gastrectomy (LTG)

32.4.1 Technical Notes

Placement of the patient, the first steps in the gastric dissection and closure of the duodenal stump are carried out as described above for LSG. The extent of lymphadenectomy for proximal tumors corresponds to a D2 clearance, including the anterior aspect of the splenic hilum. Dissection of the gastrocolic ligament is wider than in LSG. Short gastric vessels are divided with the ultrasound scalpel, and dissection proceeds to the diaphragmatic crus, dividing the phreno-esophageal membrane and vagal nerves.

Group 2 (left paracardial) nodes are resected. The esophagus is transected by an EndoGIA 45 linear stapler, blue reload. The whole stomach is inserted into an endo-bag and temporarily placed on the liver surface.

32.4.2 Anastomosis According to Orringer

Reconstruction of digestive continuity is carried out by means of a side-to-side esophago-jejunal anastomosis, according to Orringer, on a Roux-en-Y transmesocolic loop [22].

The second jejunal loop is transected with a linear stapler (white vascular cartridge).

An opening in the transverse mesocolon is created by harmonic scalpel.

The second jejunal loop and the esophageal stump are prepared and opened on the antimesenteric side of the jejunal loop at about 5 cm from its distal margin and on the posterior wall of the esophagus. The 45-mm linear stapler, usually loaded with a blue cartridge, is introduced through the left trocar and inserted first into the jejunal opening and then into the esophageal one. No suspension sutures are used between the esophagus and the jejunum, in order to gain freedom of movement. A side-to-side esophago-jejunal anastomosis according to Orringer is then created by firing the stapler, after which the patency of the anastomosis is verified. A naso-jejunal tube is delicately passed through the anastomosis and the opening is sealed by a double layer of 3/0 running suture.

The jejuno-jejunal side-to-side stapled anastomosis at the foot (70 cm) of the anastomotic loop, created as previously described, accomplishes Roux-en-Y restoration of the digestive tract. Minimal enlargement of the umbilical incision is needed to withdraw the bag containing the specimen. A drain is placed in Morrison's pouch near the duodenal stump. Closure of the port incisions ends the operation.

End-to-Side Esophago-jejunal Anastomosis

In 1999, Azagra described a conventional anastomosis created by using a circular stapler [3]. A large umbilical port (33 mm) is placed to allow passage of the 25-mm anvil. An incision is made in the anterior wall of the distal esophagus, a purse string suture is performed, and the anvil is slipped through the opening into the esophageal lumen with the aid of Babcock grasping forceps, prior to esophageal distal transection. The shaft of the circular stapler is then introduced into the afferent jejunal loop along its antimesenteric border through an enlargement of the left upper quadrant port by placing a wound protector or into the 33-mm trocar cannula. The shaft is clinched to the anvil, the stapler is fired, and an end-to-side esophago-jejunal anastomosis is created. The jejunal stump is closed by a 30-mm endoscopic linear stapler, and the anastomosis is checked with methylene blue instilled through the naso-gastric tube.

Hand-assisted laparoscopic total gastrectomy simplifies the technique by allowing the anastomosis to be created through a hand port [23, 24].

Oro-gastric Insertion of the Anvil in Mechanical End-to-Side Esophago-jejunal Anastomosis

The OrVilsystem (Covidien Surgical) is a ready-to-use anvil-delivery device that is designed to allow transoral insertion of the anvil into the abdominal esophagus, similar to the insertion of an orogastric tube through the mouth. In the OrVil system, the orogastric tube is connected to the center rod of the anvil, so that the anvil is transorally delivered into the esophagus, guided by the orogastric tube. The tube is easily removed from the anvil by cutting the connecting thread. The tilted anvil head of the OrVilTM system facilitates passage of the anvil through the mouth and upper esophagus, and automatically untilts for parallel closure when combined with a stapler. Intracorporeal laparoscopic double-stapling esophago-jejunostomy is performed using a 25-mm circular stapler, which can be combined with the OrVilTM system [25].

32.5 Robotic Approach to Minimally Invasive Gastrectomy

32.5.1 Robotic-assisted Minimally Invasive Gastric Surgery

Even if widely accepted, laparoscopic surgery has several limitations and disadvantages, such as limited range of instrument movement, amplification of hand tremor, two-dimensional imaging, and unnatural positions for the surgeons. Robotic surgery, performed through a remote console controlling a robotic cart (Robotic Surgical System, da Vinci Intuitive Surgical, Mountain View, CA, USA), is superior to conventional laparoscopic surgery according to several investigators for the following reasons: it has a tremor filter, can scale motions, has three-dimensional imaging, and offers a stable operative platform and improved dexterity by means of an internal articulated EndoWrist that allows seven degrees of freedom. These characteristics are especially important when precise lymph node dissection is required for surgical treatment of gastric cancer [26-28]. Nevertheless, robotic gastrectomy has also its disadvantages, including a field of view that is smaller than the laparoscopic view, longer operating time, and higher costs.

32.5.2 Robotic Set-up

The robotic and optic systems are setup by the first assistant, who works between the patient's lower limbs. Electric cables connect the robotic system to the surgeon's console. After a self-test, the arms of the EndoWrist are wrapped with covers and fixed by supports. A 3D high-resolution image is selected and a 12-mm cannula is inserted in the periumbilical trocar for open laparoscopy and optic binocular endoscopy (R0).

The pneumoperitoneum is instituted at 12 mmHg (T1 in Fig. 34.1). Two robotic trocars of 7/8 mm are inserted bilaterally in the subcostal space on the anterior axillary line (R1 and R2). Then, two trocars of 10/12 mm are inserted in the upper quadrants, below the robotic ports, the right one on the right subcostal space for liver retraction and the left one between the camera port and the left robotic port for additional retraction and insertion of endostaplers or clip appliers (T5). This additional port must be carefully placed to avoid conflict with the robotic arms. After port placement, the robotic cart is installed from the patient's head.

32.5.3 Robot-assisted LSG

The first steps are carried out under conventional laparoscopy: omentectomy, coloepiploic detachment, opening of the lesser sac, gastroduodenal dissection, and ablation of infrapyloric nodes (stations 4 and 6). Then, the second jejunal loop is prepared to allow the fashioning of a side-to-side stapled anastomosis at the foot of the Roux en-Y loop.

At this point, the robotic system is installed and lymphadenectomy begins on the anterior aspect of the hepatic artery (station 12a nodes). Once the right gastric artery is divided, the suprapyloric nodes are removed (station 5). The assistant retracts the stomach, applies clips, and operates the stapler to transect the duodenum.

Lymphadenectomy is completed by ablation of station 8, 9, and 11p nodes followed by division of the left gastric artery, with removal of nodes of station 7 and of stations 1 and 3 along the lesser curvature. The stomach is transected by linear stapler to obtain a four-fifths gastrectomy, placing the specimen temporarily on the liver surface. A 70 cm Roux-en-Y jejunal limb is chosen for restoration of the digestive tract. A transmesocolic gastro-jejunal anastomosis is fashioned with a linear cutting stapler on the posterior wall of the gastric stump. The access openings are closed by robotic running suture.

32.5.4 Robot-assisted LTG

In robot-assisted LTG, the dissection approaches the diaphragmatic crus with division of the phrenoesophageal membrane, resection of stations 1 and 2, and division of the vagal nerves. Due to the robot's dexterity, as an alternative to Orringer's anastomosis it is possible to perform a hand-sewn purse string suture on the esophagus and to complete an end-to-side esophago-jejunal anastomosis with the circular stapler, as previously described.

References

1. Goh PMY, Tekant Y, Kum CK et al (1992) Totally intra-abdominal laparoscopic Billroth II gastrectomy. Surg Endosc 6:160
2. Kitano S, Iso Y, Moriyama M, Sugimachi K (1994) Laparoscopy-assisted Billroth I gastrectomy. Surg Laparosc Endosc 4:146-148
3. Azagra JS, Goergen M, De Simone P, Ibañez-Aguirre (1999) Minimally invasive surgery for gastric cancer. Surg Endosc 13:351-357
4. Uyama I, Sugioka A, Fujita J et al (1999) Laparoscopic total gastrectomy with distal pancreatosplenectomy and D2 lymphadenectomy for advanced gastric cancer. Gastric Cancer 2:230-234
5. Japanese Gastric Cancer Association (2011) Japanese Gastric Cancer Treatment Guidelines 2010 (ver. 3). Gastric Cancer 14:113-123
6. National Comprehensive Cancer Network. Clinical Practice Guidelines in Oncology. Gastric Cancer. V.2.2010. http://www.nccn.org/professionals/physician_gls/PDF/gastric.pdf
7. Ohtani H, Tamamori Y, Noguchi K et al (2010) Meta-analysis of laparoscopy-assisted and open distal gastrectomy for gastric cancer. J Surg Res doi:10.1016/j.jss.2010.04.008
8. Huscher CG, Mingoli A, Sgarzini G et al (2005) Laparoscopic versus open subtotal gastrectomy for distal gastric cancer: Five-year results of a randomized prospective trial. Ann Surg 241:232-237
9. Mochiki E, Kamiyama Y, Aihara R et al (2005) Laparoscopic assisted distal gastrectomy for early gastric cancer: Five years' experience. Surgery 137:317-322
10. Lee JH, Yom CK, Han HS (2009) Comparison of long-term outcomes of laparoscopy-assisted and open distal gastrectomy for early gastric cancer. Surg Endosc 23:1759-1763

11. Pugliese R, Maggioni D, Sansonna F et al (2010) Subtotal gastrectomy with D2 dissection by minimally invasive surgery for distal adenocarcinoma of the stomach: results and 5-year survival. Surg Endosc 24:2594-2602
12. Shinoara T, Kanaya S, Taniguchi K et al (2009) Laparoscopic total gastrectomy with D2 lymph node dissection for gastric cancer. Arch Surg 144:1138-1142
13. Sakuramoto S, Kikuchi S, Futawatari N et al (2009) Laparoscopy-assisted pancreas- and spleen-preserving total gastrectomy for gastric cancer as compared with open total gastrectomy. Surg Endosc. Surg Endosc 23:2416-2423
14. Kitano S, Shiraishi N, Uyama I et al; Japanese Laparoscopic Surgery Study Group (2007) A multicenter study on oncologic outcome of laparoscopic gastrectomy for early cancer in Japan. Ann Surg 245:68-72
15. Tanimura S, Higashino M, Fukunaga Y et al (2008) Laparoscopic gastrectomy for gastric cancer: experience with more than 600 cases. Surg Endosc 22:1161-1164
16. Adachi Y, Shiraishi N, Shiromizu A et al (2000) Laparoscopy-assisted Billroth I gastrectomy compared with conventional open gastrectomy. Arch Surg 135:806-810
17. Hyung WJ, Song C, Cheong JH et al (2007) Factors influencing operation time of laparoscopy-assisted distal subtotal gastrectomy: analysis of consecutive 100 initial cases. Eur J Surg Oncol 33:314-319
18. Okabe H, Obama K, Tanaka E (2009) Intracorporeal esophagojejunal anastomosis after laparoscopic total gastrectomy for patients with gastric cancer. Surg Endosc 23:2167-2171
19. Kim SG, Lee YJ, Ha WS et al (2008) LATG with extracorporeal esophagojejunostomy: is this minimal invasive surgery for gastric cancer? J Laparoendosc Adv Surg Tech A18:572-578
20. Huscher C, Mingoli A, Sgarzini G et al (2007) Totally laparoscopic total and subtotal gastrectomy with extended lymph node dissection for early and advanced gastric cancer: early and long-term results of a 100-patient series. Am J Surg 194:839-844
21. Pugliese R, Maggioni D, Sansonna F et al (2009) Efficacy and effectiveness of suture bolster with Seamguard. Surg Endosc 23:1415-1416
22. Orringer MB, Marshall B, Iannettoni MD (2000) Eliminating the cervical esophagogastric anastomotic leak with a side-to-side stapled anastomosis. J Thorac Cardiovasc Surg 119:277-288
23. Chau CH, Siu WT, Li MK (2002) Hand-assisted D2 subtotal gastrectomy for carcinoma of stomach. Surg Laparosc Endosc Percutan Tech 12:268-272
24. Usui S, Ito K, Hiranuma S et al (2007) Hand-assisted laparoscopic esophagojejunostomy using newly developed purse-string suture instrument "Endo-PSI." Surg Laparosc Endosc Percutan Tech 17:107-110
25. Jeong O, Park YK (2009) Intracorporeal circular stapling esophagojejunostomy using the transorally inserted anvil (OrVil) after laparoscopic total gastrectomy. Surg Endosc 23:2624-2630
26. Kim MC, Heo GU, Jung GJ (2010) Robotic gastrectomy for gastric cancer: surgical techniques and clinical merits. Surg Endosc 24:610-615
27. Song J, Oh SJ, Kang WH et al (2009) Robot-assisted gastrectomy with lymph node dissection for gastric cancer: lessons learned from an initial 100 consecutive procedures. Ann Surg 249:927-932
28. Pugliese R, Maggioni D, Sansonna F et al (2008) Robot-assisted laparoscopic gastrectomy with D2 dissection for adenocarcinoma: initial experience with 17 patients. J Robotic Surg 2:217-222

Standard and Extended Lymphadenectomy: Technical Notes

33

Franco Roviello, Giovanni Corso, and Daniele Marrelli

Abstract

Surgical procedures for the dissection of the various lymph nodes stations differ depending on the location and stage of the gastric tumor. The guidelines of the Japanese Gastric Cancer Association recommend D2 (standard) lymphadenectomy for the treatment of advanced gastric carcinoma. However, an emerging surgical approach to the treatment of gastric tumors is the D3 (extended) lymphadenectomy, indicated for advanced cancers and in patients in good general health who are under 75 years of age. In this chapter, we discuss the D2 standard and D3 extended surgical techniques for the treatment of advanced gastric carcinoma.

Keywords

Gastric cancer • Lymphoadenectomy • D2 • D3 • Surgical procedure • Long term survival • Prognosis • Japanese classification

33.1 Introduction

The Japanese Gastric Cancer Association (JGCA) guidelines define and recommend D2 lymph node (LN) dissection for most gastric cancers. Limited lymphadenectomy, i.e., D1+ LN dissection, is indicated for selected patients with stage T1 cancers. D1+ dissection refers to the removal of level 1 stations plus station 7 (left gastric artery), with the addition of station 8a (common hepatic artery), and 9 (celiac artery) [1, 2]. Gastrectomy with D1 is indicated for T1N0 tumors limited to the mucosa (M) and for differentiated submucosal (SM) tumors < 1.5 cm in diameter. Submucosal tumors that do not meet this condition should be treated by gastrectomy with D1+ [2, 3].

Following publication of the 13th edition of the Japanese Classification of Gastric Carcinoma (JCGC), in June 1999, the standard for advanced carcinomas has been the D2 dissection [4]. Indeed, gastric cancer patients who underwent R0 surgery with standard D2 lymphadenectomy were found to have better long-term survival [5]. The more recent, extended lymphadenectomy, D3 dissection, is indicated also in advanced gastric cancer, as shown in a selected sub-group of these patients who had longer survival after this procedure [6]. Clearly, adequate knowledge of LN classification is essential in gastric cancer in order to correctly perform a D2 standard or D3 extended lymphadenectomy, as defined by the JCGA.

F. Roviello (✉)
Dept. of Human Pathology and Oncology,
Section of General Surgery and Surgical Oncology,
Translational Research Laboratory,
University of Siena,
Siena, Italy

In the late 1980s, Keiichi Maruyama and colleagues at the National Cancer Center Hospital in Tokyo created a computer program, known as the "Maruyama program," that analyzed a large series of gastric cancer patients treated by extended lymphadenectomy (i.e., D2 or more). The program estimates the rate of metastasis in each of the 16 main LN stations. The Maruyama program has been used to assess Japanese, German, and Italian populations and found to be highly accurate [7-9]. It provides a highly valuable tool for surgeons in pre-operative or intra-operative planning, as a convenient means of rationally determining an adequate lymphadenectomy for the treatment of gastric cancer.

In this chapter, we discuss the D2 standard and D3 extended surgical techniques for the treatment of advanced gastric cancer.

33.2 D2 Standard Lymphadenectomy and Lymph Node Stations

In patients with advanced gastric carcinomas, D2 dissection depends on the tumor's location.

Upper third. D2 classification of these tumors includes the following LN stations: right (station 1), and left (station 2) paracardial, lesser curvature (station 3), short gastric, right and left gastroepiploic vessels (stations 4sa, 4sb, 4d), left gastric artery (station 7), common hepatic artery (anterosuperior group station 8a), celiac artery (station 9), and proximal splenic artery (station 11p). Lymphadenectomy along the splenic hilum (station 10) and distal splenic artery (station 11) should be performed in case of T4 tumors.

Middle third. For gastric tumors located at this site, the D2 LN stations are: right (station 1), and left (station 2) paracardial, lesser curvature (station 3), short gastric, right and left gastroepiploic vessels (stations 4sa, 4sb, 4d), supra- and infra-pyloric (stations 5, 6), left gastric artery (station 7), common hepatic artery (anterosuperior group, station 8a), celiac artery (station 9), proximal splenic artery (station 11p), and hepatoduodenal ligament (along the hepatic artery, station 12a). Lymphadenectomy along the splenic hilum (station 10) and distal splenic artery (station 11) should be performed in cases of T3–T4 tumor with macroscopic lymphatic metastases.

Lower third. The D2 classification for antral/pyloric gastric tumors comprises the following: right paracardial group (station 1), lesser curvature (station 3), right gastroepiploic vessel (station 4d), supra- and infra-pyloric (stations 5, 6), left gastric artery (station 7), common hepatic artery (anterosuperior group, station 8a), celiac artery (station 9), proximal splenic artery (station 11p), hepatoduodenal ligament (along the hepatic artery, station 12a).

33.3 Lymph Node Stations in D3 Extended Lymphadenectomy

Similar to the D2 classification, LNs of the D3 groups are ranked according to tumor location.

Upper third. Suprapyloric (station 5) and infrapyloric stations (station 6), common hepatic artery (posterior group, station 8p), hepatoduodenal ligament (posterior hepatic artery, station 12p), middle para-aortic (station 16a2,b1), infradiaphragmatic (station 19), and esophageal hiatus (station 20).

Middle third. Common hepatic artery (LN posterior group; station 8p), splenic hilum (station 10), hepatoduodenal ligament (posterior hepatic artery, station 12p), retropancreatic (station 13), superior mesenteric vein (station 14v), and middle para-aortic (station 16a2,b1).

Lower third. Left gastroepiploic vessels (station 4sb), common hepatic artery (posterior group, station 8p), hepatoduodenal ligament (posterior hepatic artery, station 12p), retropancreatic (station 13), superior mesenteric vein (station 14v) and middle para-aortic (station 16a2,b1).

33.4 D2 Lymph Node Dissection: Surgical Procedure

The JGCA guidelines for gastric surgery spell out the correct approach to standard lymphadenectomy [10].

The D2 dissection, in T3-T4a tumors only, begins with a bursectomy, with removal of the superior gastro-colic ligament and the pancreatic capsule. Mobilization of the stomach exposes LN stations 4d (right gastroepiploic) and 4sb (left gastroepiploic) through the greater gastric curvature

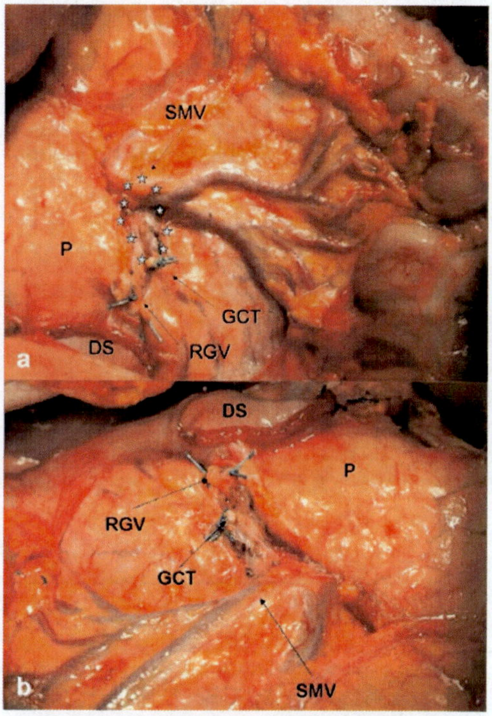

Fig. 33.1 Dissection of station 14. **a** Skeletonization of the gastrocolic trunk (*GCT*, Henle's trunk), superior mesenteric vein (*SMV*), pancreas (*P*), and duodenum (D). *Stars* encircle lymph nodes of station 14v; **b** duodenum section (*DS*), dissection of the GCT and the right gastroepiploic vein (*RGV*)

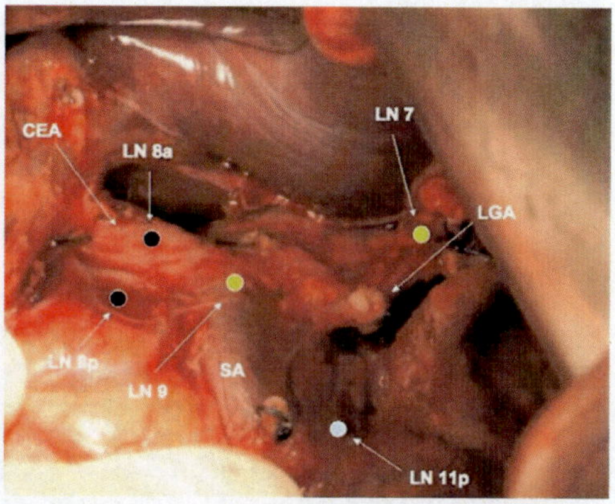

Fig. 33.2 Dissection of stations 7, 8a, 8p, 9, and 11p. Isolation and sectioning of the left gastric artery (*LGA*) and removal of station 7, with exposure of the celiac trunk (*CT*) and lymphadenectomy of station 9. This procedure exposes the branches of the CT, i.e., the common hepatic artery (*CEA*) and the splenic artery (*SA*), with removal, respectively, of stations 8a (anterior), 8p (posterior), and 11p (splenic proximal)

toward the lower pole of the spleen. Particular attention should be paid to the head of the pancreas. The middle colic and superior mesenteric veins, the gastrocolic trunk, and the right gastroepiploic vein are exposed: in tumors with apparent metastasis to the n.6 nodes, station 14v (superior mesenteric vein) is dissected (Fig. 33.1a). Station 6 (infrapyloric) is exposed after elevation of the stomach, allowing the exposure and subsequent ligation of the right gastroepiploic vessels. Duodenal transection aids in the dissection of station 6 (Fig. 33.1b).

The next step is the isolation of the gastroduodenal, common hepatic, and proper hepatic arteries, allowing dissection of stations 5 (suprapyloric) and 12a (left hepatoduodenal). The procedure continues with skeletonization of the common hepatic artery and dissection of stations 8a and 8p, LNs around the celiac artery (station 9), and those along the proximal splenic artery (station 11p). This is followed by separation and removal of the LNs along the left gastric artery (station 7), as shown in Fig. 33.2 Station 1 (right paracardial) is dissected along with the upper-third of the lesser curvature. In a total gastrectomy, en-bloc resection of the stomach facilitates dissection of station 2 (left paracardial). This surgical step completes the standard D2 lymphadenectomy.

33.5 D3 Lymph Node Dissection: Surgical Procedure

Extended D3 lymphadenectomy requires complete mobilization of the duodenum, which is accomplished with the Kocher maneuver. This provides access to the para-aortic node (PAN) stations. PAN dissection implies the resection of LNs between the level of the celiac axis and the left renal vein (station 16a2) and of nodes between the left renal vein and the inferior mesenteric artery (station

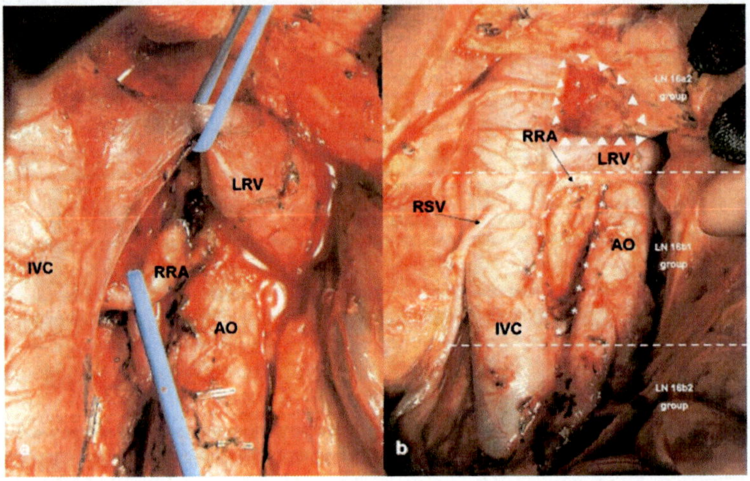

Fig. 33.3 Dissection of station 16. **a** Exposure of the aorta (*AO*), inferior vein cava (*IVC*), left renal vein (*LRV*), and right renal artery (*RRA*); **b** *arrowheads* indicate station16a2, and *stars* station 16b1. The arrow points to the right spermatic vein (*RSV*)

16b1). The left upper lateral nodes (station 16a2-lat) are not generally dissected, except in cases of upper-third tumors or macroscopic LN involvement (Fig. 33.3a, b) [6]. It is important to note that the above-mentioned Kocher maneuver broadly exposes LN stations 8p and 12p; this procedure also facilitates a complete D2 lymphadenectomy.

D3 lymphadenectomy is usually indicated for advanced tumors (cT2–T4) in patients in good general health and under 75 years of age [11].

33.6 Conclusions

D2 lymphadenectomy represents the standard surgical procedure for advanced gastric carcinoma. The technique has proven to be safe when conducted in specialized centers and is associated with a low risk of post-operative complications and mortality. D3 lymphadenectomy requires removal of the PAN, stations. This procedure is an emerging technical approach especially indicated for patients with upper-third gastric cancers. It has an acceptable morbidity rate and no increase in mortality compared to earlier approaches.

References

1. Shimada Y (2004) JGCA (The Japan Gastric Cancer Association). Gastric cancer treatment guidelines. Jpn J Clin Oncol 34:58
2. Japanese Gastric Cancer Association (2011) Japanese Gastric Cancer Treatment Guidelines. Gastric Cancer 14:113-123
3. Nakajima T (2002) Gastric cancer treatment guidelines in Japan. Gastric Cancer 5:1-5
4. Aiko T, Sasako M (1998) The new Japanese Classification of Gastric Carcinoma: Points to be revised. Gastric Cancer 1:25-30
5. Roviello F, Marrelli D, Morgagni P et al (2002) Survival benefit of estende D2 lymphadenectomy in gastric cancer with involvement of second level lymph nodes: a longitudinal multi center study. Ann Surg Oncol 9:894-900
6. Roviello F, Pedrazzani C, Marrelli D et al (2010) Super-extended (D3) lymphadenectomy in advanced gastric cancer. Eur J Surg Oncolo 36:439-446
7. Kampschöer GH, Maruyama K, van de Velde CJ (1989) Computer analysis in making preoperative decisions: a rational approach to lymph node dissection in gastric cancer patients. Br J Surg 76:905-908
8. Bollschweiler E, Boettcher K, Hoelscher AH et al (1992) Preoperative assessment of lymph node metastases in patients with gastric cancer: evaluation of the Maruyama computer program. Br J Surg 79:156-160
9. Guadagni S, de Manzoni G, Catarci M (2000) Evaluation

of the Maruyama computer program accuracy for preoperative estimation of lymph node metastases from gastric cancer. World J Surg 24:1550-1558
10. Japanese Gastric Cancer Association (1998) Japanese classification of gastric carcinoma - 2nd English edn. Gastric Cancer 1:10-24
11. Sano T, Sasako M, Yamamoto S et al (2004) Gastric cancer surgery: morbidity and mortality results from a prospective randomized controlled trial comparing D2 and extended para-aortic lymphadenectomy—Japan Clinical Oncology Group study 9501. J Clin Oncol 22:2767-2773

Subject Index